Behavior of Exotic Pets

Behavior of Exotic Pets

Edited by

Valarie V. Tynes
Veterinary Behavior Consultant
Sweetwater, Texas, USA

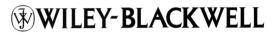

A John Wiley & Sons, Ltd., Publication

This edition first published 2010
© 2010 Blackwell Publishing Ltd

Blackwell Publishing was acquired by John Wiley & Sons in February 2007. Blackwell's publishing programme
has been merged with Wiley's global Scientific, Technical, and
Medical business to form Wiley-Blackwell.

Registered office
John Wiley & Sons Ltd, The Atrium, Southern Gate, Chichester, West Sussex, PO19 8SQ, United Kingdom

Editorial offices
9600 Garsington Road, Oxford, OX4 2DQ, United Kingdom
2121 State Avenue, Ames, Iowa 50014-8300, USA

For details of our global editorial offices, for customer services and for information about how to apply
for permission to reuse the copyright material in this book please see our website at www.wiley.com/wiley-blackwell.

Library of Congress Cataloging-in-Publication Data

Behavior of exotic pets / edited by Valarie V. Tynes.
    p. ; cm.
    Includes bibliographical references and index.
    ISBN 978-0-8138-0078-3 (pbk. : alk. paper)   1. Exotic animals–Behavior.   2. Exotic animals—Diseases—Diagnosis.
3. Exotic animals—Diseases—Treatment.   4. Wildlife diseases.   5. Pet medicine.   6. Wild animals as pets.
I. Tynes, Valarie V.
    [DNLM: 1. Animals, Domestic—psychology.   2. Behavior, Animal.   3. Mental Disorders—veterinary.
SF 756.7 B419 2010]
    SF997.5.E95B44 2010
    636.088′7—dc22
                                                                                                          2010001845

A catalogue record for this book is available from the British Library.

Set in 10/12 pt Minion by MPS Limited, A Macmillan Company
Printed in Singapore by Ho Printing Singapore Pte Ltd
1 2010

Contents

Contributors

Julia Albright MA, DVM, Dipl. ACVB
Animal Behavior Clinic
Department of Clinician Sciences
College of Veterinary Medicine
Cornell University
Ithaca, New York

Marcelo Alfredo Aba MV, MSc, PhD
Professor in Endocrinology
Endocrinology Lab, Department of Physiopathology
Faculty of Veterinary Sciences
Universidad Nacional del Centro de la Provincia de
Buenos Aires
Tandil, Buenos Aires Province
Argentina

Manuel Berdoy MPhil, DPhil
Oxford University Veterinary Services
University of Oxford
Oxford, UK

Carolina Bianchi DVM
Fellow of CONICET
Endocrinology Lab, Department of
Physiopathology
Faculty of Veterinary Sciences
Tandil, Buenos Aires Province
Argentina

Megan J. Bulloch PhD
Quest University Canada
Squamish, British Columbia

Verónica Cavilla DVM
Fellow of CONICET
Endocrinology Lab, Department of Physiopathology
Faculty of Veterinary Sciences
Tandil, Buenos Aires Province
Argentina

Sharon L. Crowell-Davis DVM, PhD, DACVB
Department of Anatomy and Radiology
College of Veterinary Medicine
University of Georgia
Athens, Georgia

Ricardo de Matos LMv, Dipl. ABVP (Avian)
Department of Clinical Sciences
College of Veterinary Medicine
Cornell University
Ithaca, New York

Susan G. Friedman PhD
Department of Psychology
Department of Special Education
Utah State University
Logan, Utah

Paul M. Gibbons DVM, MS, Dipl. ABVP (Avian)
Specialist, Exotic Animal Service
Animal Emergency Center & Specialty Services
Milwaukee, Wisconsin

Anne Fullerton Hanson PhD
Los Altos, California

Lore I. Haug DVM, MS, DACVB, CPDT, CABC
Texas Veterinary Behavior Services
Sugar Land, Texas

Paul E. Honess BSc, PhD
Primatologist
Department of Veterinary Services
University of Oxford
Oxford, UK

Naomi Latham BSc, DPhil
Zoology Department
University of Oxford
Oxford, UK

YeunShin Lee BA, MS, PhD
Lecturer
Center for Animal Welfare
Department of Animal Science
University of California—Davis
Davis, California

Heather Mohan-Gibbons MS, RVT, CPDT, ACAAB
Collected Wisdom Animal Behavior, LLC
Milwaukee, Wisconsin

Terry Norton DVM, Dipl. ACZM
Director and Veterinarian
Georgia Sea Turtle Center
Jekyll Island, Georgia

A. Dawn Faircloth Parker DVM, MBA
Behavior and Zoo Consulting
San Francisco Bay area, California

Paul Raiti DVM
Beverlie Animal Hospital
Mt. Vernon, New York

Lynne M. Seibert DVM, MS, PhD, Dipl. ACVB
All Creatures Behavior Counseling
Kirkland, Washington

Debra M. Shier PhD
San Diego Conservation Research
Division of Applied Animal Ecology
Escondido, California

Jennifer L. Sobie PhD
Department of Animal Sciences
University of Illinois
Urbana, Illinois

Wailani Sung MS, PhD, DVM
First Regional Animal Hospital
Chandler, Arizona

Valarie V. Tynes DVM, Dipl. ACVB
Premier Veterinary Behavior Consulting
Sweetwater, Texas

Sarah E. Wolfensohn BSc, MA, VetMB, CertLAS, FIBiol,
DipECLAM, MRCVS
Supervisor of Veterinary Services
Department of Veterinary Services
University of Oxford
Oxford, UK

Foreword

Finally here is a reference book for all of us who, for one reason or another, wish to educate ourselves about species, other than dogs and cats, that find their way, as pets, into our homes, or those of our friends or our clients. The appeal of so-called exotic pets runs the gamut of birds that talk to us, to those that represent an appealing sample of real nature, to those that might set us apart from our friends and neighbors. Of course, the term exotic pets is actually a misnomer; parrots, ferrets, gerbils, rats, chinchillas, and the like are abundant in nature whereas the Beagle, Black Lab, or Siamese is nowhere to be found outside our homes. Exotic pets are "exotic" because we know little about them as members of households. This is where this book offers so much valuable information; exotic pets will become less exotic, at least in terms of helping us provide the best environment, care, and medical–behavioral oversight.

For the 17 species or groups of species covered, there is a fairly uniform style in first discussing the natural history of the species in the wild, including communication, diet, reproduction, and parental care. In all chapters there is a section on prevention of problem behaviors, and when appropriate, evaluation, and treatment of behavior problems. Chapters are written by authorities on the species covered with welcome oversight by the editor to assure uniformity in chapter style; I found this particularly appealing for dealing with so many diverse species. When considering exotic pets ranging from parrots to canaries, snakes, lizards, guinea pigs, and llamas, coming up with meaningful universal principles of behavior modification, pharmacology, and welfare has to be challenging, but in the last three chapters this material is masterfully handled. Here is a text that one can turn to as a reference on a particular pet species or as a background for exotic pets in general.

In virtually all chapters there is something to say about the uniqueness of the pet discussed. Setting the tone for the style of coverage, the chapter on parrots and other **psittacines** spends more than half of the chapter on parrots in nature. Many readers will find it interesting that parrot mimicry vocalizations actually have an adaptive role in allowing the vocalizer to scare away predators by mimicking mobbing birds or by mimicking a predator to protect territory from conspecifics. In our homes parrots are preadapted to mimic us, even if the conversation is a bit one-sided. Feather picking or plucking, arguably the most important problem behavior in these birds as pets, is discussed in detail.

The chapter on **passerines**, your basic canary or zebra finch, also provides a great overview of these birds in nature. Fortunately, caregivers of pet passerines are generally spared the visual trauma of plucked-out feathers; other problems, aggression and lack of song are dealt with. While canaries and finches are pretty problem free, the chapter is a great source for understanding where these common pets fit in nature.

Snakes are masterfully handled in a chapter that, again, goes into basic behaviors that are important to understand in adopting a snake into an urban setting. The authors remind us that as the essence of the caduceus, snakes are a symbol of healing. Paradoxically, they can also symbolize the introduction of evil. Whatever a person's orientation, snakes obviously make a great pet for those who learn about their biology and normal behavior in nature. The authors provide an insight into the unique sensory capacities of snakes, especially the vomeronasal organ, the use of which is the key to understanding tongue flicking. The culinary orientation of feeding in snakes, as in eating a whole mouse, is explained along with avoiding problems and the necessity of a postprandial hot spot to help in digestion. If you, or a client, plan to adopt a snake, be sure to read this chapter.

A **turtle, tortoise, or terrapin** would seem like a very easy pet to keep. But do not let the slow movement or seemingly immortal life-span—often surpassing that of humans—fool you. They are, according to the authors, the most high maintenance of all reptiles. Reading this chapter is essential to know what you, or your client, are getting into. These tortoises and turtles are filled with scent glands—along the carapace, along the chin, and in the cloaca—something you might not expect, but then, when you think of it, how else are such slow-moving males and females going to get together. A long section on husbandry in this chapter is necessary because poor husbandry is the primary factor in illness.

Lizards are another group of potential pet species where, in nature, chemosensory information plays a critical role. The vomeronasal organs are essential for chemoreception, as are an array of specialized organs for dispensing chemical scents. Much of the discussion is devoted to husbandry, and wisely so. These creatures require considerable knowledge of species-specific requirements; in fact, most behavior problems stem from inappropriate husbandry.

The chapter on **ferrets** says straight on that "ferret" in Latin means "little thief." Despite this untrustworthy name, these are quite popular pets. One appeal is their tendency to dance or play, especially when excited. Another plus is their ease in litter box training. With ferret behavior problems one can use some of the behavior modification approaches commonly used with dogs and cats.

Rabbits, believe it or not, are the most popular urban mammalian house pet after dogs and cats. The author of this chapter gives us an overview of the origin of the rabbit as a pet and source of food, going back 3000 years to the time of the Phoenicians. Several behavioral traits of wild rabbits help in understanding their odd bits of behavior as a pet; engaging in urine spraying, coprophagy, and nursing young only once or, at the most, twice a day.

Guinea pigs as the prototypical pocket pet have been around for centuries, going back 3000 years to the Central Andean native Americans. Like other chapters this one is filled with interesting insights into their natural behavior. If the behavioral image of a guinea pig is one of tranquility, this is not far off. The guinea pig makes for a relatively easy-to-care-for pet, and this chapter provides the essentials for creating a welcoming home.

No other species kept as a pet is represented in such a broad spectrum of human activities as the **mouse**. Intimately associated with hominid dwellings around the time that modern humans evolved, over 200,000 years ago, the mouse is now known for its role as a favorite pocket pet, a persistent pest in our attics and walls, and as the mainstay of modern medical–biological research. Whether one is a laboratory investigator, a family veterinarian treating murine pocket pets, or just interested in understanding a bit of the wild fauna living in our neighborhoods, this chapter will enrich your understanding of mice.

The common **rat**, that has become a favorite pet of elementary classrooms, a common inhabitant of household attics and a staple of laboratory research in studies of general biology, is commonly known as the Norway rat. Another quirk of scientific nomenclature is that *Rattus norvegicus* did not originate in Norway, but rather in the plains of northern China. Learn more about this bit of natural history, along with a thorough review of the rat's well-known biology and behavior in this chapter. In fact, so much is known that the authors provide a table of online resources of rat biology and behavior. There is much in this chapter that should be of value to classroom teachers as well as parents who wish to take advantage of the pet rat as a bridge for teaching introductory biology.

Gerbils have the well-deserved reputation of being an adorable pocket pet, although the pocket is probably the least suitable housing for this exotic pet. Under problem behaviors, which are relatively minor, the authors remind us that gerbils are escape artists. Here is a pet where seizures are fairly common; interestingly, early handling seems to prevent most seizures. Adopters of gerbils will find the natural history and general biology well worth reading.

Hamsters, which are becoming an increasingly popular pet, are represented by primarily four species. Managing pet hamsters is made easier by reading this chapter to learn about some unique aspects of hamster behavior as well as their intriguing natural history. Maternal infanticide and cannibalism, common in pet hamsters, and probably normal in the wild hamster, might be disconcerting to the unsuspecting adopter, especially children. The authors discuss ways to reduce this behavior, and other problems, through appropriate management.

One of the most recently introduced exotic pets is the **chinchilla**, a native of the Andean mountains. In fact, the domestication of this pet is thought to have started in the 1920s in California, catching on as a pet in the 1960s. While growing in numbers as a pet in urban settings, chinchillas are classified as endangered in the wild state. In reading this chapter one gets the feeling that of the small pets, chinchillas take the most thought and planning to avoid problems.

Of the several species of **prairie dogs**, the black-tailed is the standard pet. Almost all pets are captured from wild so here is one exotic pet that has had no selective breeding, making it truly a wild type. According to the authors, if captured when young and given lots of gentle handling, they seem to imprint onto their caregivers. And they are easily housetrained. The leading behavior problem seems to be chewing: electrical cords, precious wood sculptures, rugs, window screens, furniture, and the like. The home needs to be prairie-dog proofed.

As exotic as a **camelid** might seem to be as a pet, actual domestication of camelids began some 4000–5000 years ago from native species in the Andes. An interesting bit of camelid history is that old world camels are actually new camelids, having evolved from the older camelids in the new world thanks to courageous animals crossing the Bering Land Bridge a few million years ago. While the most popular camelid pet is the llama, the authors cover the behavior and biology of all the domesticated camelid species. This chapter, like all chapters in this book, provides the essentials needed for adequate husbandry and management.

One has to believe that those who keep **hedgehogs** appreciate having a truly unusual pet; certainly the spiny pelage is not what you think of as pet-able. But these pets, once habituated, and provided with the appropriate home, are friendly, entertaining, and educational. They are easily tamed to ride around in your hand and sit beside you. The spines are only for self-defense, especially when they roll into a spiny ball. Here is another pet that has not been domesticated by selective breeding; all pets are captured from the wild. For those interested in a hedgehog, this chapter has the essential information needed to make both the pet and the caregiver happy.

About the only type of pet not mentioned in the above discussion is a marsupial. The role of a marsupial pet is beautifully fulfilled by the **sugar glider**, coming to us from Australia. The pet is so named because the webbing between their fore and hind limbs that allows them to glide from tree branches down a hundred feet or more to lower branches. And they love sugary sweet sap and nectar of the trees in Australia where they originated. Like some of the other newer pets, sugar gliders are naturally friendly when habituated; they have not been domesticated by selective breeding. The author provides a complete description of

the necessary husbandry and three-dimensional enclosure needed for a pet that finds it natural to scurry, jump, and glide through its environment.

In closing here is a volume that veterinarians attending to family pets or zoo animals, animal behaviorists, pet store managers, and, of course, exotic pet caregivers will find useful. The species covered are those that can be amicably maintained in a home or paddock. Those that should not be kept as pets—monkeys, chimpanzees, wolves, cheetah, and the like—are left out.

Benjamin L. Hart, DVM, PhD, DACVB
Distinguished Professor Emeritus
School of Veterinary Medicine
University of California, Davis

Acknowledgments

I realize that I am not being very creative or original when I say that a project of this sort could never have been accomplished without the encouragement, assistance, and support of many, many people. I want to thank all of the editors at Wiley-Blackwell who worked with me on this project. I am especially grateful to Katy Loftus for her patience and for always being so gracious about answering my numerous questions.

Identifying authors for a project of this type was a challenging endeavor. I am very proud of and grateful for the hard work and dedication to the project that was shown by this diverse group of scientists. This book could not possibly contain the depth and breadth of knowledge that it holds without them, and I am forever indebted to each and every one of them.

At risk of this sounding like an Oscar acceptance speech, I feel that it is only fair that I acknowledge the pioneering group of individuals who, if not for them, our specialty college, the American College of Veterinary Behaviorists would not even exist. We owe an enormous debt to these eight people; R.K. Anderson, Bonnie Beaver, Sharon Crowell-Davis, Benjamin Hart, Katherine Houpt, Elizabeth Shull, Victoria Voith, and Thomas Wolfle, who worked so hard to lay a foundation that allowed many such as myself to pursue advanced studies in the field of behavior. Thanks to their dedication and hard work, this field and the interest in it continues to grow. In addition, several of these people and others have served a very important role in mentoring me and encouraging me over the years. Bonnie Beaver, Karen Overall, and Peter Neville were some of the first behaviorists whom I met. I am extremely grateful for their encouragement and support of my interest in behavior. Their passion for the field has served as a constant source of inspiration for me. I also owe a great debt to Ben Hart for accepting me into his residency program and then serving as such a kind and patient mentor.

Several of my dear friends and colleagues provided valuable assistance by reading chapter drafts and giving constructive criticism. The book is definitely better for their contributions and I thank them for their time, as well as their friendship: Laurie Bergman, Lore Haug, Heather Mohan-Gibbons, Paul Gibbons, Lisa Nelson, Lynn Seibert, and Fon Chang.

Kristin Gieseker and Catherine Kelley both generously opened their homes to me and allowed me to photograph their pets. I also want to thank Millie Sanders with the Texas Ferret Lovers Rescue, who allowed us to intrude on her and her ferrets, and take pictures.

I also want to take this opportunity to acknowledge my husband Michael for his many photographic contributions, to this book, as well as many of my other previous projects. He never ceases to offer encouragement and support, no matter how much these projects distract me from "family time." I truly could not have done this without him!

Dedication

I admit that much of what I have managed to accomplish so far in life is simply due to the fact that I had the immense good fortune to be born to two people who believed that one of the most valuable things they could give their children was a good education. They saw to it that not only was the good education received in school, but that it was given at home as well. My parents made a point of introducing my brother and me to the natural world and all of its wonders. Thanks to them, I learned to love and respect all living things, not just those typically considered lovable. I owe more than I can ever repay for their constant love, encouragement, and support. Thus, it is to my parents, Gloria and Edward Vaughn, that I dedicate this book, with much love and gratitude.

1

Psittacines

Lynn M. Seibert and Wailani Sung

Introduction

Currently, there are over 9000 documented species of birds living on Earth.[1] Birds are among the most popular companion animals in the United States. Psittacine birds, in particular, are appealing companions because of their social behavior, exotic plumage, and vocal mimicry ability. There are over 300 different species of birds in the order Psittaciformes living in various parts of the world. They are found mainly in tropical and sub-tropical forests located in Central and South America, Australia, Southern Asia, New Guinea, New Zealand, and Central Africa, occupying habitats ranging from grasslands to mountain ranges to arid plains. The percentage of households in the United States keeping pet birds was estimated to be 3.9% in 2007, with the total number of pet birds estimated to be 11,199,000.[2]

Common characteristics of psittacine birds are hooked beaks with a downward curved upper maxilla that fits over an upward curved lower mandible and a thick, muscular tongue. They have a zygodactyl toe arrangement, with the second and third toes projecting forward and the fourth toe and hallux projecting backward.[2] These specialized feet allow them to maintain a good grip on branches and enable them to hang upside down or sideways. While climbing, psittacine birds use both their feet and beak for grasping.

The order Psittaciformes includes the families Loriidae, Cacatuidae, and Psittacidae. The birds belonging to this order are more commonly referred to as psittacines. The family Cacatuidae includes all cockatoo species and the cockatiel. The family Loriidae includes the lories

and lorikeets. The family Psittacidae includes Amazons (*Amazona* spp.), pionus parrots (*Pionus* spp.), macaws (*Ara, Cyanopsitta,* and *Anodorhynchus* spp.), conures (*Aratinga, Cyanoliseus,* and *Pyrrhura* spp.), rosellas (*Platycercus* spp.), budgerigars (*Melopsittacus* spp.), grass parakeets (*Neophema* spp.), African gray parrots (*Psittacus* spp.), Cape, Jardine's, Ruppell's, Meyer's parrots (*Poicephalus* spp.), lovebirds (*Agapornis* spp.), hanging parrots (*Loriculus* spp.), ring-necked parakeets (*Psittacula* spp.), and fig parrots (*Opopsitta* and *Psittaculirostris* spp.).

Psittacine birds are highly social. In their natural habitats, they typically live in large social groups with complex intraspecific interactions. Their daily activity patterns include flying, foraging, resting, and self-maintenance, as well as interactions with other members of the group. In captive settings, it is not uncommon for psittacine birds to develop abnormal behaviors. In order to provide suitable captive environments and effectively manage undesirable behaviors of captive pet birds, there must first be an understanding of natural psittacine behavior.

Flock behavior

Psittacine birds form complex social groups called flocks. Flock formation serves to reduce predation pressure, facilitate cooperative foraging, improve reproductive success, and strengthen territorial defense.[3] Birds travel to different areas to locate adequate food, and flocking increases the efficiency of food-searching activities. Flocking provides security for group members and allows them to forage more efficiently in a shorter amount of time. There is increased safety within a large flock such that individuals located in the center of the group are less likely to fall victim to predators.[3]

Flock size can vary depending on the availability of certain resources, such as food or nesting sites. Species that rely on small clumped food sources, such as fruit trees, tend to live in small diurnal feeding flocks. Galah cockatoos (*Cacatua roseicapilla*) and budgerigars (*Melopsittacus undulatus*) utilize widely dispersed food resources and typically form larger flocks.[4] A large roosting flock will often separate into smaller foraging flocks during the day. This may be a strategy adapted to minimize intraspecies competition for food.[5]

The parrots' day consists of a cyclic pattern of flying, vocalizing, foraging for food, resting, grooming, and social interactions.[6,7] Most flocks are active soon after sunrise, but tend to decrease their activities during the warmer periods of the day.[6] In the evening with decreased light available for foraging, birds engage in intraspecies social activities and focus on predator avoidance.[8]

Flock hierarchy

Within any complex social group, a system must evolve that enables flock members to determine allocation of resources and coexist with minimal aggression. Overt aggression directed at members of the flock would interfere with flock activities and increase the risk of injury and mortality within the flock. The formation of a dominance hierarchy promotes stable, predicable interactions between flock members. A dominance relationship is said to exist when a consistent pattern of dominance–submissive postural signaling occurs between two individuals within the group. The higher-ranking individual will exhibit assertive behavior toward the subordinate, and the subordinate will passively defer, reducing the incidence of overt aggression. Dominant (assertive) or submissive (subordinate) behavioral responses are determined by the outcomes of previous interactions between the individuals involved.[3] Once a dominance relationship has developed, it functions to decrease aggressive encounters between flock members, reducing competition and conferring priority of access to limited resources to higher-ranking individuals. The following behaviors were exhibited by assertive members of a cockatiel flock: turn threat, beak gape, peck threat, beak spar, peck, wing flapping, sidle approach, slow advance, and rushing and flight approach.[9] Birds exhibiting submissive or appeasement behaviors typically crouch, fluff their feathers, wag their heads, lift a foot, or avoid assertive flock members.[3]

The individuals with higher rank may benefit from preferred access to food resources, roosting sites, nests, and mating opportunities.[3] Hardy noted that aggression occurred more frequently during feeding, bathing, or seeking roosting sites.[6] Seibert and Crowell-Davis found that higher-ranking males in a captive flock of cockatiels had greater access to mates and preferred nest boxes.[9] They also noted that males were more aggressive than females, and females were more aggressive toward other females than males. While dominance relationships are critical to flock success and stability, the existence of cross-species dominance relationships has not been investigated.

Diet

In the wild, parrot diets are dependent upon the environment. Parrots are opportunistic foragers that primarily consume fruits, nuts, and seeds.[7,10,11] They have high-energy requirements due to their foraging and reproductive efforts. They may occasionally ingest insects while consuming their staple diets. Keas (*Nestor nobalis*) inhabiting the alpine region of New Zealand are the only parrots known to be omnivorous. Their diet includes plants, seeds, fruits, insects, and carrion.[12,13] Lories and lorikeets have special dietary requirements. In their natural setting, lories and lorikeets feed on fruits, seeds, blossoms, buds, and berries; they also have a specialized tongue that allows them to collect pollen and nectar from flowers.[14]

Parrots will include seasonally available items in their diets. Scarlet macaws have been observed feeding on seeds, fruits, leaves, flowers, and bark from 43 different plant species in Costa Rica. Some of the food items are non-native plants introduced in the local area for agricultural purposes.[11,14]

Reproduction

Male birds display certain ritualized behaviors during courtship. Male budgerigars display head bobbing during courtship.[15] Other psittacine courtship behaviors consist of bowing, head pumping, hopping, wing flicking, flapping, tail wagging, and strutting.[16] Male cockatoos may erect the crest feathers during a courtship display, along with opening the wings and spreading the tail feathers. When the cockatoo crest is erected during times of non-breeding, it may be an indication of excitement or arousal. Psittacine birds also use vocalizations specific to courtship. Budgerigars sing a warble song to synchronize reproductive behavior between the breeding pair. Male budgerigars have been found to warble at a higher rate than females.[4]

There are many reproductive systems used by avian species. The type of system used is dependent on ecological and social factors.[1] To briefly summarize, the different systems are:

- *Polyandry*—A female forms pair bonds with multiple males. Both females and males provide parental care.
- *Polygynandry*—Males and females both pair with multiple partners. They form a communal nest and all individuals participate in raising the offspring.

- *Polygyny*—A male breeds with multiple females. The female is responsible for raising the offspring. The male may not provide any parental care.
- *Monogamy*—A single male and single female form a pair bond for breeding and raising the offspring through the season. This is one of the most common mating systems in the avian world.

Within a monogamous reproductive system, several different breeding strategies can be employed to ensure the survival of offspring.

- *Territorial breeding*—A pair defends an established territory that contains the nesting site, or food and other resources.
- *Colonial breeding*—All mating pairs position their nests in a colony. This strategy is chosen when there are limited nesting sites near a food resource. Cooperative defense against predators is a key characteristic of colonial breeding.
- *Cooperative breeding*—The breeding pair has helpers, who may be individuals from their previous brood, who assist in feeding and protecting the offspring.

Pair bonding

Pair bonding is defined as a mutual attachment between a male and a female for the purpose of reproduction. Members of a bonded pair show preferential affiliative behaviors toward their mate, characterized by allopreening, beak touching, and allofeeding. Bonded pairs will often mutually exclude other individuals from these interactions. Males have been known to regurgitate to their partners as part of their courtship, but this behavior may also function to strengthen and maintain the pair bond.[12] Bonded pairs have also been observed to engage in aggressive behavior in defense or support of the mate.[6]

Allopreening usually occurs between breeding pairs or preferred associates and provides mutual benefits to the performer and recipient.[3] The preening is often directed to the head and areas of the body that the recipient cannot easily reach. For a bonded pair, the physical interaction of allopreening serves to strengthen their relationship. Allopreening occurs most frequently when pair bonds are first formed or after the pair has been separated. Solicitation of allopreening, with feathers fluffed and head bowed or withdrawn, can also be used for appeasement in the event of an aggressive act.

Monogamy is the formation of a pair bond that lasts through the breeding season. Parrots that form serial monogamous bonds may remain with one partner throughout the breeding season but may take part in extra-pair copulations.[9,17] After the breeding season, some pairs may stay together throughout the year.[6] More experienced pairs typically have a higher reproductive success than newly

formed pairs.[4,18] Budgerigars often maintain the same pair bond from one breeding season to the next, whereas green-rumped parrotlets (*Forpus passerinus*) frequently have different mates from season to season.[4] Certain species of parrots have adapted to different social systems at different times of the year. They may pair bond during the breeding season, then form family groups when their chicks become fledglings.

Nesting

During the breeding season, parrots nest in tree cavities. While they do not create holes in trees, they can and do modify the cavity or entrance by chewing with their beaks. Most parrots have individual nests that they defend against intruders and predators.

Some species, such as the monk parakeet, engage in communal nesting. They are colonial breeders and are the only parrots that build nests.[1] Each pair has a separate entrance into the nest. It is not uncommon for monk parakeet breeders to have a helper.

Pink cockatoos (*Cacatua leadbeateri*) sometimes displace Galah cockatoos (*Eolophus roseicapillus*) from their nests after eggs have been laid. The pink cockatoos may raise Galah cockatoos along with their own young. Galahs raised by pink cockatoos produce contact calls of pink cockatoos and associate with the foster species, even when exposed to their own species.[4]

Parental care

Hatching occurs asynchronously. In some clutches, the eldest can be several days older than the youngest hatched. Newly hatched psittacines are altricial, meaning that they are born naked, blind, weak, and helpless. They are unable to maintain their body temperature and rely upon the parents to keep them warm. Chicks are completely dependent upon the parents for food and protection from predators until they fledge and leave the nest. Due to the huge parental investments required for reproductive success, psittacine parents often engage in cooperative biparental care of offspring. Males often provide for the female and the chicks.[18] In some species of cockatoos, the males have been observed to assist with incubation of eggs.[4] As the chicks develop, the parent's nest attendance declines.[18]

Social interactions with the parents and clutch mates are necessary for vocal learning and social development. Budgerigars raised in isolated groups can eventually learn normal behavior and vocalizations once they rejoin a flock.[4] However, individual chicks raised in total isolation continued to display aberrant behaviors even after exposure to other birds.

Different species engage in a variety of parental care strategies. Meyer's parrots (*Poicephalus meyeri*), and several other psittacine species, place their juveniles together in a communal nursery area.[19] Parents continue to care for their own fledglings, and fledglings recognize and respond to contact calls from their own parents.

Once old enough to leave the nest, juvenile parrots form large foraging groups. Young psittacine birds have been observed to engage in different forms of group play. They beak wrestle, push each other with their feet or chase each other on foot or in flight. Some juvenile keas exhibit object play with a stone, stick, or any small object that they can grasp and toss in the air.[12]

Vocal communication

Avian vocal communications are comprised of different types of calls (short, innate, stereotyped vocalizations), and songs (longer complex vocalizations that are learned) used to convey specific messages. Parrots use contact calls for flock members, alarm calls for predators, flight calls, calls to indicate that food has been located, and more. Other vocalizations are used to indicate particular social relationships within the species or to identify potential mates.[20] Psittacine birds are generally silent during the day while they are feeding. Vocalizations are associated with roosting and flying from foraging sites.[1,5,6]

Vocal mimicry is an innate part of a bird's vocal development. It enables juveniles to learn the calls and songs required for communication with flock mates. While songbirds have critical periods for song learning, psittacine birds exhibit vocal plasticity in which they can learn new vocalizations throughout their lifetime. Adult budgerigars can learn and imitate complex sounds.[21]

Vocal mimicry can be utilized in predator defense, and nest and territory defense.[20] When there is a threat to a nest or an individual, the threatened individual can give the mobbing call of another species. Birds of the other species will be attracted to the call and mob the predator. If an intruder approaches a nest or territory, the threatened individual can mimic the call of a predator and frighten the intruder.

A study by Masin, Massa, and Bottoni on fledgling Meyer's parrots showed that young chicks exhibit vocal learning while they are in the nest.[19] By the time of weaning, the chicks exhibited 100% similarity with the father's vocalizations. Chicks raised without vocal context produced subsongs that were simpler and more monotonous than chicks raised with a vocal tutor.

A contact call is a distinct vocalization that a bird makes when attempting to establish the location of other members of the flock. Contact calls are one of the most common calls observed within a flock of parrots.[22] These calls can be very loud and carry for great distances. Parrots can discriminate contact calls between family members and non-members and use different contact calls for different social companions.

Vocal mimicry and plasticity enable juveniles to learn the calls and songs required for communication with other flock members. Juveniles mimic adults and learn from auditory feedback of their own calls. Amazon parrots roost in communal groups each night comprising 50–200 birds. Each group has its own dialect, and flock members only respond to calls within their own dialect.[22] Juveniles must learn this dialect before dispersal in order to interact with members of its flock.

Vocal plasticity also allows adult parrots to learn vocalizations that help maintain bonds within a flock, which is particularly relevant for species in which individuals change flocks several times in their lifetime, such as the Galahs.[4] Psittacine birds can selectively learn to mimic the vocalizations of the individuals with whom they are closely bonded.[23]

The range of hearing for psittacine birds includes frequencies from 1 kHz up to 4 kHz. Budgerigars have the ability to discriminate and remember complex vocalizations that occur in the range in which they hear best.[24] Auditory feedback is important for young birds to learn the appropriate songs. If budgerigars are deafened, they vocalize less and have contact calls that differ from the calls of normal siblings.[25] Adult birds also need auditory feedback in order to maintain the learned songs.

Non-vocal communication

Non-vocal communication consists of signals and displays. A signal is a behavior that changes the behavior of the recipient in a manner that benefits the sender. A display is a ritualized signal that conveys a specific message to the recipient. Displays are used by psittacine birds during courtship rituals.

Plumage and color also play a role in communication. Bird vision is considered tetrachromatic because they can visualize both near ultraviolet (UVA) and ultraviolet (UV) wavelengths.[15] They have the ability to see UV wavelengths because they possess a UV-sensitive cone in their retina. Parrots can also see fluorescence, which occurs when short wavelength light is absorbed and re-emitted. When the light is re-emitted, it occurs in longer wavelengths.[15,26] Certain Australian parrots, such as certain cockatoos, rosellas, blue-winged parrots, and budgerigars, have been found to possess a yellow fluorescent pigment in their feathers undetectable to the human eye.

Budgerigars are sexually dimorphic parrots that live in the arid regions of Australia. Several studies that involved altering the fluorescence of male budgerigars[15] demonstrated that alterations in reflectance in the UVA waveband affected female choice of mates. Budgerigars also possess fluorescent yellow plumage in contrast with UV reflecting blue plumage on their heads, which is used during courtship displays.[26] Hausmann et al. examined 108 species of birds and found that significantly more UV reflective plumage is found in body regions associated with active courtship display.[26] In parrots, there are twice as many species with fluorescent plumage in areas used for courtship displays, than non-displayed areas on their body.

Birds may have adapted the use of UV signals for many reasons.[26] It can be used to signal over short distances. Birds can signal with less risk of being exposed to mammalian predators since most predatory species cannot perceive UV light. UV signals contrast sharply against foliage. They may also be an indication of good health since they are created by feather microstructure rather than pigmentation. The UV signals are also iridescent which may help to augment courtship displays.

Diagnosis and treatment of common behavior problems of psittacine birds

Complaints about behavior can arise when pet birds struggle to cope with inappropriate environmental conditions, when social interactions are poor in quantity or quality, or when caregivers misconstrue normal parrot behaviors. Early adverse experiences can also influence later behavior, particularly those that occur during sensitive developmental periods. Conditions associated with some captive breeding programs, such as early separation from clutch mates, maternal and paternal separation, hand weaning practices, and inadequate socialization, can have long-term consequences on coping styles, neuroendocrine responses to stress, neural circuitry, and social competence.[27] The impressive cognitive capabilities of parrots may also be a factor in the development of behavior problems, because of the lack of adequate intellectual and occupational challenges in captive environments.[28,29]

Many parrots are kept as single-housed birds, making the human caregiver the sole target of social contact. Problem behaviors reported by owners of psittacine companion parrots include aggression and biting, feather picking and self-inflicted injuries, social avoidance of family members, excessive vocalization, destructive behavior, fears and phobias, inappropriate sexual behaviors, overeating, and failure to accept new diets.

Behavioral evaluation

The diagnosis of a primary behavioral problem requires establishing a doctor–patient–client relationship, obtaining a thorough behavioral history, performing a physical examination and appropriate diagnostic testing, evaluating the nutritional status of the bird, evaluating the environment, and observing the behavior of the bird within the environment, including interactions with caregivers and family members.[30] Important historical information that should be collected during a behavioral evaluation is listed in Table 1.1.[31]

Behavior symptoms include feather picking, mutilation, screaming, aggression, and avoidance behaviors. Symptoms

Table 1.1 Historical information during a behavioral evaluation

Early history: source of the bird, type of weaning
Housing: size and style of cage, perching areas, list of cage contents
Object enrichments: toys (style, number, rotation)
Locations of cages and play areas
Feeding schedule and foraging opportunities
Photoperiod: sleeping arrangements and schedules
Confinement schedule: time in cage, out of cage, alone
Primary caregiver interactions: time spent with bird, nature of interactions
Family member interactions
Presence of other species
Bathing
Training and commands: methods used
Reaction to new objects or people
Play behavior
Physical exercise and locomotor activities
Sexual behaviors
Air and lighting quality
Recent changes to environment
Description of a typical day for the bird

should not be mistaken for diagnoses. A list of differential diagnoses should be developed based on diagnostic testing and the behavioral history. Specific information about the behavioral complaint or complaints should include a detailed description or videotape of the behavior, age of onset and any particular events associated with the onset of the behavior, temporal or seasonal patterns, and an estimated or recorded frequency of the behavior. It is also important to determine if the behavior is more likely to occur in the presence of particular individuals, or in specific locations. The caregivers' response to the behavior and the outcomes of previous interventions should be detailed. For aggression complaints, document who (the victim), where (the location), and what (the specific behaviors of the bird) for each episode, as well as the outcome of each episode.

General treatment considerations

Environment

The environment should, to the extent possible, allow for the expression of species-typical natural behaviors, and accommodate the natural time budgets for these activities. Attention to foraging opportunities, sleep patterns, physical activities, and social interactions is important in the treatment of behavioral disorders in birds.

The majority of psittacine birds kept as pets are from tropical to semi-tropical regions where the typical photoperiod would include approximately 12 hours of light and 12 hours of dark. Sleep and rest occupy the majority of the 24-hour time period when time budgets are measured in the wild.[32] Budgerigars studied under conditions of constant illumination spent an average of 38% of a 24-hour period in sleep states.[33] Half-moon conures (*Aratinga canicularis*) under similar experimental conditions spent 57% of the 24-hour period sleeping or drowsing.[34]

Sleep is essential for mental and physical health. Sleep deprivation has been suspected as a risk factor for increased reproductive activities, fears or anxiety, stereotypies, and aggression or irritability. A minimum of 12 hours of uninterrupted sleep in a quiet, dark area away from household activities is recommended for any bird that is presented for behavioral abnormalities.

Foraging activities and food handling occupy a significant proportion of a parrot's waking hours.[35] When pet birds are fed pelleted or seed diets *ad libitum* from a dish, the time budget required for feeding activities is drastically altered. This has been postulated to contribute to the development of abnormal behaviors. In a study of wild crimson rosellas, young birds spent an average of 67% of their active time in foraging and feeding activities.[36] In captivity, a variety of feeding techniques can be used to encourage foraging, or food searching, such as placing non-perishable foods in multiple locations around the cage or mixing non-edible items with the food (Figure 1.1). Placing food on clean areas of the cage floor and adding branches, leaves, or shavings is another option. Foraging devices and puzzle feeders are commercially available or can be easily constructed.[37] Attention to safety, as well as adequate nutrition, is important when incorporating foraging enrichment strategies.

In addition to food-oriented activities, additional strategies can be used to address deficiencies in the captive environment. Captive environments are rarely able to accommodate all species-typical activities (reproductive behavior, flight, flock interactions), but substitutions can focus on providing acceptable alternative activities to occupy the time budget. For any problem parrot, recommendations should focus on creating appropriate intellectual stimulation (training opportunities), providing exercise (flying, flapping, swinging, running, climbing), beak activity (chew toys, branches) (Figure 1.2), and positive social interactions. Effects of social enrichment were documented in a laboratory study involving orange-winged Amazon parrots. Isosexual pair housing of young Amazon parrots resulted in greater use of enrichments, fewer bouts of prolonged screaming, less time spent preening, and less inactive time, than singly housed control birds.[38]

Behavior modification

Behavior modification uses operant conditioning techniques to strengthen the occurrence of desirable behaviors and diminish the occurrence of undesirable behaviors. With operant conditioning, behaviors are goal-directed and controlled by their consequences, or controlling stimuli. Operant conditioning paradigms can involve positive reinforcement, negative punishment, positive punishment, and

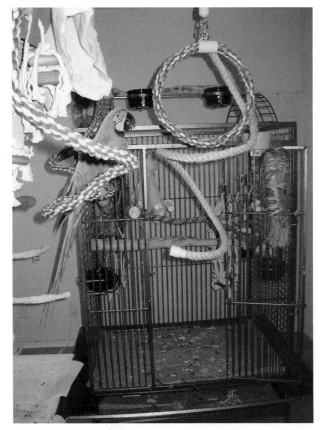

Figure 1.1 A cage containing a variety of foraging devices and toys.

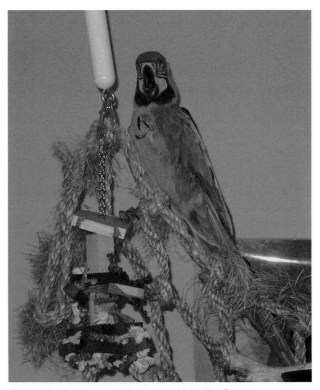

Figure 1.2 A macaw exercising on a stand outside of its cage.

negative reinforcement.[39] For a detailed discussion of the meaning of these terms and their application, see Chapter 18.

Desensitization, counter-conditioning, and flooding are all techniques commonly used to modify behavior. These techniques, their advantages and disadvantages, and instructions for their application are covered in detail in Chapter 18.

Training parrots to understand and comply with simple requests (commands) can build confidence, reduce fear, and facilitate predictable interactions between bird and human. Commands can be practical (step up, stay, quiet), or promote physical activity (dance, swing, turn around), and will serve to increase the caregiver's ability to communicate effectively and predictably with the parrot, and allow for the intellectual stimulation associated with learning new commands.

Pharmacotherapy

Pharmacological treatment options for behavioral disorders in birds are detailed in Chapter 19. Medication can be used to prevent self-harm, improve quality of life, or facilitate responses to the behavior modification plan.[30]

Fears and phobias

Fear responses in psittacine birds involve characteristic vocalizations, defensive postures, avoidance, escape attempts, frantic behavior, displacement behaviors, and aggression. A variety of factors contributes to fear responses in psittacine birds. Parrots are prey species, many of which do not have long histories of domestication, and some of which suffer from socialization or developmental deficits. Housing conditions, environmental stressors, and sleep deprivation can also contribute to fear responses.

The effects of environmental enrichment on fear responses to novel objects in orange-winged Amazons (*Amazona amazonica*) were evaluated.[40] Physical enrichments included swinging ladders and spiral boings. Foraging enrichments included fruit cages, toy boxes, and treat baskets. Parrots housed in enriched environments were significantly less fearful of novel objects compared to parrots housed in barren environments.

The effects of rearing conditions on the development of fear were studied in Nanday conure chicks (*Nandayus nenday*).[41] Four different treatment groups were raised in either enriched environments (with other chicks, soft toys, and sensory stimulation) or restricted environments, and were either exposed to early handling or were not handled beyond the feeding routine. Both handling and environmental enrichment were found to significantly reduce fear of novel objects.

Treatment of fears and phobias involves identifying sources of fear, and removing or minimizing contact. Frightened birds should be removed from high traffic areas and allowed to explore new objects and places on their own schedule. A sleeping cage that allows for security and uninterrupted sleep can be vital for fearful parrots.

Caregivers should avoid reinforcing (giving excessive verbal comfort or attention to) behaviors consistent with fear. Positive reinforcement training should focus on building confidence through acquisition of new commands and skills.

Gradual desensitization can be used when the stimuli that elicit fear or anxiety can be identified and manipulated for controlled exposures. Fear can result from a variety of stimuli, many of which may not be apparent to the human caregivers.[42] Fear can also occur as a result of interactions or associations with humans. In a case report of a Goffins cockatoo (*Cacatua goffini*) diagnosed with a conditioned fear response of the primary caregiver, desensitization and counter-conditioning were used successfully to improve the relationship and reduce the fear.[43] Anti-anxiety medications can be used in severe cases of fear or phobias, but limited data is available regarding efficacy and safety.

Feather plucking and self-mutilation

Feather picking may not be the most prevalent behavior problem affecting companion psittacine birds, but it is the most common complaint for which the veterinarian is consulted. The plumage serves multiple functions, including flight, insulation, protection from physical trauma, protection from UV radiation, waterproofing, and visual communication.[44] After foraging, grooming occupies the largest amount of a wild bird's time budget. Self-preening and allopreening (preening of another individual) function to maintain feather condition, provide comfort or de-arousal, and strengthen social bonds.[45]

Feather picking disorder, or behavioral feather picking, is characterized by self-initiated feather removal or damage, and/or self-inflicted damage to soft tissues, in the absence of an identifiable primary medical explanation[46–51] (Figures 1.3 and 1.4). In addition to aesthetic consequences, feather chewing or plucking can result in abnormal feather development, hemorrhage from damaged blood feathers, follicular damage, discomfort, and loss of insulation. Consequences of soft tissue mutilation might include hemorrhage, secondary infections, and penetration of body cavities.

A variety of medical differentials or risk factors should be investigated including organopathies, infectious diseases, internal and external parasites, seasonal hormonal changes, dermatological conditions, toxin exposures, malnutrition, food sensitivities, conditions causing pain or discomfort, and neoplasia.[46–48] In a review of dermatohistopathology findings for 408 feather picking and self-mutilating birds, paired biopsies from affected and non-affected skin were evaluated.[52] Inflammatory skin disease was diagnosed based on the histological presence of inflammation in both

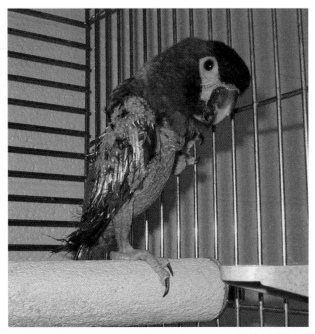

Figure 1.3   A macaw with severe feather damage due to feather picking.

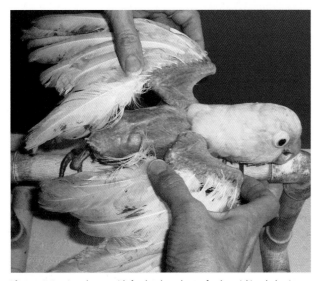

Figure 1.4   A cockatoo with feather loss due to feather picking behavior.

affected and unaffected skin samples. Macaw species and Amazon species were most likely to be diagnosed with inflammatory disease. Traumatic skin disease was diagnosed by the absence of inflammation at both affected and unaffected biopsy sites. Traumatic skin disease was reported in cockatoos and African gray parrots. Traumatic skin disease and inflammatory skin disease were reported with approximately equal frequencies in conures, eclectus parrots, Quaker parrots, cockatiels, and caiques.

There are many suggested risk factors for feather picking disorder, but none scientifically proven to cause feather picking in pet birds. Possible environmental factors include inadequate bathing, mechanical injury or skin irritation,

poor air quality, toxin exposure, abrupt changes, and sleep deprivation.[47] Possible behavioral risk factors include lack of stimulation, lack of control or unpredictability, lack of foraging opportunities, confinement, crowding, social incompatibility, and social isolation. Individual factors include chronic hormone induction, species, gender, neurotransmitter abnormalities, and individual differences in coping styles.[51] A single retrospective study has identified several significant risk factors for feather picking in pet parrots: species (African gray parrots), gender (female), and lack of play behavior.[53] Additional species predispositions have been reported based on clinical impressions, including conure, macaw, and cockatoo species.[50]

Treatment considerations should include attention to nutrition, general health, social interactions, photoperiod, housing, and air quality, and control of reproductive behaviors. Special attention should be given to foraging enrichment and stress reduction.[50,51] Foraging and physical enrichments were shown to prevent and improve feather picking behavior in laboratory-housed orange-winged Amazon parrots and in African gray parrots.[54,55]

Neurochemical abnormalities should be considered, particularly in cases of chronic feather picking. Feather picking disorder has been compared to trichotillomania, an impulse control disorder of humans.[56] Medications used to treat compulsive or impulsive behavioral disorders in other species may be helpful in treating persistent feather picking or self-mutilation problems in psittacine birds. Selective serotonin reuptake inhibitors are the treatment of choice based on treatment responses in a variety of species. Successful adjunctive use of medication for the treatment of feather picking has been reported using fluoxetine, paroxetine, clomipramine, naltrexone, gabapentin, amitriptyline, and haloperidol.[57–63] Hormone therapies may also prove useful. Pharmacological interventions are described in detail in Chapter 19.

Reproductive behavior problems

The onset of puberty, ranging from 6 months to 6 years depending on the species, may be associated with a variety of behavioral complaints. Behavior problems associated with hormonal changes may include screaming, or frequent contact calling, aggression or territorial defense of cage and nesting sites, intolerance of handling, irritability, favoring one person, sexual displays, frequent regurgitation, panting, and masturbation.[64]

While species differences exist, typical environmental cues that trigger reproductive behaviors include changes in day length, temperature, or rainfall, the presence of nesting sites, and the presence of potential mates. Caregivers that stroke their birds over the back or tail can also stimulate sexual behavior and should be advised to discontinue any forms of handling that stimulate the bird.[65] Seasonal variations in temperature, photoperiod, and food supply are typically absent in captive environments, which can result in chronic hormone stimulation.[66]

Persistent sexual behaviors in pet psittacine birds create challenges for behavioral management as well as physical health. Potential medical concerns for females include dystocia, cloacal prolapse, pathologic fractures, and coelomitis. In male birds, orchitis and cloacal prolapse are possible.[67] General treatment recommendations should include decreasing the photoperiod, providing more dark time, removing potential or perceived nesting areas, and reducing the fat content of the diet. Hormone therapy, such as leuprolide acetate, may also be indicated.[68] However, species differences in sensitivity to leuprolide acetate are possible as well as variations in effects based on the timing of administration during the reproductive cycle.[69]

Aggression

The postulated causes of human-directed aggression (lunging, charging, pecking or striking, or biting) in psittacine birds include play and exploration, instrumental or conditioned aggression, territoriality, fear, mate-related and sexually induced aggression, and redirected aggression.[70]

Play and exploration

Parrots use their beaks like hands to explore the environment. Juveniles of several psittacine species have been observed to engage in social play in the wild. Play behaviors included clawing, play biting, and mock fighting. Treatment of play aggression includes provision of chew toys, regular opportunities for appropriate play and interactions, and positive reinforcement (rewards) for appropriate play behavior. Corrections for play biting are often unsuccessful. Caregivers should be instructed to discontinue interactions if mouthing becomes excessive.

Fear aggression

Fearful behavior in psittacine birds may involve aggression if the bird is otherwise unable to extricate itself from the stressful situation. Caged birds that are unable to fly or prevented from escaping may choose aggression when flight or avoidance is not an option. Caregivers should receive instructions about how to recognize postures that are consistent with fear, and how to avoid eliciting these responses. Safety considerations are important for both the caregiver and the bird. Forcing unpleasant exposures is seldom helpful and tends to worsen fear responses and aggressive behaviors. Desensitization and counter-conditioning is often successful in cases of fear aggression.[40]

Instrumental or learned aggression

For birds that do not desire to interact (to be petted or handled at particular times or by particular individuals),

biting is often a highly effective means of avoiding contact. If the bird can successfully use aggression to avoid certain activities, then negative reinforcement of aggression is possible. Caregivers should respect the preferences of the bird regarding interactions and avoid activities that elicit aggressive responses. Birds can be taught with positive reinforcement to comply with caregiver requests.

Territorial aggression

Many avian species establish, maintain, and protect access to particular areas in their natural habitats. Aggression may be directed against any intruder, regardless of familiarity. The bird is often normal and friendly when taken away from the vicinity of the cage. Treatment will require that the cage be moved away from high traffic areas to reduce the incidence of territorial displays. Otherwise, negative reinforcement of aggressive displays can influence the severity of the problem. The bird can be taught to step up on a hand-held perch, rather than a hand, to allow removal from the cage.

Gradual desensitization and counter-conditioning for approaches to the territory (cage) can be effective. The bird is allowed to have a special treat or offered verbal praise as individuals gradually approach the cage area from a comfortable distance. If the bird shows signs of defensive behaviors, the approacher stops and resumes once the bird has settled. Alternatively, the caregiver can work with the bird in a neutral area at a comfortable distance from the cage, and then gradually move the training sessions closer to the cage.

Sexual aggression

Lack of suitable conspecific mates and seasonal hormonal changes can result in sexual behaviors directed at a preferred human. Sexual behaviors may involve a combination of the following: regurgitation, masturbation, excessive contact seeking, guarding, and aggression directed at other individuals when the preferred individual is present. Problem onset may coincide with the species' natural breeding season, with lengthening daylight, or at random times when conditions support breeding behavior (households with unnatural photoperiods, presence of breeding birds, and stimulation of the bird by the caregiver).

Treatment suggestions include allowing non-preferred family members to participate in feeding and maintenance care when possible and avoiding any forms of handling that stimulate the bird to engage in sexual behaviors. Gradual desensitization and counter-conditioning for approaches to the bird when it is with its preferred person or in the nesting area can be attempted.

Hormonally mediated behaviors can be extremely frustrating for caregivers. Hormone therapies can be used to facilitate behavior modification by minimizing sexual and aggressive behavioral responses and increasing the success of the behavior modification program.

Excessive vocalization

Differences in noisiness exist between species and in caregiver tolerance of noise. It is considered normal for most parrots to vocalize loudly several times a day for up to 15–20 minutes.[66] Causes of excessive vocalization include operantly conditioned attention-seeking behavior, fear-induced vocalizations, excessive contact calling, distress or injury, and lack of opportunity to engage in acceptable behaviors, or lack of environmental enrichment.

Caregiver influence on excessive vocalization behavior of psittacine birds should always be considered. Typical human responses to screaming often serve to reinforce the behavior. Yelling at the bird, running into the room to scold the bird, shaking the cage, or picking up the bird to return it to the cage can all be construed as reinforcing if the bird's goal was to get attention. It is likely that actions intended to be punishing may actually be reinforcing.

Screaming by a bird that is seeking attention should be ignored by all family members. As unacceptable behaviors are being extinguished via removal of the reinforcer (attention), caregivers should also establish and maintain appropriate behaviors by engaging the bird in regular training sessions, rewarding the bird during quiet times, and encouraging and reinforcing acceptable vocalizations, such as singing, whistling, or talking.

Negative punishment of excessive vocalization can also be effective. When screaming occurs, the caregiver should turn around, leave the room, close the door, or cover the cage. Removal of attention and stimulation (time-out) should be enforced just long enough for the bird to settle.

Environmental and behavioral strategies should focus on creating environments in which the bird and caregiver can be successful. If the caregiver diary indicates a pattern to the vocalization problem, then feeding, playtime, or training sessions can be scheduled just before the bird's "loud times." Preemptive strategies can be highly successful in reconditioning undesirable behavioral responses that occur with predictability.[64]

Fear or distress calls should never be ignored, nor should contact calls. When contact calls become persistent, behavior modification techniques can be applied. Parrots in impoverished environments may be predisposed to excessive vocalizations, and appropriate environmental enrichments are indicated.

Conclusions

In their natural environments, parrots are presented with endless activities and challenges related to survival, social interactions, and reproductive success. A thorough understanding of natural psittacine behaviors, social structure, and reproductive strategies helps to establish recommendations for captive housing and care. The prevalence of serious behavioral problems in captive psittacine birds raises important questions regarding the suitability of some species as captive companions, appropriate guidelines for breeding programs and chick rearing, and the possibility of preventive counseling strategies for caregivers of psittacine birds.

Acknowledgments

All photos in this chapter courtesy of Lynne M. Siebert.

References

1. Elphick C, Dunning Jr JB, Sibley DA. *The Sibley Guide to Bird Life and Behavior*. New York: Chanticleer Press, Inc, 2001.
2. AVMA. *US Pet Ownership and Demographics Sourcebook*. Schaumburg: AVMA, 2007.
3. Wilson EO. *Sociobiology: The New Synthesis*. Cambridge: The Belknap Press of Harvard University Press, 1975.
4. Farabaugh SM, Dooling RJ. Acoustic communication in parrots: Laboratory and field studies of budgerigars, *Melopsittacus undulates*. In: Kroodsma DE, Miller, EH, eds. *Ecology and Evolution of Acoustic Communication in Birds*. Ithaca: Cornell University Press, 1996;97–117.
5. Chapman CA, Chapman LJ, Lefebvre L. Variability in parrot flock size: Possible functions of communal roosts. *The Condor* 1989;91:842–847.
6. Pizo MA, Simão I. Daily variation in activity and flock size of two parakeet species from southeastern Brazil. *Wilson Bull* 1997;109(2):343–348.
7. Hardy JW. Flock social behavior of the orange-fronted parakeet. *The Condor* 965;67:140–156.
8. Berg KS, Brumfield RT, Apanius V. Phylogenetic and ecological determinants of the neotropical dawn chorus. *Proc R Soc B* 2006;273: 999–1005.
9. Seibert LM, Crowell-Davis SL. Gender effects on aggression, dominance rank, and affiliative behaviors in a flock of captive adult cockatiels (*Nymphicus hollandicus*). *J Appl Anim Behav Sci* 2001;71(2):155–170.
10. Ragusa-Netto J. Feeding ecology of the Green-cheeked parakeet (*Pyrrhura molinae*) in dry forests in western Brazil. *Braz J Biol* 2007;67(2): 243–249.
11. Vaughan C, Nemeth N, Marineros L. Scarlet Macaw, Ara Macao, (Psittaciformes: Psittacidae) diet in Central Pacific Costa Rica. *Rev Biol Trop* 2006;54(3): 919–926.
12. Diamond J, Bond AB. *Kea, Bird of Paradox*. Berkeley: University of California Press, 1999.
13. Emery NJ. Cognitive ornithology: The evolution of avian intelligence. *Phil Trans R Soc B* 2006;361:23–43.
14. Low R. *Lories and Lorikeets*. New York: Van Nostrand Reinhold Company, 1977.
15. Pearn SM, Bennett ATD, Cuthill IC. Ultraviolet vision, fluorescence and mate choice in a parrot, the budgerigar *Melopsittacus* undulates. *Proc R Soc B* 2001;268:2273–2279.
16. Sparks J, Soper T. *Parrots A Natural History*. New York: Facts on File, 1990;58–94.
17. Emery NJ, Seed AM, von Bayern AMP et al. Cognitive adaptations of social bonding in birds. *Phil Trans R Soc B* 2007;362:489–505.
18. Wilson KA, Field R, Wilson MH. Successful nesting behavior of Puerto Rican parrots. *Wilson Bull* 1995;107(3):518–529.
19. Masin S, Massa R, Bottoni L. Evidence of tutoring in the development of subsong in newly-fledged Meyer's Parrots *Poicephalus meyeri*. *Ann Braz Acad Sci* 2004;76(2):231–236.

20. Baylis JR. Avian vocal mimicry. In: Kroodsma DE, Miller EH, Ouellet H, eds. *Acoustic Communication in Birds*. Vol. 2. New York: Academic Press, 1982;51–83.

21. Watanabe A, Eda-Fujiwara H, Kimura T. Auditory feedback is necessary for long term maintenance of high-frequency sound syllables in the song of adult male budgerigars (*Melopsittacus undulatus*). *J Com Physiol A* 2007;193:81–97.

22. Wright TF, Wilkinson GS. Population genetic structure and vocal dialect in an amazon parrot. *Proc R Soc B* 2000;268:609–616.

23. Kavanau JL. *Behavior and Evolution: Lovebirds, Cockatiels and Budgerigars*. Los Angeles: Science Software Systems, Inc, 1987.

24. Brauth SE, McHale CM, Brasher CA et al. Auditory pathways in the budgerigar: I. Thalamo-telencephalic projections. *Brain Behav Evol* 1987;30:174–199.

25. Dooling RJ, Gephart BF, Price PH et al. Effects of deafening on the contact call of the budgerigar, *Melopsittacus undulates*. *Anim Behav* 1986;35:1264–1266.

26. Hausmann F, Arnold KE, Marshall NJ et al. Ultraviolet signals in birds are special. *Proc R Soc B* 2002;270:61–67.

27. Latham NR, Mason GJ. Maternal deprivation and the development of stereotypic behaviour. *Appl Anim Behav Sci* 2008;110:84–108.

28. Van Hoek CS, ten Cate C. Abnormal behavior of birds kept as pets. *J Appl Anim Welfare Sci* 1998;1(1):51–64.

29. Pepperberg IM. Cognitive and communicative abilities of grey parrots. *Appl Anim Behav Sci* 2006;100:77–86.

30. Seibert LM, Landsberg GM. Diagnosis and management of patients presenting with behavior problems. *Vet Clin N Am Small Anim Prac* 2008;38:937–950.

31. Welle KR, Wilson L. Clinical evaluation of psittacine behavioral disorders. In: Luescher AU, ed. *Manual of Parrot Behavior*. Oxford: Blackwell Publishing, 2006;175–194.

32. Wirminghaus JO, Downs CT, Symes CT et al. Vocalizations and behaviours of the cape parrot *Poicephalus robustus*. *Durban Mus Novitates* 2000;25:12–17.

33. Ayala-Guerrero F. Sleep patterns of the parakeet (*Melopsittacus undulatus*). *Physiol Behav* 1989;46(5):787–791.

34. Ayala-Guerrero F, Perez MC, Calderon A. Sleep patterns in the bird *Aratinga canicularis*. *Physiol Behav* 1987;43(5):585–589.

35. Echols MS. The behavior of diet. *Proc Annu Conf Assoc Avian Vet* 2004;267–270.

36. McGrath RD, Lill A. Age-related differences in behavior and ecology of crimson rosellas during the non-breeding season. *Aust Wildlife Res* 1985;12:299–306.

37. Bauck L. Psittacine diets and behavioral enrichment. *Sem Avi Exotic Pet Med* 1998;7(3):135–140.

38. Meehan CL, Garner JP, Mench JA. Isosexual pair housing improves the welfare of young Amazon parrots. *Appl Anim Behav Sci* 2003;81:73–88.

39. Smith I. Basic behavioral principles for the avian veterinarian. *Proc Annu Conf Assoc Avian Vet* 1999;47–55.

40. Meehan CL, Mench JA. Environmental enrichment affects the fear and exploratory responses to novelty of young Amazon parrots. *Appl Anim Behav Sci* 2002;79:75–88.

41. Luescher AU, Sheeham L. Rearing environment and behavioral development of psittacine birds. *Proc Annu Conf Assoc Avian Vet* 2004;297–298.

42. Wilson L, Luescher AU. Parrots and fear. In: Luescher AU, ed. *Manual of Parrot Behavior*. Oxford: Blackwell Publishing, 2006;225–231.

43. Seibert LM, Sung W, Crowell-Davis SL. Animal behavior case of the month: Fear in a Goffins cockatoo. *J Am Vet Med Assoc* 2001;218(4):518–520.

44. Cooper JE, Harrison GJ. Dermatology. In: Ritchie BW, Harrison GJ, Harrison LR, eds. *Avian Medicine: Principles and Application*. Lake Worth: Wingers, 1994:607–639.

45. Bergman L, Reinisch US. Comfort behavior and sleep. In: Luescher AU, ed. *Manual of Parrot Behavior*. Oxford: Blackwell Publishing, 2006; 59–62.

46. Burgmann PM. Common psittacine dermatological diseases. *Sem Avi Exotic Pet Med* 1995;4(4):169–183.

47. Koski MA. Dermatological diseases in psittacine birds: An investigational approach. *Sem Avi Exotic Pet Med* 2002;11(3):105–124.

48. Nett CS, Tully TN. Anatomy, clinical presentation, and diagnostic approach to feather picking pet birds. *Compendium* 2003;25(3):206–218.

49. Jenkins JR. Feather picking and self-mutilation in psittacine birds. *Vet Clin N Amer Exotic Anim Prac* 2001;4(3):651–667.

50. Rosskopf WJ, Woerpel RW, eds. Feather picking and therapy of skin and feather disorders. In: *Diseases of Cage and Aviary Birds*. 3rd ed. Baltimore: Williams and Wilkins, 1996;397–405.

51. Seibert LM. Feather picking disorder in pet birds. In: Luescher AU, ed. *Manual of Parrot Behavior*. Oxford: Blackwell Publishing, 2006;255–265.

52. Garner MM, Clubb SL, Mitchell MA et al. Feather picking psittacines: Histopathology and species trends. *Vet Pathol* 2008;45:401–408.

53. Briscoe JA, Wilson L, Smith G. Non-medical risk factors for feather picking in pet parrots. *Proc Annu Conf Assoc Avian Vet* 2001;131.

54. Meehan CL, Millam JR, Mench JA. Foraging opportunity and increased physical complexity both prevent and reduce psychogenic feather picking by young Amazon parrots. *Appl Anim Behav Sci* 2003;80:71–85.

55. Lumeij JT, Hommers CJ. Foraging enrichment as treatment for pterotillomania. *Appl Anim Behav Sci* 2008;111:85–94.

56. Bordnick PS, Thyer BA, Ritchie BW. Feather picking disorder and trichotillomania: An avian model of human psychopathology. *J Behav Ther Exp Psy* 1994;25(3):189–196.

57. Seibert, LM. Animal behavior case of the month: Toe chewing in a cockatiel. *J Am Vet Med Assoc* 2004;224(9):1433–1435.

58. Martin KM. Behavioral approach to psittacine feather picking. *Proc Annu Conf Assoc Avian Vet* 2004;307–312.

59. Seibert LM, Crowell-Davis SL, Wilson GH et al. Placebo-controlled clomipramine trial for the treatment of feather picking disorder in cockatoos. *J Am Anim Hosp Assoc* 2004;40:261–269.

60. Turner R. Trexan (naltrexone hydrochloride) use in feather picking in avian species. *Proc Annu Conf Assoc Avian Vet* 1993;116–118.

61. Doneley B. Use of gabapentin to treat presumed neuralgia in a Little Corella (*Cacatua sanguinea*). *Proc Annu Conf Assoc Avian Vet: Australasian Committee* 2007;169–172.

62. Eugenio CT. Amitriptyline HCl: Clinical study for treatment of feather picking. *Proc Annu Conf Assoc Avian Vet* 2003;133–135.

63. Iglauer F, Rasim R. Treatment of psychogenic feather picking in psittacine birds with a dopamine antagonist. *J Small Anim Prac* 1993;34:564–566.

64. Seibert LM, Graham J. That time of the year? Seasonal reproductive disorders in birds. *Proc Annu Conf Assoc Avian Vet* 2004;219–227.

65. Van Sant F. Problem sexual behaviors of companion parrots. In: Luescher AU, ed. *Manual of Parrot Behavior*. Oxford: Blackwell Publishing, 2006;233–245.

66. Wilson L, Lightfoot TL. Concepts in behavior: Section III. Pubescent and adult psittacine behavior. In: Harrison GJ, Lightfoot T, eds. *Clinical Avian Medicine*. Vol. I. Palm Beach: Spix Publishing, 2006;73–84.

67. Speer B. Sex and the single bird. *Proc Annu Conf Assoc Avian Vet* 2003;331–343.

68. Ottinger MA, Wu J, Pelican K. Neuroendocrine regulation of reproduction in birds and clinical applications of GnRH analogues in birds and mammals. *Sem Avi Exotic Pet Med* 2002;11(2):71–79.

69. De Witt M, Westerhof I, Penfold LM. Effects of leuprolide acetate on avian reproduction. *Proc Annu Conf Assoc Avian Vet* 2004;73–74.

70. Welle KR, Luescher AU. Aggressive behavior in pet birds. In: Luescher AU, ed. *Manual of Parrot Behavior*. Oxford: Blackwell Publishing, 2006; 211–218.

2

Passerines

Wailani Sung

Introduction

Man has enjoyed the companionship of caged birds since the time of Alexander the Great.[1] The type of birds people keep in captivity ranges from small finches to large macaws. Small songbirds are popular because they are easy to maintain in captivity, are colorful, and due to their small size can be kept in a confined space. Certain birds, like the canary, are highly prized for their lovely song.

Over half of all living birds make up the order Passeriformes. Passerines belong within the order Passeriformes. Within the passerine family, they can be further subdivided into the Oscines and Suboscines. Some birds have a specialized vocal apparatus that enables them to sing. These birds are classified as Oscines. The popular small caged birds found in most local pet stores are mostly oscine birds. Within the Oscines, there are about 70 families of songbirds. The birds in this group have the most highly developed and complex songs.

The most well-known captive oscines are canaries (*Serinus canaria*), Gouldian finches (*Erythrura gouldiae*), and zebra finches (*Taeniopygia guttata*). They belong in the broad category of birds known as finches and finch-like birds. The different families of finches include Fringillidae, Passeridae, Estrildidae, and Ploceidae. Finches and similar species are found throughout the world. Estrildidae includes the zebra finch and Gouldian finch, along with waxbills, manikins, and munias. The common characteristics they all share are small size, brightly colored plumage, pleasant song, and a hard, broad bill. They have a foot pattern with three toes pointing forward and one pointing back.

While they do not demand attention and care to the extent that their psittacine cousins do, captive passerines can also exhibit behavioral problems due to inadequate care and husbandry. Zebra finches have been studied extensively by researchers around the world and much is known regarding their behavior. A generalized overview of basic passerine behavior will be presented here using the zebra finch as a model. Known differences in behavior between zebra finches and other songbirds will also be presented.

Colony activity

Zebra finches are socially monogamous birds that live in colonies in Australia's open grasslands. These areas tend to be sparsely populated with trees and bushes. Each zebra finch colony has 1–2 trees in which they gather for social activities. These "social trees" are where they congregate for resting, preening, allopreening, and singing.[2] All members of the flock participate in social activities. Even breeding pairs gather on the social trees. The fact that breeders will leave their nests unoccupied to engage in social activities attests to how important interactions with conspecifics are. Nests may be left alone for as long as 1–2 hours.[2]

Flock behavior

Flocks are formed to decrease predation pressure, increase foraging opportunities, and increase reproductive success. Flocks are coordinated by the calls of flock members. The finch's day begins around sunrise with distance calls. Once they hear the calls, finches start flying in to gather in one area. From this area, they then leave in small foraging flocks consisting of 2–10 birds. After foraging for a few hours, the flock takes a break in a nearby tree or bush. They separate into small groups for social activities, which include resting, preening, singing, and courting. Later in the day, the birds form into flocks again and forage for several more hours before sunset. At the end of the day, all the small foraging flocks congregate again in one area before returning to their roosting nests.

In the non-breeding season, feeding flocks can number up to 350 birds.[2] Flocks are composed of adult pairs and immature individuals. In the breeding season, the flock may only number about 10–20 individuals. The breeders may join the feeding flock for less than an hour after leaving the roost. After the breeding season is over, the foraging flock increases in size again.

Feeding behavior

The finches feed primarily on grass seeds. Each seed is dehusked before it is ingested. The zebra finch forages mainly on the ground for seeds. They have been seen on occasion to pick the seeds from standing grass heads. Birds in the wild are constantly foraging for more food to keep up with the high cost of survival and reproduction.

Breeding behavior

The breeding period of the zebra finch can last from 8 to 15 months. Zebra finches in all parts of Australia, except central Australia, typically are seasonal breeders. There tends to be a peak in breeding in the spring and a decline in the winter months. The zebra finches in central Australia are non-seasonal breeders and rely on other factors to time their breeding, such as rainfall and increased seed production. Gouldian finches also tend to limit breeding to certain times of the year, usually when the dry season occurs.

Zebra finches are monogamous and remain together for the rest of their lives. Once a male and female form a pair bond, they always remain together except when incubating or brooding. In the non-breeding season, the pair has a roosting nest, where they sleep at night. During the breeding season, the pair builds a separate breeding nest in thorny or prickly bushes. In contrast, Gouldian finches build nests in the hollows of Eucalyptus trees.[3] The parents of both finches and canaries engage in biparental care. Both males and females participate in nest building, incubation, brooding, and feeding the nestlings.[2,3] Like many avian species, finches have altricial young. The young are completely dependent upon the parents to provide food and warmth until they fledge.

Zebra finches are indeterminate layers, which means they can control the number of eggs they lay.[2] If an egg is removed, they can lay another egg to replace the lost egg. As the female continues to lay eggs, her constant contact with the eggs provide negative feedback to the ovarian follicles. This stops follicular growth, which signals an end to the egg laying process.[2] Zebra finches typically can have 2–7 eggs in each clutch. The female starts to incubate the eggs after the fourth egg is laid. The breeders incubate the eggs for 11–15 days before the chicks are hatched. The eggs can be left for a few hours each day while the breeders engage in social activities. Sometimes the eggs are also left unattended if the parents fend off intruders or if predators approach the nest.

The zebra finches nest in colonies throughout the year. Therefore they utilize a colony breeding strategy.[2] The colony breeding strategy is most likely selected when there is a limited number of nesting sites and a need for security.[4] In the Australian plains, trees and bushes are limited in number. Multiple nests will be built on trees and bushes within a certain area. Colony breeding provides more safety because there are more birds looking out for predators. Another advantage is that colony members may learn the location of different food resources.

The mating behavior of breeders in a colony can become synchronized as the season progresses. Environmental cues, such as rainfall, food availability, as well as other social factors may play a role in synchronization. When captive males were exposed to playbacks of birds singing in their colony, they sang more frequently. The females were also stimulated by the males' courtship sounds. The playback influenced the rate at which the females became physiologically ready for fertilization. These sounds encouraged the females to lay eggs at a faster rate. The females that were exposed to elevated song rates also had larger clutches than control females.[5] Another interesting finding was that the females produced larger clutches for the preferred males that sang most frequently and had the longest songs.[5]

Synchronized breeding improves the reproductive success of colony members in several different ways. The advantages are the possibility of more offspring and decreased loss due to predation. Females that are stimulated earlier in the season can produce larger clutches when the females are at a heavier body weight. They can possibly have another clutch before the end of the season.[5] Also, the more chicks present in one area, reduces the probability that any individual female's chicks gets eaten by predators.[5] In zebra finches, once the juveniles are fledged, the breeders can have another clutch in as early as 34 days.[2]

Zebra finches can become opportunistic breeders, which means they can continue breeding if all the necessary conditions are present. The females' gonads can remain in a permanently activated state.[5] This is in contrast to seasonal breeders. Seasonal breeding females need to be cued by several factors, such as male courtship, nest site, rainfall, habitat conditions, and so on, before she is ready for copulation and reproduction.[5]

Canaries are seasonal breeders.[6] They typically mate in the spring around March or April. Sometimes their breeding period can extend into August.[6] They are photoperiod-dependent breeders. The lengthening daylight provides a cue to stimulate courtship and mating behaviors.[7] In males, the increasing daylight produces an increase in testicular size, whereas the female canaries do not experience any size changes in their gonads. This indicates that females may need more than just increasing photoperiod in order to start breeding. Other environmental cues, such as food supply, population density, presence of nest sites, presence of a mate, temperature, humidity, and songs, may also be necessary.[7] When female canaries were exposed to playbacks of male songs, they gathered more string for nest building. They also laid more eggs when they heard a large repertoire of syllables compared to a smaller repertoire.[8]

The seasonal changes also bring about modifications in the canary's song. Many other temperate zone bird species also exhibit seasonality in their song behavior.[6] During the breeding season, the male canary sings a "stable" song. The stable song contains highly stereotyped syllable types with constant repertoire size. It remains the same throughout the breeding season. At the end of the breeding season, the males' gonads go into regression. During this time period, the testosterone levels decrease, which affect the male's behavior. They experience a full feather molt and singing stops for the next 4–6 weeks.[7]

The male canaries usually resume singing in October. The stable song then changes into an unstable song associated with non-breeding.[6] The non-breeding canary sings significantly shorter songs. These songs have a decreased number of syllable repetitions and a lower repetition rate. This behavior occurs similarly in other photoperiod-dependent breeders.[6] The non-stable songs contain more non-repeated syllables. At this point, the song gets slightly modified. Some syllables may be dropped and new syllables may be incorporated. These new syllables will be re-integrated into a new repertoire in the next breeding season.[6] Therefore the song repertoire changes on a yearly basis. Canaries add to their song repertoire as they age; the older the canary, the larger the song repertoire.

Bond formation

A pair bond is the formation of a mutual attachment between a male and female individual. In this pairing, aggressive behavior is reduced while sexual behavior is increased.[9] Once a pair bond has formed, the pair engages in exclusive allopreening and partner defense. A partner invites allopreening by fluffing out the feathers around the head and throat.[10] Partners must have tactile contact in order to form a pair. Visual and auditory or auditory contact alone is not enough for the male and female to form a bond.[9] They must be able to touch and most importantly allopreen in order to cement their bond. Allopreening can also occur between parents and offsprings. Siblings will also allopreen each other. The allopreening behavior usually stops when the males develop their sexually dimorphic feathers, around 40 days of age.[2]

Once a pair bond has formed, both male and female will defend their partner against approaches from same sex rivals.[2] The amount of time one bird spends near another individual is a good indicator of sexual preference.[11] Zebra finches are considered a "contact" species, in which partners remain in close contact with each other. The pair maintains a close spatial proximity when engaged in foraging activities.[9] Even in the non-breeding seasons, the pairs can be found perched or squatting in physical contact with each other.

Zebra finches can form pair bonds as early as 50–60 days of age.[2] Pair bonds can develop even before the males develop their full adult plumage. The finches can start breeding as young as 2–3 months of age.

Courtship behavior

In many passerine species, the male engages in an elaborate courtship display. Zebra finches do not display complex courtship behaviors. There are a few different courtship strategies that the males may engage in. One strategy is to approach the female and perform exaggerated greetings. An alternate strategy is to approach the female and direct several song phrases at her. The third strategy is most direct and usually exhibited by males in an existing pair bond; the male jumps directly onto the back of the female and starts copulation.[2]

Female preference

When a female finds a male attractive, she indicates her preference for that particular male in one of three ways. She approaches the male, engages in copulation, or exhibits nesting behavior. If the female is not interested in the male, she will fly away. In the zebra finch, a female may express her interest by performing a head tail twist greeting.

The female solicits copulation by crouching in a horizontal position and quivering her tail.[11] It has been noted that if the male zebra finch sings a long, complex song, he can induce the female to perform the copulation display.[11]

A large repertoire of songs from male canaries can cause the females to gather more nesting material.[8] This is an indication that the female prefers that particular male. If the female finds the mate attractive, she invests more in her offspring. She provides more often for the nestling and produces larger clutches. She may also deposit more androgens and immunoglobulins in her yolks. These two factors provide several benefits for a nestling. The immunoglobulins will boost a nestling's immune response. The androgens can affect the growth rate, begging rate, competitiveness, and mortality.[12]

Other factors that might influence a female's preference for a particular male include familiarity, complex song, and plumage. Familiarity has a definite influence on a female's choice for a mate. Female zebra finches have been found to prefer their mates' songs and father's songs over other males. The female is most likely influenced by early learning experiences. She may choose the song that sounds most familiar to her. The female's preference for her father's song may be counterintuitive. However, it may function solely as a social preference rather than a preference for mating with the father.[8] When a female zebra finch is removed from the nest before day 25, she does not show a preference for her father's song. This is an indication that a female's preference for certain songs is learned and not innate.[13]

Though familiarity is important to female zebra finches, it does not appear to have a strong influence on female Gouldian finches. It has been shown that female Gouldian finches do not always associate with males of the same color morph as themselves.[3] Researchers found that red-headed females had a preference for red-headed males. However, black-headed females associated with both red-headed and black-headed males. The yellow-headed females were the most accepting. They did not exhibit a color preference among the males. The females also preferred males that had longer pintail feathers.[3] It is interesting to note that the male Gouldian finches also had preferences for certain females. They preferred females that had the same head color morph as themselves.

In many songbird species, song complexity plays an important role in influencing a female's preference for a mate. The females show a distinct preference for long complex songs, which they learn through early exposure.[14] In one study, when a large repertoire of male canary songs was played to the female canaries, they laid eggs at a faster rate than when they heard a shorter repertoire.[5] The female canaries also showed preference for songs with certain elements, such as high syllable repetition rates and faster tempos.[15,16] These elements are difficult for the males to produce. The females may use these factors to determine the quality of their suitors.[16]

Males that can sing long complex songs are more attractive to females because they may be more genetically and physically fit compared to males that are unable to produce these complex songs. The high vocal center is an area of the brain associated with the production of complex signals. This area is very vulnerable to developmental stress. So if a male can produce an attractive song, it is an indication that his brain is well developed. This is a trait that he can pass to his offspring. Therefore, the ability to produce long elaborate songs may be a good indicator of a male's brain capacity.[17] The development of a long complex song is an indication of a male's overall fitness.[18]

If the relative song quality between two male rivals is similar, the female may base her choice on other factors, such as the appearance of male plumage and other morphological traits to determine mate quality.[19] When researchers altered the chest bars of male zebra finches, it affected the female's choice of mates. The females preferred males with symmetric chest bars.[19] Asymmetric chest bars may indicate to the females that a particular male may have poor feather quality or poor overall health.

Aggression

In certain avian social groups, such as chickens and psittacines, a dominance hierarchy has evolved to allow flock members to live together with minimal agonistic interactions.

A dominance relationship occurs when a higher ranking bird exhibits assertive behavior toward the subordinate and the subordinate passively yields. Aggression among conspecifics typically occurs over resources, such as food, nest material, shade, roosting, mates, nests, and perches at nest entrances. Examples of agonistic behaviors are bill fence, chase, bill gape, fly at, and active supplants.[2,9] The winner of agonistic encounters usually adopts a more horizontal posture while the loser retreats, loses its balance, or flies off. Postures associated with submission, such as food begging, feathers fluffed out, or squatting, do not prevent attacks from dominant individuals.[2]

In a flock of free-living banded birds, Zann did not find a stable dominance hierarchy.[2] A linear order existed among the birds but it changed on a daily basis. It has been observed that in captivity, certain individuals exhibit more aggressive behaviors toward other birds. The aggressive birds initiate and win more fights.[2] A study performed on zebra finches in a laboratory setting found that dominant males interfered with song and courtship activities of subordinate males.[9] The status of a male can be affected by the presence or absence of his partner. He is usually much more aggressive and assertive when the female is present.

Male zebra finches direct more agonistic behavior toward other males prior to the formation of the pair bond. This agonistic behavior may help strengthen the pair bond.[9] After a male has fended off a rival and returns to his partner, they engage in beak touching activity. Female–female aggression increases after pair-bond formation, but at a lower intensity compared to the rate of male–male aggression. This may be an indication that males may invest more energy in competition to gain access to females. On the other hand once the bond is formed, the females will fight to defend their bond from other female rivals.[2]

Communication

Vocalizations

Zebra finches have 12 distinct vocalizations. Vocalizations can be separated into calls and songs. Calls are usually short, stereotyped vocalizations that are innate to the animal, such as alarm calls, flight calls, distance calls, contact calls, begging calls, and so on. Songs are the more complex vocalizations that need to be learned.[4]

In zebra finches, the distance call is one of the most important and commonly used vocalizations. It is a vocal signal that transmits over long distances. The distance call may convey specific information to only certain flock members, since calls differ between the colonies, individuals, and sexes. Contact calls are used mostly by pair-bonded individuals to keep track of each other. Both males and females can emit these short monophasic calls.[9]

Songs are composed of a series of different sounds. These different sounds are called syllables. The order of the syllables in a song is referred to as syntax. Once formed, syntax is highly stable.[20] The acoustic properties of the syllables are known as phonology.[20] Each song contains repeatable phrases of syllables. So a bird not only needs to learn the syllables of the song, it also needs to learn to place them in an appropriate pattern to produce an attractive song.

The primary function of male songs in passerines is to attract a mate.[4,16] Some passerines also use songs to defend a breeding territory.[4] In zebra finches and canaries, only the males sing long complex songs.[11,21] The male's song production reaches a peak before egg production commences.[5] The nestlings acquired songs by listening to their father's songs.[22] Song learning consists of two stages. The first stage is the sensory phase. In this phase of learning, the nestlings listen to their fathers and try to memorize his song. The father provides the sensory model of the song to the chicks. Male zebra finches can start to sing around 25–35 days of age.[21] The sensitive period of song learning occurs between 35 and 65 days of age. When male and female zebra finches are exposed to songs during this phase, it influences their preference for certain songs.[22] This early exposure may provide both sexes with a basic reference with which to compare all other songs. When finches retuned their syllables, they selected the original tutor syllables as models over unfamiliar ones.[20]

The second stage of song learning is the sensorimotor phase. In this phase, the nestlings try to reproduce the songs they hear. Auditory feedback is essential for the sensorimotor learning phase.[21] The nestlings sing and listen to their songs. Then they make the necessary adjustments to match their songs to their model song.[20,23,24] Some fledglings may join a flock as early as 35 days.[2] They can then learn songs from other members of the flock.[22] Young males can learn song elements from other adults whom they maintain closest proximity to within a flock.[25] Only two-thirds of wild males have similar songs to their fathers.[2] This is due to the fact that they can incorporate other elements learned from conspecifics into their song.

Crystallization occurs when the song becomes stable and stereotyped usually around 90 days of age.[20] The crystallized song is not an exact copy of the tutor's song due to individual variation.[20,24] Auditory feedback is also needed to maintain the crystallized song.[21] Without auditory feedback, songs can become altered over time. This is an indication that adult zebra finches must have internal reference in order to maintain their song.[20]

Two types of songs are usually produced, a directed and an undirected song.[2,26] The directed song is used in courtship and is intended for the female. This song has a faster tempo and contains more syllables.[26] Undirected songs may have multiple functions, such as sexual advertisement and mate guarding. This song is usually not directed at any particular individual. Female zebra finches were found to choose their mate's directed song more often over their mate's undirected song. The females also preferred an unfamiliar male's directed song over his undirected song.[27] There must be a component in the directed songs that females can discern and find attractive.[27]

Zebra finches are age-limited learners, whereas canaries are open-ended learners. The songs of age-limited birds do not vary much after their first year of life. In open-ended learners, they continue to learn and vary their song structure upon each successive year.[21]

Sex differences in vocalizations

Female canaries rarely sing and when they do their songs are simple compared to the males.[21] There is sexual dimorphism in these birds' brains. The telencephalon in male songbirds is larger than in females. Testosterone is also needed for song development. Zebra finches that were castrated as juveniles developed abnormal songs.[21] Female zebra finches also have smaller forebrain nuclei. They lack some structures in the brain that are needed for complex song production.[21] Therefore the females are simply unable to produce songs similar to males.

Non-vocal communication

Communication can also occur through active visual cues. A display is a ritualized signal that sends a specific message. A signal is behavior performed by the sender that changes the behavior of the recipient in such a manner as to benefit the sender.[4] In the wild, the zebra finch nestlings have developed a prominent pattern of black markings in the mouth. The markings are displayed when the nestlings open their mouth wide while begging from the parents. Apparently, the markings encourage the parents to start feeding their offspring. Some nestlings from domesticated strains of zebra finches no longer develop these mouth markings. The black marks start to fade around the time they fledge.

Canary parents have a tendency to feed the chicks in closest proximity but may alter this strategy based on the chick's signal. The largest chicks tended to be the ones closest to the parents. These chicks usually get fed first. However, if the smallest chick was the hungriest, parents directed significant more feedings to the smallest chick, even though it was not closest to the parent. The parents were reacting to the small chicks begging signal that indicated its need.[28]

Sexual dimorphism

Plumage pattern can be a form of communication. It can signal the gender or age of a bird. In finches and canaries, the males are the more brilliantly colored birds. Typically, juvenile birds are a more drab color compared to their parents. Juvenile zebra finches have gray feathers and black bills.[29] They start developing secondary sexual plumage around 35–40 days of age. At this time, the bill color changes from black to red.[29] The males develop specific feathers on the throat and flanks. The adult plumage is completely developed by days 55–60. The adult colors will intensify until 90–100 days of age.[2]

Adult male zebra finches have black and white chin stripes with black breast bands. They have orange cheek patches and white spotted flank patches.[29] Males have a deeper red-colored bill than females. Females appear dull in comparison to a male. They do not have any chin stripes or cheek patches or spotted flank patches. However, some females can develop small breast bands.[29]

In Gouldian finches, the sexual dimorphism is much more dramatic due to the male's brightly colored plumage. The males have brighter body plumage and longer pintail feathers than the females.[3] The tail is black and white with a deep blue rump.[30] They have bright green wings and back with a yellow belly. Their breast is violet–purple color with an azure blue collar bordering the head mask. These traits are all expressed with continuous variations across a population. The females are duller in coloration. Juvenile Gouldian finches are a dull green brown color. The males do not develop the brightly colored plumage until after they molt their juvenile plumage. In this species, both sexes can exhibit three different colored head morphs: black, yellow, and red. These head morphs occur naturally in the wild.

Color signals in birds

Birds have a tetrachromatic color vision system. Birds are sensitive to wavelengths from 320 nm in the ultraviolet (UV) spectrum up to 700 nm.[31] They possess four cone types that enable them to see UV sensitive (UVS), short wavelength sensitive (SWS), medium wavelength sensitive (MWS), and long wavelength sensitive (LWS). Color-based signaling is common in birds. Plumage color can be an indicator of sex and physical condition.[31,32]

UV reflectance is associated with human visible feather colors—blues, greens, yellows, and reds. The zebra finch has long wave reflecting carotenoid and melanin-pigmented plumage.[31] The UV spectrum may serve as a private communication channel that birds can utilize.[32] In studies that removed UV reflectance, it was found that the female's choice of mates was affected. In another study, in which females were offered males to choose from, the males with all UV cues removed were chosen the least compared to males with a normal full spectrum (UV+).[31] Removing the UV cues somehow altered the appearance of the males. This change was found least desirable by the females. UV cues also affected female preference in Gouldian finches. Females were found to prefer males with more intense UV/blue head collars.[3]

The zebra finch's red beak color has long wavelength reflection. It has little reflection at short or medium wavelength. One study, in which a filter removed the color red from the visible spectrum, showed that the female mate choice can be altered. Males presented through this filter were preferred less by the females. Removal of the UV spectrum had the least effect on female mate choice. This leads us to assume that the female may pay more attention to a certain color in the male's visible spectrum compared to his UV spectrum.[31]

Color may also affect a bird's disposition and agonistic behavior. In Gouldian finches, there are three colors of head morph: red, black, and yellow. The most common head morph in the wild is black (70%). The red head morph occurs in 30% of the wild population. The yellow head morph is rare and occurs about 1 in 3000–5000 birds. It has been found that the red-headed males were more aggressive. They are dominant over the black- and yellow-headed males.[30] Even when head color was altered, the red-headed males were more aggressive toward the other color morphs. The red-headed males instigated altercations more often. They also prolonged aggressive interactions (i.e., active supplants). The head color morphs showed linear hierarchy. The red-headed males dominated over black-headed males who in turn, dominated over yellow-headed males. The advantages of being a red-headed male were: preferred access to food, nest sites, and females.

However, there was a cost to being a red-headed male. Red-headed males had testosterone levels that were 5 times greater than normal.[33] Black-headed males had lower testosterone levels. The red-headed males also had elevated corticosterone levels. A red-headed male was more susceptible to stress produced by housing conditions and breeding. They did not have normal immunocompetency. On the opposite end of the spectrum, the black-headed males demonstrated reduced stress response and immunosuppression in socially competitive environments.[30] This may be the main reason why there are more black-headed individuals in the wild populations.

It was also interesting to note that within the red-headed morphs, the males that had a more intense red color (more longwave) dominated the less intensely colored males.[30] The red color may operate as a classic dominance trait. Variations in red carotenoid-based signals may play an important role in dominance-related interactions in a number of species. The red color has affected interactions in other species including humans, indicating that red may add to a general intimidation value in agonistic encounters.

Behavior problems in passerine birds

Canaries and zebra finches have been bred in captivity for the past several 100 years.[1] A new generation of birds can be created in a relatively short period of time, as short at every 90 days in the zebra finch.[2] Therefore, it has been relatively easy for people to select for certain color mutations and alter the general appearance of certain birds. The common domesticated canary looks far different from the first captive canaries. There are numerous breeds of domestic canaries. Several color mutations have occurred in zebra finches. Although their general appearance may be different, their overall behavior has not altered greatly from their wild ancestors. Pet birds have adapted to living in captivity, but if certain conditions are not met, they can still suffer from inadequate care and exhibit behavioral problems.

While behavioral problems are not as common in passerine birds as they are in psittacine birds, they still occur. Most of the behavior problems reported by owners can be addressed using the knowledge we have on normal passerine behavior. Information on how to do a proper behavioral evaluation in psittacine birds is covered in Chapter 1, and these principles can be easily applied to passerines as well. The basic principles of behavior modification are explained in Chapter 18. General treatment considerations for passerine birds include focusing on various aspects of their husbandry and natural behavior that contribute to overall behavioral health.

Environment

A good environment that allows a bird ample room to fly around and exhibit species typical behaviors is always best. Passerines are social creatures and would prefer to be housed with other social birds rather than be alone. The cage should not be placed in areas of high traffic or have exposure to drafts, aerosol, or fires.

Most of the wild passerine birds live in areas where they have approximately 10–12 hours of daylight. Caregivers should strive to keep their birds on this schedule, either covering the cage or placing the cage in a dark room at night for 10–12 hours of undisturbed sleep.

Foraging

In the wild, finches spend a large portion of each day foraging for seeds. They forage primarily on the ground but sometimes directly from the grass heads[2]. Caregivers can provide some of the food in a puzzle toy or foraging containers to provide environmental enrichment. The bird will have to manipulate the toy in a certain manner in order to obtain the food rewards. Owners can also spread the food on the floor of the cage. They can mix the seeds with a non-edible, non-toxic substrate that the birds will have to pick through to get the seeds. Allowing birds to work for their food, more closely simulates the amount of time they would spend foraging in the wild.

Enrichment

Providing enrichment is crucial to keeping a pet bird well adjusted to living in a confined environment. Toys can be found in different sizes and textures. The toys should be rotated on a daily or weekly basis. There should be enough toys in the cage or aviary if there are multiple birds housed together.

Aggression

In the wild, agonistic encounters usually occur over potential mates, defense of mates, or over resources. Due to their small size and ease of maintenance, some owners may place too many birds in a cage or aviary. This can lead to overcrowding problems. Aggression can occur between birds fighting for preferred resources within a confined space. Since they are living in a confined area, the losers of these altercations may not have any safe area for escape. It is very important not to place too many birds in a confined area without providing outlets for escape. If multiple birds are kept together, multiple nests and feeding areas should be provided to decrease altercations over resources. The cage or aviary should be large enough to accommodate places for nests at various levels, provide access to food and water, and other areas where the birds can gather for socialization. The environment should also contain perches of various sizes and textures to keep the birds' feet healthy.

Another aspect to keep in mind is that even though these birds are social, they may prefer not to interact with birds from different species. For certain species, living with other species that do not exhibit the same social behaviors may be a source of social stress.

Stress can lead to an increase in aggression and corticosterone levels. Increased corticosterone levels can be detrimental to a bird's health.

Reproductive behavior problems

Early learning experiences can influence how a bird interacts with conspecifics and caregivers. If the caregiver is interested in having a breeder bird, they should then limit the amount of attention they give to the juveniles. It has been shown that juvenile zebra finches can form bonds as early as 50 days.[2] If the caregiver desires a breeder, then the juvenile bird should be provided with appropriate companions at that time. Some hand-raised birds or solitary birds may form inappropriate bonds with their caregivers. They can become sexually imprinted on the caregivers. Sexual imprinting occurs when a bird directs courtship and mating behaviors preferentially to an individual that exhibits traits similar to the parental individuals with which it was raised.[34] These birds are not sexually interested in interacting with conspecifics. Even after they have been presented with appropriate mates, these birds show a preference for people.

Some species have also adapted to non-seasonal breeding and can have several clutches year round. For owners who are not interested in having multiple clutches throughout the year, one method to discourage the pair from continuing to breed is to disrupt their photoperiod by providing decreased daylight and lengthening the dark period. Another method is to replace the newly laid eggs with ceramic or plastic eggs. The pair will sit on the eggs for several weeks after which they will go into their non-breeding stage and the false eggs can be removed.

Feather picking

Feather picking is not a common problem in passerines. Some caregivers have been known to mistake a female's brood patch for signs of a behavior problem. Most feather loss in passerines can be attributed to changes related to reproduction, such as picking the feather for a brood patch or to line the nest, or may be a sign of an underlying health problems. Therefore, a complete physical exam and appropriate diagnostics should be the first steps taken when presented with a passerine with feather loss.

Though rare, some passerines may start feather picking as a result of stress. Overcrowding, lack of appropriate stimulation or foraging opportunities, or lack of social interactions are some of the reasons that can cause a bird to pick its feathers. Correcting some of the underlying issues can improve or resolve the bird's behavior. Resolving the problem is more likely if environmental changes are made as soon as possible after the problem is first noted.

Lack of song

It is important for owners who want a bird for its impressive vocal qualities to choose the appropriate gender. The females do not possess the same capabilities of males for song production. The males may need to have a potential mate in order for them to continue singing or be motivated to start singing. These males should also have been exposed to male songs during their sensitive period. Other males do not have to be present. Zebra finches can learn from tape recordings.[20] Simply playing a recording for finches and canaries at the critical time in development can produce a male with a wonderful song repertoire.

Conclusion

Passerines are social creatures that live in flocks with multiple individuals. Their daily lives are filled with constant activities. Captive birds often are not provided with enough stimulation in their environment. Finches and canaries have been known to live to 5–10 years of age in captivity. In order for these songbirds to live to the fullest extent of their lives, we need to provide them with environments and activities that keep them physically and mentally stimulated. A comprehensive understanding of passerine behavior will enable us to provide the best care for our beloved songbirds.

References

1. Dorst J. *The Life of Birds, Volume II*. New York: Columbia University Press, 1974.
2. Zann RS. *The Zebra Finch*. Oxford: Oxford University Press, 1996.
3. Pryke SR, Griffith SC. The relative role of male vs. female mate choice in maintaining assortative pairing among discrete colour morphs. *J Evol Biol*. 2007;20(4):1512–1521.
4. Elphick C, Dunning Jr JB, Sibley DA. *The Sibley Guide to Bird Life and Behavior*. New York: Chanticleer Press, Inc, 2001.
5. Waas JR, Colgan, PW, Boag, PT. Playback of colony sounds alters the breeding schedule and clutch size in zebra finch (*Taeniopygia guttata*) colonies. *Proc R Soc B* 2005;272(1561):383–388.
6. Voigt C, Leitner, S. Seasonality in song behaviour revisited: Seasonal and annual variants and invariants in the song of the domesticated canary (*Serinus canaria*). *Horm Behav* 2008;54:373–378.
7. Bentley GE, Audage NC, Hanspal EK et al. Photoperiodic response of the hypothalamo–pituitary–gonad axis in male and female canaries, *Serinus canaria*. *J Exp Zool* 2003;296(A):143–151.
8. Searcy WA, Yasukawa K. Song and female choice. In: Kroodsma, DE, Miller, EH, eds. *Ecology and Evolution of Acoustic Communication in Birds*. Ithaca: Cornell University Press, 1996;454–473.
9. Butterfield PA. The pair bond in the Zebra finch. In: Crook, JH, ed. *Social Behaviour in Birds and Mammals*. London: Academic Press Inc, 1970;249–278.
10. Wilson EO. *Sociobiology: The New Synthesis*. Cambridge: The Belknap Press of Harvard University Press, 1975.
11. Clayton NS. Assortative mating in zebra finch subspecies, *Taeniopygia guttata guttata* and *T.g. castanotis*. *Phil Trans R Soc B* 1990;330(1258):351–370.
12. Gilbert L, Williamson KA, Hazon N et al. Maternal effects due to male attractiveness affect offspring development in the zebra finch. *Proc R Soc B* 2006;273(1595):1765–1771.
13. Riebel K. Early exposure leads to repeatable preferences for male song in female zebra finches. *Proc R Soc B* 2000;267(1461): 2553–2558.
14. Wright TF, Brittan-Powell EF, Dooling RJ et al. Sex-linked inheritance of hearing and song in the Belgian Waterslager canary. *Proc R Soc B* 2004;271(6):S409–S412.
15. Zollinger SA, Suthers RA. Motor mechanisms of a vocal mimic: Implications for birdsong production. *Proc R Soc B* 2004;273: 483–491.
16. Drăgănoiu TI, Nagle L, Kreutzer M. Directional female preference for an exaggerated male trait in canary (*Serinus canaria*) song. *Proc R Soc B* 2002;269(1509):2525–2531.
17. Airey DC, Castillo-Juarez H, Casella G et al. Variation in the volume of zebra finch song control nuclei is heritable: Developmental and evolutionary implications. *Proc R Soc B* 2000;267(1457):2099–2104.
18. Buchanan KL, Leitner S, Spencer KA et al. Developmental stress selectively affects the song control nucleus HVC in the zebra finch. *Proc R Soc B* 2004;271(1555):2381–2386.
19. Swaddle JP, Cuthill IC. Female zebra finches prefer males with symmetric chest plumage. *Proc R Soc B* 1994;258(1353):267–271.
20. Funabiki Y, Funabiki K. Song retuning with tutor model by adult zebra finches. *Develop Neurobiol* 2007;68(5):645–655.
21. Brenowitz EA, Kroodsma DE (1996) The neuroethology of birdsong. In: Kroodsma, DE, Miller, EH, eds. *Ecology and Evolution of Acoustic Communication in Birds*. Ithaca: Cornell University Press, 1996;285–304.
22. Riebel K, Smallegange IM, Terpstra, NJ et al. Sexual equality in zebra finch song preference: Evidence for a dissociation between song recognition and production learning. *Proc R Soc B* 2002; 269(1492):729–733.
23. Janata P, Margoliash D. Gradual emergence of song selectivity in sensorimotor structures of the male zebra finch song system. *J Neurosci* 1999;19(12):5108–5118.

24. Liu W, Gardner TJ, Nottebohm F. Juvenile zebra finches can use multiple strategies to learn the same song. *Proc Natl Acad Sci USA* 2004;101(52):18177–18182.

25. Mann NI, Slater, PJB. Song tutor choice by zebra finches in aviaries. *Anim Behav* 1995;49:811–820.

26. Huang Y, Hessler NA. Social modulation during songbird courtship potentiates midbrain dopaminergic neurons. *PLoS One* 2008; 3(10):1–8.

27. Woolley SC, Doupe AJ. Social context-induced song variation affects female behavior and gene expression. *PLoS Biol* 2008; 6(3):0525–0537.

28. Kilner R. When do canary parents respond to nestling signals of need? *Proc R Soc B* 1995;260(1359);343–348.

29. Price DK. Sexual selection, selection load and quantitative genetics of zebra finch bill colour. *Proc R Soc B* 1996;263(1367):217–221.

30. Pryke SR, Griffith SC. Red dominates black: Signaling among head morphs in the colour polymorphic Gouldian finch. *Proc R Soc B* 2006;273(1589):949–957.

31. Hunt S, Cuthill IC, Bennett ATD et al. Is the UV waveband a special communication channel in avian mate choice? *J Exp Bio* 2001;204:2499–2507.

32. Hausmann F, Arnold KE, Marshall NJ et al. Ultraviolet signals in birds are special. *Proc R Soc B* 2002;270:61–67.

33. Pryke SR, Astheimer LB, Buttemer WA et al. Frequency-dependent physiological trade-offs between competing colour morphs. *Biol Lett* 2007;3(5):494–497.

34. Freeberg TM. Culture and courtship in vertebrates: A review of social learning and transmission of courtship systems and mating patterns. *Behav Proc* 2000;51:177–192.

3
Snakes

Heather Mohan-Gibbons and Paul Raiti

Introduction

No creature has elicited a broader range of human emotions than the snake. It has symbolized the introduction of evil into the world; and paradoxically, it is also the symbol of healing and modern medicine. In some cultures, snakes are revered because they represent good luck and longevity. In countries such as India, snakes are not killed because of their predation upon rodents. Snakes are an essential component of the natural world and deserve to receive the same conservation status as the environments they inhabit. Snakes have been used as models for human seizure disorders and malignant diseases. Snakes venom extracts are currently being utilized for the treatment of hypertension, thromboembolism, and coagulation disorders.

History

There are approximately 2500 species of snakes distributed in almost all ecosystems. Endemic snakes are absent from Ireland, the Antarctic, and Hawaii; however, snakes have been introduced to Hawaii. The most widely distributed reptile on the planet is the yellow-bellied sea snake. Approximately 12% of all snakes are highly venomous to man. Snakes do not possess limbs or external ears. All snakes are predators and occupy habitat types which are broadly divided into arboreal, ground dwelling, fossorial, aquatic, and semi-aquatic.

Snakes belong to the order Squamata (possessing scales) which also includes lizards. The origin and history of snakes is controversial due to some of their unique adaptations. There is an absence of well-defined paleontological evidence determining clear origin, so there are several hypotheses. Many agree that snakes, lizards, and amphisbaenians (wormlike tropical lizards) have a shared ancestor. One hypothesis is that snakes are separated from

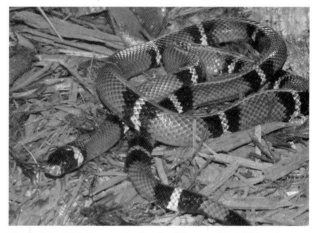

Figure 3.1 Clinically normal milksnake. (Courtesy of Paul Gibbons.)

varanids; a second is that they share more in common with gekkonids; and a third is that they evolved from burrowing lizards.[1]

Colubrids and boids are the most common types of snakes kept in captivity. Examples of colubrids are ratsnakes, kingsnakes, milksnakes, garter snakes, and gopher snakes (Figure 3.1). Most colubrids are oviparous (egg layers). Others such as water snakes and garter snakes are viviparous (live bearers). Boids are considered more primitive than colubrids and include boas and pythons (Figure 3.2). Boas (i.e., boa constrictor, rainbow boa, tree boas) are viviparous. Pythons (i.e., green tree python, royal python, Burmese python) are oviparous.

Senses and communication

Reptiles rely heavily on visual and chemosensory cues.[2] Snakes possess tactile, kinesthetic, radiant heat, and vibrational receptors. Ophidian eyes are unique among reptiles

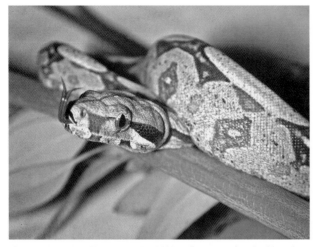

Figure 3.2 Clinically normal red-tailed boa. (Courtesy of Paul Gibbons.)

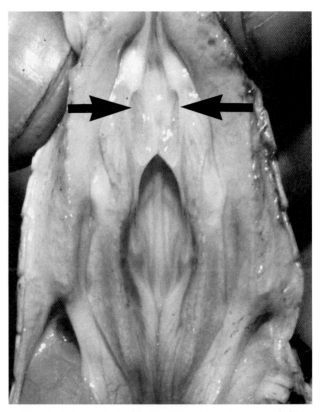

Figure 3.3 Openings (arrows) to the vomeronasal ducts in the roof of the mouth of a boa constrictor. (Courtesy of Paul Raiti.)

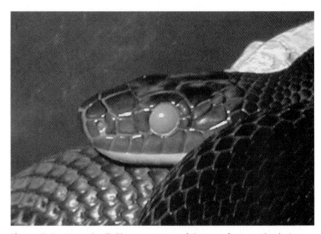

Figure 3.4 Normal milk-like appearance of the eye of a ratsnake during the shedding process. (Courtesy of Paul Raiti.)

in that they possess hard lenses which are incapable of changing shape for visual accommodation; instead, the lens is moved forward or backward due to changes of pressure in the posterior chamber.[3] Diurnal snakes possess circular pupils and nocturnal snakes possess vertical pupils. Chemical cues are also used and are very efficient as they remain after the animal has passed, work day or night, and are effective over large areas.[2]

Snakes have two main chemosensory systems, olfactory and vomeronasal.[2] Each nasal cavity is lined by ciliated epithelium which is sensitive to volatile odorants.[4] The olfactory nerve (Cranial Nerve I) transmits signals to the olfactory bulbs located in the telencephalon.[4] Each vomeronasal organ (Jacobson's organ) consists of a pit lined with sensory epithelium located in the roof of the snake's mouth (Figure 3.3).[4] There is no anatomical communication with the nasal cavity. Fluid, produced by the Harderian gland located posteromedial to the eye, drains from the lacrimal duct into the vomeronasal duct where it provides nourishment for the vomeronasal organ.[4] The vomeronasal organs are innervated by the trigeminal nerve (Cranial Nerve V). Snakes and lizards exhibit a behavior of tongue flicking, which is used to bring the chemical cues of the environment into the ducts within the mouth.[4] Tongue flicking patterns will change with environmental conditions such as exploring, social context, feeding, and defense.[4] For example, an increase in tongue flicking behavior is common when something novel is presented to the snake or when the snake is placed into a cage of a conspecific.[4] Receptivity of males to female pheromones for courtship and copulation, male to male combat, trailing to find communal hibernaculums, post-hibernation aggregation, and trailing prey all depend on the tongue and vomeronasal organs.[2]

Pheromones are chemicals produced by individuals that effect a change in the physiology or behavior of conspecifics.[2] The major sites of pheromone production are the epidermal lipid glands located on the dorsolateral skin of females.[2] Prior to shedding, the skin becomes opaque due to the formation of lymph between the old and new layers (Figure 3.4) and snakes can appear "blue."[5,6] Shedding, in particular, increases the release and deposition of pheromones to stimulate reproductive behavior,[7] so this can be an ideal time to introduce snakes for mating.

Reptiles possess a variety of other glands whose secretions are used in communication. Male and female snakes have paired cloacal glands located in the base of the tail.

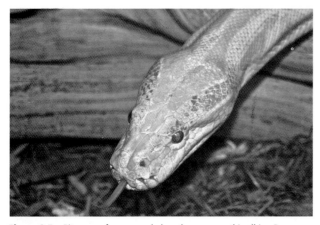

Figure 3.5 Pit organs form a row below the nares on this albino Burmese python. (Courtesy of Heather Mohan-Gibbons.)

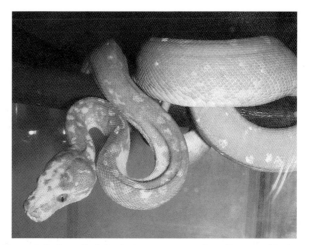

Figure 3.6 Pre-strike behavior in a green tree python. (Courtesy of Paul Raiti.)

Suggested functions of these glands include attracting mates, aggregation cues, and defense.[2] During handling, snakes commonly express these glands which emit a musky odor. Snakes passively mark the environment by simply moving through it leaving olfactory cues on their trails.

The burrowing blind snake uses its cloacal glands to help avoid injury while obtaining prey. Their diet consists of termites and ants. When attacked by ants, these snakes cover themselves with secretions from their cloacal glands that have been found to repel several species of ants.[2]

Boas, pythons, and pit vipers possess specialized receptors called pit organs (thermal pits) that detect radiant heat (Figure 3.5).[8] These organs are capable of detecting temperature changes as low as 0.003°C (0.01°F).[8] Pit organs are innervated by the trigeminal nerve (Cranial Nerve V) and are important in triggering and guiding the strike toward prey.[8] Snakes that do not possess pit organs rely more on cutaneous thermoreceptors for feeding behavior.[8]

Hunting behavior in snakes can be divided into three phases: (1) pre-strike, (2) strike, and (3) post-strike. Pre-strike involves assessing the prey type and decreasing the distance between the snake and the prey for optimal strike distance (Figure 3.6). Depending on the kind of snake, pre-strike behavior is determined by visual cues, chemical cues, vibrations, and infrared receptors.[4] Tongue flicking carries scent particles to the vomeronasal organs. Snakes with their tongues removed are not able to locate prey (Figure 3.7a and b).[4] Strike is the actual attempt to capture prey when it is in the right location. Post-strike involves killing and swallowing the prey head-first and is determined by chemical and tactile cues.[4]

Snakes exhibit numerous antipredator behaviors. Examples are freezing, tail rattling, mimicry of head with tail, flight, striking, voiding cloacal secretions, death feigning, flattening, hissing, writhing, biting, and gliding (Figure 3.8).[3] If a captive snake is routinely displaying these behaviors, then the animal's husbandry and environment needs to be evaluated to ensure proper welfare.

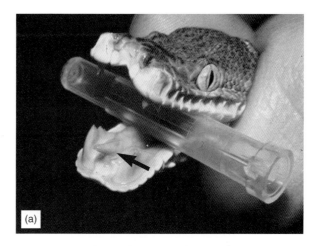

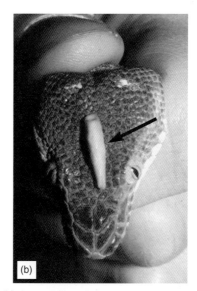

Figure 3.7 (a) This emerald tree boa was presented for anorexia. Oral examination revealed a granuloma encasing the tongue (arrow). (Courtesy of Paul Raiti.) (b) After removal of the lingual granuloma, the snake resumed feeding. (Courtesy of Paul Raiti.)

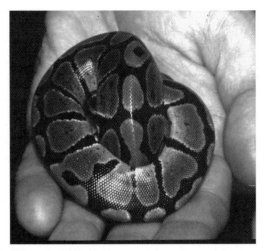

Figure 3.8 Defensive "balling" behavior in a royal python. (Courtesy of Paul Raiti.)

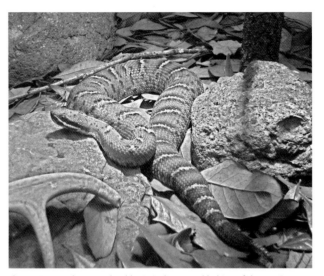

Figure 3.9 Substrates should mimic the natural habitat of the species to provide adequate texture and environmental enrichment. (Courtesy of Paul Gibbons.)

Husbandry

To ensure the reptile has proper welfare and husbandry, one should consider applying the "Five Freedoms" to snakes as a guideline. The reader is encouraged to refer to Chapter 20 for more information about the Five Freedoms. All are important in creating the right living conditions and ensuring proper welfare for the life of the captive snake.

Substrate

Substrates need to be non-toxic, easy to clean, easy to replace, and non-irritant. There is no universal substrate that can be used for all snakes. Selection of substrate should attempt to replicate the niche that the snake occupies in its natural setting (Figure 3.9). Fossorial snakes from xeric habitats such as sand boas do better on a substrate of fine grade sand which provides security, allows ambush predation, and prevents buildup of excessive humidity in the enclosure. Water snakes do well on a substrate of gravel above shallow water in addition to a large water bowl for soaking and consuming fish. Other substrate examples are newspaper, wood chips, mulch, and wood shavings. Newspaper, although not aesthetically pleasing, is the most cost effective, easy to clean, and readily available material.[9] It is appropriate for most ground-dwelling snakes.

Heat sources

Snakes are ectothermic meaning that body temperature is dependent upon heat obtained from the environment; however, snakes actively control body temperature by a process called behavioral thermoregulation.[10] Ectothermy is energetically less costly than endothermy because it consumes less oxygen.[11] This has permitted reptiles to exploit niches where birds and mammals could not survive. The hypothalamus and pineal gland are integral components of behavioral thermoregulation. Heliothermy is the process of basking and thigmothermy is the process of absorbing heat from warm surfaces.[10] Behavioral thermoregulation determines habitat selection and prey availability.[12] Snakes also possess regional heterothermy in which temperature variations of different regions of the body have been identified.[11]

Temperature affects growth, development, gestation time, survival rate of neonates, metabolism, digestion, ecydysis, the immune system, behavior, locomotion, tongue flicking, prey capture, defensive behavior, and regional heterothermy.[13] Establishing a temperature gradient is essential for snakes to thermoregulate. This is accomplished by providing a lower temperature on one side and a higher temperature on the opposite side of the enclosure. The snake is then capable of selecting its preferred temperature. A snake's activity within the enclosure is a function of ambient temperature and the snake's metabolic requirements over a 24-hour period. If the snake spends most of the time either avoiding or seeking heat, then the temperature gradient within the enclosure should be re-evaluated.

Snakes possess an extensive vascular system in the integument which, in conjunction with the lungs and cardiac shunting, controls heat exchange.[11] Snakes, like other reptiles, select higher temperature ranges for digestion, shedding, gamete maturation, antibody production, and gravidity.[14] Temperature is critical for normal embryogenesis. Indian python eggs incubated at 27.5°C (81.5°F) instead of 30°C (90°F) had young exhibiting changes in scalation, color, and vertebral kinking.[11] Snakes experimentally infected with *Aeromonas* species selected higher temperatures; hence, the term "behavioral fever."[15]

Examples of heat sources are incandescent bulbs, ceramic bulbs, thermal tape and pads, and infrared bulbs. Arboreal snakes should be provided with heat from above, while ground-dwelling and fossorial snakes should be provided with heat from below. All thermal sources should preferably be located outside the enclosure to avoid burns.[5,6] The use of heating stones is strongly discouraged as severe burns to reptiles have resulted in high morbidity and even death. If heat is provided from beneath, no more than 30–50% of the bottom should be covered in order to allow the snake to move to a cooler area. Ideally, heat sources should be controlled by a thermostat to prevent overheating and a separate thermometer placed in the hottest area in the enclosure to measure true temperature. Acute hyperthermia kills snakes quickly; prolonged hypothermia can cause degenerative changes in neurons of the central nervous system.[15] Snakes with hypothermia are ataxic and have varying degrees of motor paralysis.

Light

Visible light is essential for snakes to maintain normal circadian rhythms. The number of daylight hours is dependent on where the snake's native habitat is found. Equatorial species need 12 hours of daylight and 12 hours of darkness. Most diurnal reptiles (i.e., chelonians, lizards) require exposure to ultraviolet B light (UVB) to form vitamin D_3. The majority of captive snakes are not provided with exposure to UVB and seem to thrive and reproduce for many years. Metabolic bone disease due to calcium deficiency has not been identified in snakes which lack exposure to UVB. It is thought that whole prey provides adequate amounts of vitamin D_3. However, recent studies show that some species do increase their 25-hydroxyvitamin D blood levels when they are exposed to UVB lighting.[6] If a UVB source is used, it is important to read instructions carefully. Reptiles should be able to move freely to within 30 cm (11.8 in.) of the bulb to receive beneficial effects. Snakes should be checked daily for signs of damage to the integument from bulbs emitting UVB. Additionally, humans should refrain from looking directly at UVB bulbs. Fluorescent bulbs produce less UVB with time and should be replaced every 6 months. Burger[16] measured the UVB-attenuating properties of 14 different materials that are commonly used to cover enclosures. They found that the newly designed UV-transmitting acrylic shows adequate UVB meter irradiances; however, it does not allow for adequate D_3-synthesizing ability. It is recommended to use air-permeable materials between the UVB bulb and the animal to ensure proper D_3 conversion for health and normal behavior.

Water

Terrestrial reptiles ingest most of their preformed water from prey; however, all need to be provided with fresh water. The water bowl needs to be shallow but large enough for a snake to submerse its whole body. Snakes soak to promote

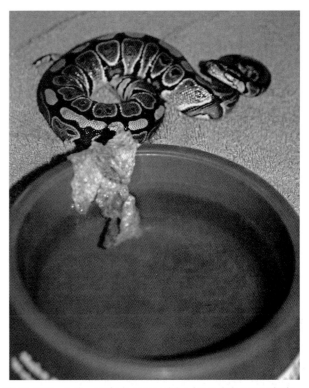

Figure 3.10   Snakes need a large enough bowl to soak their entire body and will often soak to promote shedding. (Courtesy of Paul Gibbons.)

shedding, lower body temperature, and stimulate defecation (Figure 3.10). In the wild, many arboreal snakes drink water droplets on leaves; consequently, it is recommended to mist the enclosure daily. Water bowls should be cleaned and disinfected once weekly.

Humidity and ventilation

The ambient relative humidity for snakes varies between 20% and 100% depending on the species and the climate of their natural habitat. An array of disease processes can occur if the relative humidity is too high or too low. Excessively high humidity can cause dermatitis and respiratory infections. Excessively low humidity can cause dysecdysis (difficult shedding).[5] Humidity is increased by daily misting, adding a humidifier to the room, placing damp moss on the bottom of the enclosure or in the hide box, aerating water in the tank, or by adding plants.[6] Ventilation is important for normal respiratory function. Sometimes adequate air circulation is sacrificed in an attempt to maintain heat within the enclosure so at least one side of the terrarium should be vented. Fans can be used to circulate room air.

Housing

Habitat selection in the wild depends upon various factors such as thermal preferences, availability of prey, protection from predators, suitable nesting areas, and hibernaculums for overwintering.[12] These aspects should be kept in mind when selecting an enclosure for a snake. Enclosures need to be escape-proof, non-toxic, non-porous, and easy to clean.[17] A clinical type of habitat contains a hide box, water bowl, and newspaper as a substrate. This type of housing is not aesthetically pleasing, but it does satisfy the "Five Freedoms" described in Chapter 20 and is easy to clean. Naturalistic-type habitats attempt to replicate the biotic environment of a particular species consequently minimizing stressors related to captivity.

There are many widely available pre-made cages on the market today for a diverse array of snakes. For ground-dwelling snakes, there should be a hide box on the cool side and another on the warmer side. A hide box needs to be large enough to fit the animal comfortably but not so large that it does not feel secure. Many snakes will only ingest prey inside a hide box. An arboreal setup has more height than width. There should be multiple horizontal perches at various heights so that the snake can control its distance from the heat source for effective thermoregulation.

Dimensions of the enclosure need to be large enough to accommodate the type and size of snake, and provide a temperature gradient. The largest cage possible should be provided; however, the longest side should be at least 3/4 of the snake's total body length and the shortest side should be at least 1/3 of total body length. The height for an arboreal species should be the full body length, and half the body length for terrestrial or burrowing snakes.[17]

Handling

Approaching a snake should be done in a slow, steady, and deliberate manner. Although it is true that certain species tend to have stereotypical behaviors, it should be noted that there are always exceptions. Prior to striking, a snake may retract the anterior part of the body into an "S" shape, gape, hiss, or rattle the tail. Most owners quickly become familiar with their animal's behavior. Neonates tend to be more defensive and flighty than their adult counterparts. Depending on size, snakes should be supported in two places when handled. The head is gently but firmly cradled between the thumb and index fingers.[6] The second hand supports the body at the approximate mid-point (Figure 3.11). This works well for tractable animals less than 1.5 m (4.9 ft). Snakes larger than 2 m (6.5 ft) typically require two or more handlers depending on the size of the snake. This is particularly true with boa constrictors, carpet, and Burmese pythons. The use of snake hooks is helpful for removing arboreal snakes from perches. When a snake needs to be transported, it should be placed in an escape-proof container, such as a cloth bag tied with a knot. The bag should then be placed into a secure box. Special care should be taken when a snake is presented for exam during shedding. If the old epithelium is rubbed off before the newly forming epithelium underneath has matured, scarring can result.[6,9]

Locomotion

Seven modes of terrestrial locomotion have been described in snakes:[18]

1. Lateral undulation is the most common mode of locomotion. Horizontal waves travel down alternate sides of the body axis and generate force at fixed points in the environment. The body pushes posterolaterally against these pivot points with lateral and caudal forces that combine for forward propulsion.
2. Slide pushing is similar to lateral undulation because it relies on alternating waves of body motion. It is generally employed on low-friction surfaces. It differs from lateral undulation by not using fixed points in the environment to create forward forces; instead, body waves are propagated so rapidly that they generate sufficient friction to slowly propel the body forward.
3. Concertina locomotion is used on low-friction terrestrial surfaces or within tight spaces such as burrows. It involves repeatedly establishing a stable platform with one section of the body while another section moves.
4. Sidewinding is a fairly rapid mode of locomotion most commonly employed in low-friction or shifting substrates such as sand dunes or mud. All forces against the substrate are vertical, and sections of the body are alternately lifted and moved forward, which produces series of unconnected, parallel tracks that are oriented at an obtuse angle to the direction of travel. This type of motion prevents the body from having prolonged contact with hot surfaces such as in the desert.

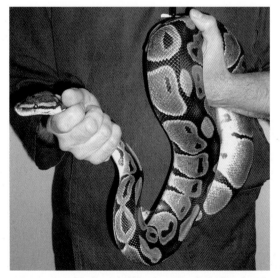

Figure 3.11 A royal python is held by supporting the body and gently controlling the head. (Courtesy of Paul Raiti.)

The sidewinder rattlesnake is probably the best known example.

5. Saltation (jumping) is used by a few short, stout snake species including the horned viper and Pacific ground boa. It is primarily a form of defensive behavior. The entire body is lifted off the substrate by a rapid straightening of the body from cranial to caudal.

6. Rectilinear locomotion differs from the above modes because it does not rely on alternating contraction of the lateral muscle bodies of the trunk. Instead, costocutaneous muscles, which run from the ribs to the ventral skin on both sides of the body act synchronously, sequentially contracting and relaxing to draw the body forward in a generally straight line. Rectilinear locomotion is most commonly employed by ground-dwelling pythons, boas, and vipers.

7. Aquatic locomotion resembles terrestrial locomotion with a few important differences. Swimming snakes produce regular axial waves that increase in lateral extent as the waves move caudally. This is contrasted by terrestrial lateral undulation in which force is applied at fixed points. Some snakes, such as the warty water snake, have anatomical adaptations that enhance their lateral surface area and ability to create propulsive forces.

Ingestive behavior

All snakes are predators consuming a wide range of prey including mammals, birds, reptiles, eggs, amphibians, insects, fish, worms, and mollusks. Food is not masticated but swallowed whole (Figure 3.12). Prey is either killed prior to ingestion by constriction or evenomation, or simply overpowered and swallowed live. Hunting behavior has been divided into two types:[3]

1. Active foragers consume prey frequently in order to maintain a positive energy balance due to the increased energy costs of foraging. Consequently, these snakes tend to be relatively slender, possess acute vision, and move quickly. Examples are ratsnakes, racers, and coachwhips.

2. Ambush foragers consume relatively less prey due to decreased energy costs associated with a "sit and wait" strategy. They consume a wider variety of prey and are stockier in build compared to active foragers. Examples are boa constrictors and ground boas.

It is normal for snakes to be anorexic during the shedding process (ecydysis) which typically lasts from 2 to 3 weeks. During this time, snakes become inactive, avoid contact, and may seek shelter in a humid area.[6,19] After shedding, snakes are usually voracious and will eat immediately.[19]

All snakes have a postprandial thermophilic response meaning they actively seek heat after eating to help the digestive process;[12] hence, the importance of providing a thermal hot spot. Suboptimal temperatures cause maldigestion, bloat, constipation, and compromise the immune system. It is thought that the success of venomous snakes found at higher altitudes is due at least in part to digestion of prey by the injected venom.[13]

Although there may be limitations on diet variability, an effort should be made to formulate the diet as much as possible after the natural diet, based on field observations. Snakes should not be fed prey from the wild as they can ingest pesticides, insecticides, and parasites.[6] A common reason snakes do not eat in captivity is that the prey offered is incorrect for the species.[5] Most snakes kept in captivity such as kingsnakes, ratsnakes, boas, and pythons will consume thawed mammals such as mice and rats. Feeding thawed food eliminates the possibility of bite wounds from live prey (Figure 3.13).[6,19] Prey should be pre-warmed to elicit a stronger feeding response particularly with boids. Since many snakes are nocturnal or crepuscular, offering food in the evenings will often stimulate a recalcitrant feeder to eat.[20] Some snakes are extremely sensitive to movement; consequently, a stronger feeding response generally occurs when there is less activity around the enclosure.[9]

Piscivorous snakes such as water snakes and garter snakes can be fed thawed fish; however, a thiamine supplement should be sprinkled on the fish prior to consumption because thiamine is inactivated by freezing.[6] Hypothiaminosis causes

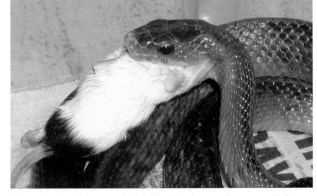

Figure 3.12 This Asian ratsnake, like all snakes, swallows prey whole. (Courtesy of Paul Raiti.)

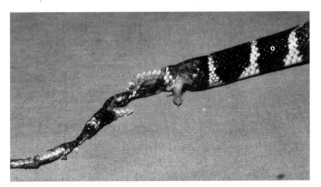

Figure 3.13 Severe rodent trauma to a kingsnake that was offered food during shed. (Courtesy of Paul Raiti.)

neurological disease (cerebrocortical necrosis) character-ized by ataxia, muscle tremors, blindness, and paralysis.[6] Treatment with parenteral thiamine in the early stages of disease can reverse neurological symptoms. Feeding of live fish prevents this problem; however, it should be noted that the feeding of live vertebrate prey to animals is prohib-ited in the United Kingdom.

Some species of snake exhibit prey ontogeny as they grow. For example, many neonates prefer tree frogs and geckoes; however, as the snakes grow to maturity, prey selection changes to small mammals and birds. To counter this problem in captivity it may be necessary to feed thawed amphibians or diminutive lizards to hatchling snakes. Another practice is called "scent transfer" whereby a thawed day-old mouse (pinkie) is rubbed against a frozen amphibian con-sequently tricking the snake into consuming mammalian prey.[21] Arboreal neonates may have to be "tease fed" by holding a thawed pinkie with forceps and coaxing the snake to strike by gently rubbing the prey item along the snake's mouth. Arboreal snakes must be perched on a branch to elicit a feeding response. Some snakes such as the green tree python, particularly juveniles and subadults, wiggle their tails (caudal luring) to attract potential prey.

Feeding frequency is based upon several factors. Hatchlings and juvenile snakes, due to their relatively higher meta-bolic rates, require more frequent feedings than adults. Hatchlings typically do not take their first meal until after the first shed because they subsist on yolk deposits. Juvenile and subadult colubrids are typically offered a thawed rodent of appropriate size once weekly. As a general rule, the diameter of the prey should be approximately the same diameter of the snake at its thickest part. Many captive snakes presented in clinical practice are overweight with some approaching obesity. Overweight snakes are prone to gout, cardiovascular disease, hepatic lipidosis, infertility, dystocia, and decreased longevity.[6,20,22] Colubrids that are feeding once weekly should defecate at the same frequency. Excretory products consist of two components: feces and urates. The fecal portion is brown in color and semi-solid to solid in consistency. Undigested hair, teeth, and claws of rodents are visible in the feces. Urates are yellow to white in color and liquid to solid in consistency.

Boas and pythons, particularly those that are arboreal, tend to have relatively lower metabolic rates than colubrids; hence, feedings should be done less frequently. Juveniles can be fed approximately every 10 days, while adults can be fed every 2–3 weeks. It is normal for adult male boids to be anorexic during the winter months. A good rule of thumb with arboreal boids is to make sure that defecation occurs by every third meal prior to the next feeding. If the snake has not defecated, it should be soaked in shallow water for several hours to stimulate peristalsis. In the author's experi-ence (PR), overfed arboreal boids are prone to regurgitation and cloacal prolapse (Figure 3.14).[23]

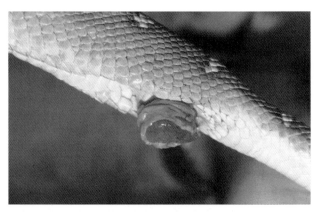

Figure 3.14 Cloacal prolapse in an emerald tree boa. (Courtesy of Paul Raiti.)

Social behavior

Snakes have traditionally been thought to be non-social animals; however, that image has been modified through the years. Current research shows that snakes are social during certain times of the year. Examples are during breeding season and in overwintering hibernaculums. In Manitoba, Canada, red-sided garter snakes have been found in aggregations of over 10,000 snakes in individual dens. Communication by pheromone production is thought to be responsible for this behavior.[4]

It is generally recommended to house snakes indi-vidually except for breeding.[5,21] Snakes sharing the same enclosure should never be offered prey simultaneously. This prevents injuries such as multiple snakes attempting to swallow the same prey item or each other.[5] The hous-ing of different species together is also discouraged due to individual husbandry and thermoregulatory needs. It should be noted that some snakes (i.e., kingsnakes) are ophiophagous (snake-eaters). In species (i.e., green tree pythons) where male combat occurs, it is crucial to be certain that prospective pairs have been sexed correctly to prevent life-threatening injuries.

Certain types of social behavior have also been shown to inhibit breeding. Male snakes that have lost a combat will have less interest in breeding a female.[24] When females are bred continually, or frequently exposed to males showing aggressive displays, both tend to lose interest in mating for a period of time. Personal observation (PR) suggests that some snakes can have individual social preferences. For example, a female may prefer a particular male for copu-lation from year to year while consistently rejecting other males. More research is needed to determine if this is merely an artifact of captivity or truly an example of mate choice. Female mate choice has been documented in other vertebrate species and probably serves to insure the great-est reproductive fitness. Currently, there is no evidence of female reptiles going into male territories and leading the mating activity.[25]

Reproductive and maternal behavior

The most comprehensive knowledge about physiological regulation of sexual behavior is based on only a few species of reptiles.[25] From those studies, three patterns of reproductive cycles have been shown to exist for snakes:

1. Associated reproductive cycles are seen in reptiles from subtropical or temperate zones where there is a long active season. Sex hormone secretion and gonadogenesis stimulate copulation, egg, and fetal development. A period of cooling followed by warming temperatures is required for successful reproduction.[24] Examples of snakes with this type of cycle are ratsnakes, pinesnakes, gopher snakes, kingsnakes, and milksnakes.
2. Dissociated reproductive cycles are associated with a short active season. Sexual behavior is not dependent upon sex hormone secretions or ovulation.[26] Insemination occurs during the fall months and females store sperm during winter until ovulation and birthing the following spring.[24] This insures that the neonates can utilize a longer active period for optimal growth. For example, the male behavior in an adult garter snake is not activated by androgen, but rather by hibernation.[27] Several studies have shown male garter snakes exhibiting strong sexual response in the spring when measured levels of androgen are low.[28] It appears that this behavior can only be stimulated by hibernation. Studies have shown that males that do not hibernate do not court females in the spring.[27]
3. Constant reproductive cycles are seen in snakes from the tropics where reproduction can occur throughout the year.

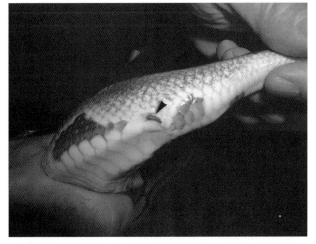

Figure 3.15 Prominent spurs in a male royal python. (Courtesy of Paul Raiti.)

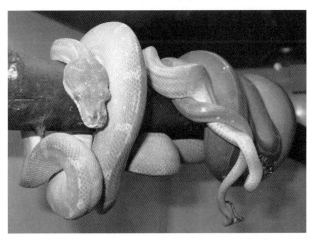

Figure 3.16 A pair of green tree pythons copulating. (Courtesy of Paul Raiti.)

Successful reproduction depends upon interactions between multiple external and internal factors. External factors consist of various climatic, physical, and social cues. For example, onset of breeding in one species of garter snake, *Thamnophis melanogaster*, appears to only occur when the female is in optimal nutritional condition.[29] Other studies on the red-sided garter snake, *Thamnophis sirtalis*, demonstrated that when light was manipulated without heat there was no effect on sexual behavior. However, when temperature was raised from 4°C (39°F) to 28°C (82°F), even in complete darkness, the females became receptive.[25] Internal factors consist of neuropeptides secreted by the pineal gland, hypothalamus, pituitary gland, and gonads.

Receptivity of female snakes begins with the release of pheromones from their epidermal lipid glands after shedding. This stimulates tongue flicking in males whereby chemical cues are transferred to the vomeronasal organs and courtship behavior begins. In colubrids this consists of biting and in boids it consists of spurring by the males. Spurs are vestigial remains of pelvic limbs that are located

on either side of the vent (Figure 3.15). Many species of male snakes will chin-rub along the length of the body of the female.[2] In garter snakes, the skin is thought to be the sole source of attraction and that males have a male-identifying pheromone that other males avoid.[30]

Behavior of the female is not required for mating to occur, as numerous accounts have shown male garter snakes actively courting dead females.[2] Boids often require the presence of multiple males competing for the female before courtship begins. All male snakes possess two copulatory organs called hemipenes located in the base of the tail. The male wraps its tail around the female's tail followed by intromission of a hemipenis into the female's cloaca (Figure 3.16). Copulation can last from minutes to several hours. This may occur periodically over several days. In red-sided garter snakes, a gelatinous plug produced by the sexual segment of the male's kidney is then deposited into the female's cloaca. This plug inhibits further copulatory attempts by other males.[31] One experiment found that females that have a plug in their cloaca or had the secretion spread upon their back, are not courted by other males as long as the substance is present.[32]

Many snakes are purchased as juvenile sexed pairs with the goal of producing offspring as the snakes mature. Acquiring "proven" pairs that are not geriatric is another option to improve the possibility of producing viable offspring. Obtaining an adult mate for a resident snake does not guarantee viable breeding, even if each snake has bred successfully in the past.

Gravidity stimulates a strong thermophilic response and reduced activity.[13] Arboreal snakes often spend more time basking and it is important to provide multiple hot spots of differing temperatures to permit choice of preferred perching site. A hide box with moistened substrate (moss) should be provided for ground-dwelling snakes. Females will spend longer periods of time inside the hide box just prior to oviposition. Ground-dwelling boas and pythons may bask upside down. It is normal for gravid snakes to become anorexic as girth increases.[5] Most gravid snakes shed several days to weeks prior to producing eggs or live young. Restlessness often occurs when delivery is imminent.

Some colubrid snakes coil loosely around the eggs; however, most females simply abandon them. Eggs must then be incubated at appropriate temperatures to ensure hatching. Pythons (i.e., green tree python, Indian python) brood their eggs by forming tight coils around them to maintain proper humidity and incubation temperature (Figure 3.17). These snakes are capable of endothermic thermogenesis whereby spasmodic contraction of skeletal muscles increases incubation temperatures by up to 5°C (9°F).[11] Most herpetoculturists remove the eggs and place them in an artificial incubator until hatching. Brooding pythons are very protective of their eggs, so caution must be used when separating eggs from the

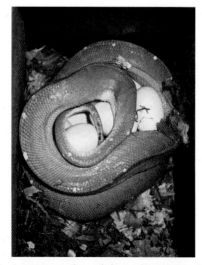

Figure 3.17 A green tree python coiled around its eggs to stabilize humidity and temperature for proper embryonic development. (Courtesy of Paul Raiti.)

female. Some herpetoculturists permit maternal incubation of python eggs; however, females that are separated from their eggs resume feeding sooner than pythons incubating their own eggs.

Female snakes have been observed consuming infertile products of conception. It is suspected this may be a form of antipredator behavior or a means of recycling lost nutrients.[33] Snakes possess sex chromosomes; consequently, sex of neonates is not affected by incubation temperature as in many chelonians and lizards. Parthenogenisis has been documented in snakes such as the Brahminy blind snake, rattlesnakes, warty water snakes, and garter snakes.[24]

Behaviorial problems

Most behavioral problems of snakes are associated with stressors secondary to inappropriate captive management. Photographs of the snake's enclosure at home can provide invaluable information to the veterinarian when addressing such issues. A thorough discussion of husbandry practices should be done prior to physical examination. Acclimatization of wild-caught snakes can be particularly difficult. Extreme fight or flight responses to perceived threats may diminish with time.

Nose rubbing during escape attempts is a sign that the snake is in a stressful environment. Attempts should be made to eliminate this behavior because it can result in rostral abrasions leading to abscessation and maxillary osteomyelitis. Provision of three of the four sides of the enclosure with a visual barrier and placement of the enclosure in a low traffic area of the home will significantly reduce stress. The addition of more hide boxes and climbing areas is also beneficial. In general, escape behavior is reduced the longer the snake is in captivity and when the snake has adequate husbandry and enrichment.

Anorexia is a non-specific sign that can be normal (e.g., during ecdysis, hibernation, or gestation, and so on), but can also be caused by poor husbandry or disease.[19] It is frequently a sign of maladaptation.[21] Snakes will not eat if their husbandry and nutrition are not appropriate for their needs.[19] Some snakes have very specialized diets such as bird eggs or mollusks which must be addressed prior to acquisition. It can also take weeks to months for wild-caught snakes to begin consuming prey regularly.[21] Unfortunately, many of these snakes never acclimate to captivity and eventually succumb to bacterial infections.

A snake may regurgitate for many reasons including size, type, and frequency of the meals, handling, inadequate husbandry, and stress related to captivity.[19,21] A diagnosis of stress-related regurgitation should only be made after a thorough diagnostic work-up has ruled out other causes (bacterial, fungal, viral, neoplasia, foreign bodies). Affected snakes typically regurgitate immediately to several hours after consumption of prey. With time and patience some of these snakes ultimately adapt to captivity. However, for this reason, purchasing captive born snakes is strongly recommended.

Gravid snakes, denied an appropriate nest box, will retain their eggs until a suitable site is found. Affected snakes can become egg bound, ultimately requiring veterinary care. For more information about reproductive problems in snakes see Johnson.[22]

Snakes are capable of developing learned behaviors particularly in regard to feeding. An association is quickly made between the owner's presence and the presentation of food; hence, care should be taken when inserting a hand in the cage even during routine cleaning. Cleaning of enclosures and feeding the animals should be done at separate times. The transfer of scent particles on the hands commonly stimulates a feeding strike. Thawed prey should be dropped into the enclosure near the opening of the hide box or presented on long tongs for arboreal snakes. It may be necessary to wear leather gloves during cage cleaning or feeding or to remove the snake from the enclosure prior to cleaning. Feeding responses are usually stronger from late afternoon to evening. Accordingly, it may be safest to clean enclosures during the day. When presenting prey to large snakes such as boa constrictors, Burmese and reticulated pythons, it is prudent for there to be at least one other experienced snake handler present. Serious injuries and human fatalities have occurred during feeding strikes by large constrictors. It is important to check with local laws regarding the legality of acquisition and maintenance of these snakes.

Pain and pain management

There are limited studies on pain perception in reptiles.[6] Identifying pain in snakes can be rather subjective and currently there is no gold standard for evaluating pain in non-human patients.[34] Many animals will not show signs of pain as a means to avoid predation. The practicioner must be familair with normal and abnormal behavior for each species. Pain may manifest itself through abnormal behavior such as lethargy, anorexia, aggression, tensing, increased respiratory rate, biting at an area on the body, rubbing a body part on a surface, withdrawl, and avoidance.[34] Little research has been done evaluating which drugs and dosages are effective for pain management for reptiles.[35,36] A variety of analgesics (NSAIDS, opioids, local anesthetics) have been used in snakes for pain relief;[34,37,38] however, only recently have controlled studies been conducted to scientifically evaluate this issue.[35] Pain management should be immediately addressed by the veterinarian whenever an injured snake is presented. The use of preemptive and multimodal analgesia should be a part of every surgical procedure.[6] It is much more effective to prevent pain than to manage pain that is already present. More evidence-based studies are needed,

but in the meantime, herpetoculturists should remain aware that while not actually painful, stress associated with captivity may also be injurious, and have a similar negative impact on the snakes' welfare and well-being.

It is the authors' opinion that venomous reptiles should only be kept by specialized facilities such as zoos, research, conservation, and venom extraction centers. For more information about venomous reptiles see Boyer.[39]

Acknowledgment

Paul Raiti would like to thank William Cermak for his assistance in the preparation of some of the photographs.

References

1. Reperant J, Rio J, Ward R et al. Comparative analysis of the primary visual system of reptiles. In: Gans C, Ulinski P, eds. *Biology of the Reptila Neurology C*. Chicago: Univeristy of Chicago Press, 1992;175–240.

2. Mason RT. Reptilian pheromones. In: Gans C, Crews D, eds. *Hormones, Brain, and Behavior: Biology of the Reptilia Volume 18, Physiology E*. Chicago: University of Chicago Press, 1992;114–228.

3. Ford NB, Burghardt GM. Perceptual mechanisms and the behavioral ecology of snakes. In: Seigel RA, Collins JT, eds. *Snakes: Ecology and Behavior*. New York: McGraw-Hill, 1993;117–164.

4. Halpern M. Nasal chemical senses in reptiles: Structure and function. In: Gans C, Crews D, eds. *Hormones, Brain, and Behavior: Physiology E*. Chicago: University of Chicago Press, 1992;423–523.

5. Funk RS. Biology and husbandry: Snakes. In: Mader DR, ed. *Reptile Medicine and Surgery*. 2nd ed. St. Louis: Saunders, 2006;42–58.

6. Mitchell MA. Snakes. In: Mitchell MA, Tully TN, eds. *Manual of Exotic Pet Practice*. St. Louis: Saunders-Elsevier, 2009;136–163.

7. Radcliff C, Murphy JR. Precopulatory and related behaviorsin captive crotalids and other reptiles: Suggestion for further research. *Int Zoo Yearb, Volume 23*, 1983; 163–166.

8. Molenaar G. Anatomy and physiology of infrared sensitivity of snakes. In: Gans C, Ulinski P, eds. *Biology of the Reptilia: Neurology C Volume 17*. Chicago: University of Chicago, 1992;367–453.

9. Boyer TH. *Essentials of Reptiles: A Guide for Practitioners*. Lakewood, CO: AAHA Press, 1988.

10. Pough H, Gans C. The vocabulary of reptilian thermoregulation. In: Gans C, ed. *Biology of the Reptilia: Physiology C, Volume 12*. London: Academic Press, 1982;17–23.

11. Bartholomew G. Physiological control of body temperature. In: Gans C, Pough FH, eds. *Biology of the Reptila: Physiology C, Volume 12*. New York, NY: Academic Press 1982;167–211.

12. Reinert HK. Habitat selection in snakes. In: Seigel RA, Collins JT, eds. *Snakes: Ecology and Behavior*. New York: McGraw Hill, 1993;201–240.

13. Peterson CR, Gibson AR, Dorcas ME. (1993) Snake thermal ecology: The causes and consequences of body-temperature variation. In: Seigel RA, Collins JT, eds. *Snakes: Ecology and Behavior*. New York: McGraw-Hill, 1993;241–314.

14. Avery R. Field studies of body temperatures and thermoregulation. In: Gans C, Pough FH, eds. *Biology of the Reptilia: Physiology C, Volume 12*. New York, NY: Academic Press, 1982; 93–166.

15. Firth B, Turner J. Sensory, neural, and hormonal aspects of thermoregulation. In: Gans C, Pough FH, eds. *Biology of the Reptilia: Physiology C, Volume 12*. New York, Ny: Academic Press, 1982; 213–274 .

16. Burger RM, Gehrmann WH, Ferguson GW. Evaluation of UVB reduction by materials commonly used in reptile husbandry. *Zoo Biol* 2007;26:417–423.

17. Varga M. Captive maintenance and welfare. In: Girling SJ, Raiti P, eds. *BSAVA Manual of Reptiles*. 2nd ed. Quedgeley, Gloucester, England: British Small Animal Veterinary Association, 2004;6–17.

18. Pough FH, Andrews RM, Cadle JE et al. Body support and locomotion. In: *Herpetology*. 3rd ed. Upper Saddle River, NJ: Pearson Prentice Hall, 2004;353–384.

19. Funk RS. Differential diagnosis. In: *Reptile Medicine and Surgery*. 2nd ed. St. Louis: Saunders-Elsevier, 2006;675–682.

20. Donoghue S. Nutrition. In: Mader DR, ed. *Reptile Medicine and Surgery*. 2nd ed. St. Louis, Missouri: Saunders Elsevier, 2006;251–298.

21. Boyer TH. Snakes. In: *Essentials of Reptiles*. Lakewood, CO: American Animal Hospital Association, 1998; 119–146.

22. Johnson JD. Urogenital system. In: Girling SJ, Raiti P, eds. *BSAVA Manual of Reptiles*. 2nd ed. Quedgeley, Gloucester, England: British Small Animal Veterinary Association, 2004;261–272.

23. Maxwell G. *The More Complete Chondro*. Rodeo, NM: ECO Herpetological Publishing & Distribution, 2005.

24. Wright KM. Breeding and neonatal care. In: Girling SJ, Raiti P, eds. *BSAVA Manual of Reptiles*. 2nd ed. Quedgeley, Gloucester, England: British Small Animal Veterinary Association, 2004;40–50.

25. Whittier J, Tokarz R. Physiological regulation of sexual behavior in female reptiles. In: Gans C, Crews D, eds. *Hormones, Brain, and Behavior*, Chicago, IL: The Unversitiy of Chicago Press, 1992;25–69.

26. Crews D, Gans C. The interaction of hormones, brain, and behavior: An emerging discipline in herpetology. In:Gans C, Crews D, eds. *Hormones, Brain, and Behavior*. Chicago, IL: The University of Chicago Press, 1992;1–23.

27. Moore MC, Lindzey J. The physiological basis of sexual behavior in male reptiles. In: Gans C, Crews D, eds. *Hormones, Brain, and Behavior Biology of the Reptilia Volume 18, Physiology E*. Chicago, IL: The University of Chicago Press, 1992;70–113.

28. Crews D. Alternative reproductive tactics in reptiles. *Bioscience*, 1983;33:562–566.

29. Garstka WR, Camazine B, Crews D. Interactions of behavior and physiology during the annual reproductive-cycle of the red-sided garter snake (*Thamnophis-Sirtalis-Parietalis*). *Herpetologica* 1982;38:104–123.

30. Gillingham JC, Dickinson JA. Postural orientation during courtship in the eastern garter snake, *Thamnophis-S-Sirtalis*. *Behav Neural Biol* 1980;28:211–217.

31. Duvall D, Schuett GW, Arnold SJ. Ecology and evolution of snake mating systems. In: Seigel RA, Collins JT, eds. *Snakes: Ecology and Behavior*. London: Academic Press, 2006;165–200.

32. Ross P, Crews D. Influence of seminal plug on mating-behavior in garter snake. *Nature* 1977;267:344–345.

33. Ross RA, Marzec G. *The Reproductive Husbandry of Pythons and Boas*. Stanford: Institute for Herpetological Research, 1990.

34. Hawkins, MG The use of analgesics in birds, reptiles, and small exotic mammals. *J Exotic Pet Med* 2006;15:177–192.

35. Sladky KK, Kinney ME, Johnson SM. Analgesic efficacy of butorphanol and morphine in bearded dragons and corn snakes. *J Am Vet Med Assoc* 2008;233:267–273.

36. Olesen M, Bertelsen M, Perry S, Wang T. Effects of preoperative administration of butorphanol or meloxicam on physiologic responses to surgery in ball pythons. *J Am Vet Med Assoc*, 2008; 233:1883–1888.

37. Schumacher J, Yelen T. *Anesthesia and Analgesia*. 2nd ed. St. Louis: Sanders Elsevier, 2006.

38. Redrobe S. Anaesthesia and analgesia. In: Girling SJ, Raiti P, eds. *BSAVA Manual of Reptiles*. 2nd ed. Gloucester: British Small Animal Veterinary Association, 2004;31–146.

39. Boyer DM. Special considerations for venomous reptiles. In: Girling SJ, Raiti P, eds. *BSAVA Manual of Reptiles*. 2nd ed. Gloucester: British Small Animal Veterinary Association, 2004;357–362.

4

Turtles, tortoises, and terrapins

Heather Mohan-Gibbons and Terry Norton

History

The order Chelonia or Testudines includes tortoises, turtles, and terrapins and is comprised of approximately 270 species,[1] one-quarter of which reside in North America.[2] Chelonians thrive in a wide range of ecosystems. Aquatic species occur in marine, brackish, and freshwater habitats, while terrestrial species reside in desert to tropical environments.[3] Understanding the natural history of a particular species of turtle maintained in captivity is critical for developing an appropriate plan for housing and husbandry. It is beyond the scope of this chapter to provide detailed information on the natural history of every chelonian species; however, there are several excellent texts and reference articles available.[2,4,5] Furthermore, there are a number of valuable texts and reference articles pertaining to chelonian husbandry, nutrition, and management in captivity, both as pets and for breeding purposes.[6-9] Chelonians require more care than many people realize and are the most intensive of all reptile groups to maintain in captivity.

Chelonians have long lifespans, often surpassing humans, and are slow to reach reproductive maturity. For example, the loggerhead sea turtle reaches sexual maturity at approximately 25–35 years of age.[10] The slow sexual maturity rates of chelonians tend to make them more susceptible to human pressure than other vertebrates. These pressures include habitat degradation and destruction, collection for commercial traffic such as the pet trade, and exploitation for food and medicinal purposes.[3]

Senses and communication

The visual spectral sensitivity of sea turtles has been investigated extensively, because of its important role in the survival of the species. The presence of lights on shore leads to hatchling misorientation as well as affecting females adversely when they come up to nest. In a visual discrimination study, the painted turtle (*Chrysemys picta*) and the yellow-bellied slider (*Trachemys scripta*) showed two types of visual receptor cells, one sensitive to red which is dominant at high intensity light, and another sensitive to blue that dominates at low light intensity.[11] For the green turtle, the eye is most sensitive in the violet to yellow visible spectrum. One study concluded that green turtles were more strongly attracted to blue light than red.[12] Witherington evaluated green turtles, hawksbill turtles, and olive ridley hatchlings and found that they were attracted to light in the near-ultraviolet to yellow region of the spectrum, and relatively indifferent to light in the yellow–orange to red region.[13,14] In contrast, loggerhead hatchlings showed an aversion to light in the green–yellow to yellow region of the spectrum. An applied husbandry recommendation that comes from this information is the utilization of a red bulb for a night time heat source so that the photoperiod is not disrupted for sea turtles. Furthermore, this information can be useful in a conservation setting by the recommendation of using a red LED flashlight or no flashlight at all when working on nesting sea turtle beaches.

Some research has been done to identify the hearing ability of turtles. Based on light microscopy on the ear structure of marine turtles, the middle ear has a thick tympanum and is poorly adapted as an aerial receptor when compared to other reptiles and mammals, but is efficient at low-frequency bone conduction hearing.[15] Semi-aquatic and terrestrial turtles can detect the direction of a tone and have been shown to use hearing to problem-solve in maze learning.[16] Of the number of species tested, turtles are most sensitive to sounds in the 200–700 Hz range.[17,18]

Reptiles have two main chemosensory systems: olfactory and vomeronasal systems.[19] In the reptiles studied thus far, the basic structure of the olfactory system appears to be the same across reptilian groups.[20] However, the presence, structure, and function of the vomeronasal gland varies greatly among reptiles.[20] Many chelonians do not have a vomeronasal gland, but instead have a homologous structure in addition to their olfactory system.[20] A vomeronasal gland has been identified in several species that may be found in the pet trade, including the European pond turtle (*Emys orbicularis*),[21] red-eared slider (*Trachyemys scripta*), Reeve's turtle (*Chinemys reevesii*),[22] and stinkpot turtle (*Sternotherus odoratus*).[23] Both the olfactory and vomeronasal systems respond to inhaled odors in turtles. Halpern reported that when the nerves are severed to the olfactory system or the vomeronasal gland, European pond turtles had impaired ability to search for food.[20] This is noteworthy because in captivity, when a chelonian has plugged nares from a respiratory infection or other causes, they often will not eat. The olfactory system may be responsible for a turtle's food preferences at a young age. For example, studies conducted on loggerhead (*Caretta caretta*) and green sea turtles (*Chelonia mydas*) found that they develop food preferences within 14 days after hatching.[24,25] When a hatchling turtle was offered a new food type that had not been in its diet previously, most would not eat it initially. However, after a 14-day feeding trial most turtles in the study no longer had food preferences.

Reptiles have a variety of glands and glandular secretions used in communication. Chemical cues are efficient, effective for long periods, and often work over large areas.[19] All families of turtles (except Testudinidae) have specialized secretory producing glands that lie medially along the junction of their carapace and plastron.[19] Analysis in green sea turtles (*Chelonia mydas*) and the common musk turtle (*Sternotherus odoratus*) revealed that the glands are holocrine and have a series of secretory lobules that are encapsulated in striated muscle.[26] The glands of three species, the common musk turtle, the loggerhead sea turtle (*Caretta caretta*), and the Kemp's ridley sea turtle (*Lepidochelys kempii*) produce a water soluble, protein rich, non-acidic secretion with a high-molecular-weight. It is unknown what purpose these glands or their secretions serve. Secretions may function as a pheromone, or because the glands are located in striated muscle, it has been hypothesized that the secretion may be expelled as a predator deterrent.[19]

The mental glands or integumentary organs found on the chin or throat of chelonians are another type of sensory gland.[27] These are holocrine glands and are found in 21 of the 69 chelonian genera in the Emydidae, Testudinidae, and Platysternidae families.[19] The holocrine glands of the chelonians in the *Gopherus* genus change size during the reproductive season and are much larger in males.[28] The male gopher tortoise (*G. polyphemus*), may travel to various burrows occupied by females within his territory. When a female tortoise comes out of her burrow, the male will bob his head up and down and follow her. Additionally, he may wipe his leg barb covered with pheromones near the female's nose

or rub the female with his chin, where the mental scent glands lie.[29]

The third location of sensory glands in chelonians is the cloaca. Female cloacal pheromones appear to play an important role in mating behavior; however, research pertaining to how these glands are used has not been conducted. A few anecdotal reports exist that suggest that cloacal secretions by females may stimulate male courtship behavior.[19] A red-foot tortoise (*Geochelone carbonaria*) mounted a skeletonized shell that had female cloacal secretions rubbed onto it. Another male tried to mount a head of lettuce that a female had just climbed over.

The only evidence for chemical communication between aquatic turtles is also anecdotal. Rathke's glands are paired exocrine organs embedded along the infra-marginal scutes or in the inguinal region on the ventral side of the shell.[19] Aquatic turtles may use cloacal discharges and the Rathke's glands for sociochemical exchanges.[19] One unproven hypothesis is that the offshore aggregation of Kemp's and olive ridley sea turtles (known as the "arribada", which means the arrival) is a response to the pheromonal attraction to the secretion from the Rathke's gland.

Although there is much to be learned about chelonian sensory behavior and communication, it is clear that it is complex and varies from species to species. Management strategies for maintaining various chelonians in captivity should strive to allow for normal sensory behaviors to be utilized.

Husbandry

Appropriate enclosures and good husbandry are critical to establishing normal behavior in captive chelonians. Unfortunately, poor husbandry and environmental conditions are the primary factors contributing to illness in captive reptiles including chelonians. In addition to the chelonian-specific husbandry information that follows, the reader is encouraged to refer to Chapter 20 for more details on animal welfare in general. The captive environment should encourage natural behaviors of a particular species, lend itself to easy maintenance, prevent escapes, and minimize stress. Enclosures and housing needs of a particular chelonian species should be based on its natural history, whether it is aquatic, semi-aquatic or terrestrial, size of the turtle, the numbers being housed, and available literature regarding successful captive maintenance of the species being considered.[30] The New York Turtle and Tortoise Society's minimal requirement recommendations for housing terrestrial chelonians is that the combined shell size of all the turtles present should not exceed one-quarter of the floor surface area of the enclosure.[31]

Chelonians tend to pace or swim in the perimeter of an enclosure or may repeatedly rub body parts such as the rostrum or limbs against clear barriers such as glass, plastic, or chain link fencing in an effort to get out since they can see through them. To avoid these behaviors and to prevent injury, it is recommended that solid barriers such as wooden fencing or other opaque surfaces be used in the construction of chelonian habitats.[30,31] It is preferred to keep terrestrial chelonians outdoors as much as possible to allow space to exercise, to exhibit natural behaviors such as digging and grazing, and to allow for exposure to unfiltered sunlight (Figure 4.1). An outdoor enclosure needs to have a perimeter fence with a securely fastened door and depending on the species, the fencing should be buried 15.2–61 cm (6–24 in.) deep so as to prevent the turtle from digging out.[31] New acquisitions for an existing collection of chelonians should be strictly quarantined for a minimum of 60 days. For more information on setting up natural habitats and hospital cages refer to the chapter on lizards (Chapter 5), and the section titled "Construction of the enclosure."

All reptiles, including Chelonia, are ectothermic and depend on environmental heat and mobility to thermoregulate. Chelonians need full spectrum lighting (UVA, UVB, visible, and infrared wavelengths) to synthesize vitamin D_3 which is important for mineral metabolism, reproduction, and normal behavior. Photoperiod can play a significant role in reproduction, as well as having beneficial psychological and behavioral effects.[8] Outdoor enclosures will allow the chelonian to thermoregulate more naturally as long as shade is available. Types of lighting, heat sources, and humidity for setting up an appropriate captive environment are all covered extensively in Chapter 5.

When chelonians are housed together, multiple shelters, hide boxes, or cage furniture should be provided for security and hiding. The hide areas should be large enough to fit the animal comfortably but not so large that they do not feel secure.[30] Hide areas can also be created with a variety of

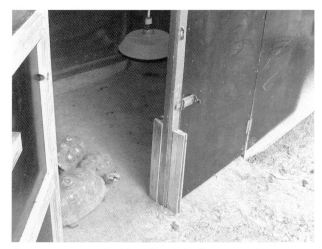

Figure 4.1 An example of an outdoor shelter for tortoises. The tortoises can go out into direct sunlight or go into the shelter for shade. On one side of the shelter, there is a low wattage ceramic heat emitter as a heat source in cooler weather. (Courtesy of Heather Mohan-Gibbons.)

materials such as dead palm fronds and other plant material. Substrate can be provided to allow the turtle to bury itself for security. Familiarity with the natural history of the particular chelonian will dictate whether it is preferred to house them singly, in pairs, or in groups. For more information on materials and how to provide shelters, refer to Chapter 5 and the section titled "Shelters."

The gopher tortoise (*Gopherus polyphemus*), California desert tortoise (*G. agassizii*), and to a lesser extent the African spurred tortoise (*G. sulcata*) are adapted for digging and maintaining a burrow in the wild. Juvenile free-roaming Florida box turtles (*Terrapene carolina*) are found more frequently in areas with leaf litter and moist substrates with high canopy coverage.[32] It is critical that the captive environment provide situations for these natural behaviors to be expressed. For more information on substrates for chelonians, refer to the Chapter 5 section on "Substrates" and those recommended for burrowing species. One of the authors (TMN) has observed captive radiated tortoises (*G. radiata*) maintain plots of grass by grazing on a small area frequently. This behavior appears to allow for new, more nutritious, and easier to digest grass to grow and be readily available. Small areas of grass can be grown indoors for behavioral and nutritional enrichment. The Georgia Sea Turtle Center, a rehabilitation center, feeds green sea turtles under their care a variety of vegetables, including romaine and other dark leafy vegetables, green peppers, and cucumbers. PVC pipe holders have been created to secure the food items to the bottom to promote the natural grazing behavior of these turtles.

Chelonians need to be provided with fresh water at all times and will use it for soaking, cooling, and drinking and, in the case of aquatic species, this may be where they spend the majority of their time. For terrestrial turtle species, the water source should be large enough for the turtle to submerge its entire body including the lower part of their shell while being stable and sturdy enough to not tip over (Figure 4.2). Soaking the turtle regularly (daily to several times per week) in a separate container of clean shallow water may be necessary for smaller enclosures (Figure 4.3). While acceptable, this is less desirable as the animal can no longer choose when to access the water source. Tortoises in the genus *Gopherus* have been observed dropping their front end downward during rainfall, so water is channeled along their scutes, along their forelimbs, and into their mouths.[33]

Aquatic turtles are even more labor intensive than terrestrial species especially as they mature. Aquatic turtles typically require a more elaborate filtration system than fish and regular water changes are often required. Installing a drain in large aquatic enclosures will allow for more efficient water changes and easier cleaning. When housing diamondback terrapins (*Malaclemys terrapin*), saltwater marsh turtles or certain sea turtle species, water salinity may need to be adjusted by adding salt. More sophisticated life

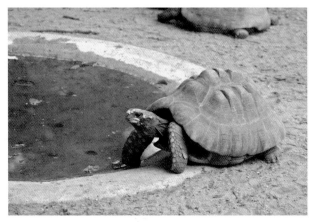

Figure 4.2   All chelonians need a water source that is stable. Containers need to be secured or buried or they will be tipped over. This water source has sides that are gradual so the tortoise can easily access deeper water for soaking. (Courtesy of Heather Mohan-Gibbons.)

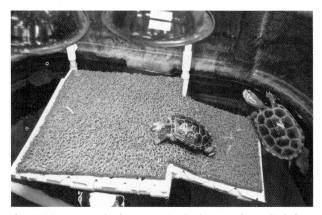

Figure 4.4   An example of an appropriate haul-out area for any kind of water turtle. This allows the turtle to completely dry off and has a heat source above to provide warmth. This one is made of PVC piping and 3 M gray matting that is used at the Georgia Sea Turtle Center for terrapins. (Courtesy of Simon Dilts.)

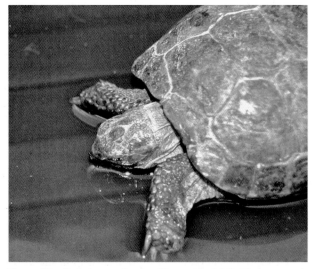

Figure 4.3   Chelonians can be placed in a soaking tub that is deep enough for them to soak and drink on a daily basis. (Courtesy of Paul Gibbons.)

support systems are needed for maintaining sea turtles and larger aquaria. Details regarding filtration systems, water quality, and management of water systems can be found in a number of sources.[8,34–36] Most aquatic turtles require a basking area with easy access so they can get in and out of the water for basking and complete drying under a heat and light source (Figure 4.4).

Hibernation may be important in some temperate chelonians because it stimulates reproductive activity in males and synchronizes ovulation in females. Hibernation may assist in maintaining normal thyroid activity and may increase life expectancy in captivity.[37] Many hibernating species cease to feed in the winter. This may end up being problematic if the turtle is not hibernated and maintained at warmer temperatures. Only healthy robust chelonians that have been eating normally should be hibernated. Recent or current illness is an obvious reason to postpone

or not institute hibernation. A thorough understanding of the hibernation process and how to simulate it in captivity is critical prior to implementing this on a particular individual or group of turtles.[31]

Locomotion

Due to the tremendous variation in size and anatomy, locomotion is not the same for all chelonians. In general, terrestrial chelonians walk slowly, with a lateral footfall pattern that provides maximum support to overcome the limitations created by the limited range of motion within the openings between the carapace and plastron, and fusion of the pelvic and pectoral girdles to the shell.[38,39] The movement of the forefoot on each side follows movement of the hind foot on the same side.[38] Tortoises walk with the plastron raised off the ground, whereas most semi-aquatic species use a lunging gait and often drag the caudal corners of the plastron on the ground.[39] Providing adequate substrate and space for the species of chelonian being maintained in captivity as described earlier is critical to keeping the feet and nails healthy and allowing for normal locomotion.

Digging is a natural behavior for some species such as the gopher tortoise (*Geochelone polyphemus*) for which they are well adapted anatomically. Gopher tortoises dig their burrows by using their front spade-like feet and strong claws. As the digging takes the burrow deeper underground, the tortoise will move backward and use its front feet to sweep the soil farther up toward the mouth of the burrow. The depth of the burrow can be 3–7 m (9.8–23 ft) and the length may be from 1 to 17 m (3.2–55.8 ft). The burrow is very important to the habitat and other wildlife because it provides shelter to 300–400 other species. The gopher tortoise is therefore considered to be a keystone species for the longleaf pine ecosystem.[29]

Semi-aquatic turtles use their webbed feet in two different types of aquatic locomotion, paddle-swimming and bottom-walking. Bottom-walking is similar to the lateral footfall pattern of terrestrial locomotion, but in paddle-swimming, the limbs move in more rapid diagonal couplets that may become irregular.[39]

Marine turtles of the families Cheloniidae and Dermochelyidae have modified forelimbs that form elongate, wing-like paddles. These modified forelimbs are moved synchronously and forward propulsion is created during both the upstroke and downstroke by adjustments in the angle of motion. Marine turtles have relatively small hind limbs that are used primarily as rudders and elevators for steering.[38] The hind limbs are also critical for moving on land and nesting.

Ingestive behavior

Visual, chemosensory, and infrared detection are important senses employed for food acquisition by a variety of reptiles. Chelonians have a number of adaptations that aid in food acquisition. For example, as small fish and amphibians approach the mata mata turtle (*Chelus fimbriatus*), it swings its head to the side. As the mouth opens, a strong sucking movement is set off by rapid depression of the hyoid, and the mouth then closes instantly upon the prey.[5] Other species have developed unique anatomical features to attract prey, such as the worm-like lure inside the bottom jaw of the alligator snapping turtle (*Macroclemys temminckii*).[40] The turtle lies motionless with its mouth wide open and twitches the lure back and forth. When a fish nips at the "worm" or touches the inside of the mouth, the powerful jaws slam shut. Many herbivorous chelonians forage for vegetation, but do not travel far, possibly due to thermal stress and/or predation.[41] For example, juvenile gopher tortoises (*Gopherus polyphemus*) have brief foraging periods and remain near their burrows.[41] In contrast, most of the sea turtle species including the herbivorous green turtle, travel long distances to reach their foraging grounds.[42]

Chelonia use a variety of senses to accurately identify food (be it plant or animal) including visual reception (eyes), mechanoreceptors (ears and integument), and chemoreception (tongue, nose, and vomeronasal organs). For example, Boyer reports that box turtles (*Terrapene* spp.) are particularly attracted to red-, yellow-, and orange-colored foods.[34]

Providing adequate nutrition is a critical part of the care of captive chelonian. However, it is beyond the scope of this chapter to provide detailed nutritional information on this group of reptiles because of the diversity and complexity of their feeding behavior and dietary needs. Briefly, chelonians can be broadly divided into herbivores (many of the tortoises, green sea turtle [*Chelonia mydas*], several freshwater turtles), omnivores (box turtles and others),

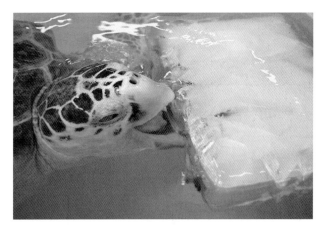

Figure 4.5 Small pieces of food can be provided in ice blocks for both foraging and enrichment opportunities for water turtles. (Georgia Sea Turtle Center, Courtesy of Amy Hupp.)

and carnivores (snapping turtles, soft shells, and others). Some species such as the green sea turtle are primarily carnivorous while occupying the pelagic life stage in the sargassum rafts as juveniles. They leave the pelagic habitats and enter benthic foraging areas at a size of 20–35 cm (7.9–13.8 in.) carapace length depending on the location. At this time, they shift to an herbivorous diet consisting of various sea grasses and algae. Many freshwater turtles demonstrate similar feeding strategies as they mature. Understanding the natural history and feeding behavior is critical to maintaining captive specimens and critical to providing a nutritionally complete diet. A combination of commercially available prepared diets, vitamin and mineral supplementation, live prey items, natural forage, and high-quality fruits and vegetables may be utilized depending on the species.

Presentation of food can be just as important as the types of food being fed. Feeding time may be the primary source of enrichment for the chelonian, especially if housed indoors. There are a variety of ways to use food as enrichment to encourage natural foraging and feeding behaviors. Some examples include placing food items in an ice block (Figure 4.5) or other non-destructible item for aquatic species, securing vegetables in a PVC pipe to encourage bottom feeding in aquatic herbivores (Figure 4.6), feeding live prey, and providing grass and non-toxic forage to encourage grazing in herbivorous chelonians (Figure 4.7). The American Association of Zoo Keepers (http://www.aazk.org) is a great resource for ideas regarding enrichment.

Social behavior

Aggression is a normal part of the behavioral repertoire of most animals and chelonians are no different. For example, in the wild, the aggressive behavior of female loggerhead sea turtles (*Caretta caretta*) ranges from passive threat displays

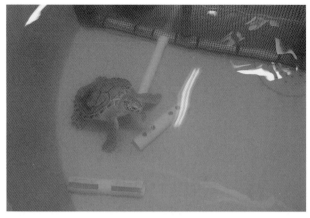

Figure 4.6   An example of a submerged enrichment device. This one offers foraging opportunities by allowing leafy greens to protrude from holes made in a sunken PVC tube at the Georgia Sea Turtle Center. (Courtesy of Amy Hupp.)

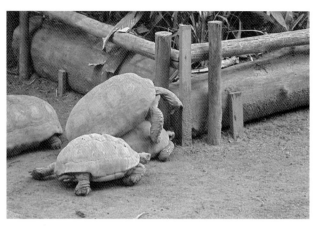

Figure 4.8   Two male tortoises followed a female, sniffing her cloacal region before one mounted her. (Courtesy of Heather Mohan-Gibbons.)

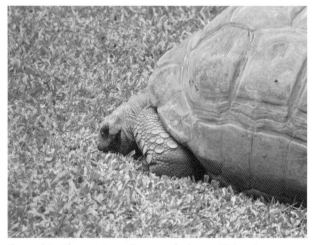

Figure 4.7   Many tortoises will graze on fresh grass. This can be one way to provide nutrition in captivity and also provide enrichment by allowing the tortoise to forage in a natural manner. (Courtesy of Heather Mohan-Gibbons.)

(e.g., head–tail circling) to aggressive combat (e.g., sparring) directed toward other females.[43]

In captivity, aggression can present a serious problem when multiple turtles are housed in the same enclosure, especially if space is limited (Figure 4.8). For example, some aquatic species, such as diamondback terrapins, may be housed with conspecifics when enough space is provided. However, other species such as snapping turtles, softshell turtles, and big-headed turtles are known to be more aggressive and should not be housed together at all.[35] Aggression is common among captive breeding male tortoises and may include shell ramming, overturning the opponent, head bobbing, open mouth threat displays, dominance threat displays (e.g., male tortoise raises its body very high off the ground), vocalizations, and biting.[44] Turtles that are housed together should be separated permanently if aggression is seen. Turtles from different geographical regions should never be housed together because of the potential for disease transmission, parasites, and increased

environmental stress. Aggression directed toward human caretakers is less common, but could be associated with previous aversive events, a response to perceived threats, or competition for resources.

Aggregation has been reported in some tortoises when the population density is high.[45] The desert tortoise (*Gopherus agassizii*) is typically solitary in the summer and spring, but may aggregate in large numbers when suitable shelters are limited in the winter.[46]

The "arribada" that occurs in ridley sea turtles is another form of aggregation. The hypothesized advantages of this nesting strategy are to saturate the area with eggs so that local predators are provided with an overabundance of food and the surplus may be left to hatch in safety. Unfortunately, this behavior has made these species vulnerable to excessive harvest of adults and eggs by humans.

Little is known about the social needs of chelonian species. It is reasonable to consider some chelonian behavior as social, and species that exhibit such behavior could benefit from social interactions. In one author's experience (TMN), those species that seem more gregarious should have interaction with conspecifics, because living in isolation for a social animal can be detrimental. Some species, however, do not appear to be at all sociable and in these species there may be no benefit gained from group living. For example, inter-male combat can be a serious problem in some species, leading to stress and injury, especially when space is limited. Until more is known about this important subject, caution should be exercised when attempting to group house multiple chelonia.

Other turtle species such as diamondback terrapins (*Malaclemys terrapin*) and painted turtles (*Chrysemys picta*) may have locally high nest density especially after a rain, but none of this is especially synchronous or coordinated.[47] One of the authors (TMN) has observed over 20 terrapins crossing a causeway in less than 1 hour, after a rain storm, in an effort to find suitable nesting sites. Unfortunately this behavior is often fatal. About 200–300 terrapins are hit during their annual nesting season from early May to early July on this one causeway in Georgia.

Reproductive behavior

Excellent husbandry, nutrition, and enclosure design and space are critical components in the development of a successful chelonian breeding program.[48] Additionally, understanding the reproductive behavior and biology of the particular species in the wild is critical. Many species of turtles breed and nest annually,[49] while others, such as several of the sea turtle species, nest every 2–3 years.[50] Seasonal annual cycles are more common in temperate zones, while turtles in tropical regions may reproduce more continuously.[51] Many species of chelonians may store sperm for variable periods of time, and in some cases potentially for many years. Furthermore, some turtles may lay multiple clutches (sometimes with different paternity) in the same season without further breeding.[49,52] Turtles that are wild caught have the potential to lay viable eggs in captivity for at least 1 year or more without exposure to a male.[53,54]

Visual, tactile, and olfactory cues may be involved in chelonian courtship depending on the species. For example the male red-eared slider (*Trachemys scripta elegans*) will visually "fan" the female by quivering his long forelimb claws in front of her in the water.[44] Male tortoises may trail behind a female sniffing the cloacal region and following her prior to mounting (Figure 4.9), suggesting that there is a pheromone or other chemical information being perceived.[19] Auffenberg found that male gopher tortoises (*Gopherus polyphemus*) will evert their swollen mental glands and bob their head rapidly.[55] This is believed to aid in wafting scent through the air. The female tortoise will rub her front leg against her chin glands before extending that leg forward to a male before mating.

One study investigating the olfactory systems effect on breeding behavior found that when both the vomeronasal and olfactory nerves were cut in the European pond turtle, all reproductive behavior stopped. When just one or the other was severed, breeding behavior was impaired 60–70%.[21] Male red-foot tortoises (*Geochelone carbonaria*) will stand facing a female with the neck extended low and swaying side to side while grunting.[56] Female green sea turtles (*Chelonia mydas*) likely signal reproductive readiness to males via chemical cues.[57] Galeotti found that Hermann's tortoises (*Testudo hermanni*) can detect their own species from others by odor alone, and males can determine both sex and sexual maturity of females by olfactory cues.[58]

In some species, visual cues appear to be used for gender recognition. Auffenberg found that when male red-foot tortoises (*Geoclelone carbonaria*) had their head colored black, they did not elicit aggression from other males.[59] When their heads were painted to resemble natural male head colors, the males were then challenged. Many other species of reptiles will expose their brightly colored integument for social displays and mating.[11]

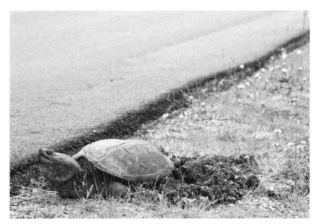

Figure 4.9   A female snapping turtle laying her eggs along a roadside in Maine. (Courtesy of Heather Mohan-Gibbons.)

Some male tortoises may demonstrate aggressive behavior while attempting to breed, potentially causing severe shell and limb trauma to the female.[20] Overzealous males can also cause severe shell and limb trauma to females during breeding. It may be necessary to separate genders in small captive environments.[60] One of the authors (TMN) has observed a male Burmese black mountain tortoise (*Manouria emys phayrei*) rub his plastron down to the bone by excessive and frequent breeding. Courtship may last several hours, copulation typically lasts a few minutes, and vocalization is common, especially in tortoises.[56] Male mud and musk turtles (Kinosternidae) touch the female's cloaca with their rostrum, then rub along her side in the region of the musk gland, and finally will bite at her head before copulating.[19] These musk glands have a dual purpose in providing gender recognition cues and anti-predator defense mechanisms.[61]

Poor reproductive performance in male chelonians may be due to a variety of causes. Underlying medical causes or physical abnormalities should be ruled out by a thorough physical examination and diagnostic work-up. Appropriate environmental stimuli may be helpful in stimulating reproductive activity. For example, a simulated rainy season may be necessary for tropical species. Removing the male and then reintroducing him to the female later may also stimulate renewed interest. The male and female should be appropriately matched according to size. Mate fidelity has not been documented in turtles.[56]

Gravid terrestrial chelonians may show increased basking, reduced feeding or foraging behavior, and increased territorial behavior.[52] Many chelonians become anorectic during late gravidity, and this may persist until egg laying. One study, in spotted turtles (*Clemmys guttata*), found that the females' energy reserves do not effect immediate reproductive output in a single nesting season.[62] However, over the 3-year study, females that remained in poor body condition either did not reproduce or laid a large number of small eggs. Females in the best condition laid a large number of large eggs. This study suggests that since female spotted turtles in poor body condition could still produce a large clutch, egg size may be the best predictor of reproductive health in this species.

Chelonians will seek out a suitable area for nest excavation, egg laying, and incubation. Many female turtles press their head and ventral side of the neck onto the ground, apparently in an attempt to detect a good nest site location.[63] In the pursuit of a suitable nesting site, some females may appear to be hyperactive. Under normal circumstances, she will often excavate a shallow nest and lay the eggs before covering them. Sea turtles may come up to nest and if a suitable nest site is not available, the female may return to the ocean and come up later that night or the next day in search of more suitable nesting habitat. Gravid captive females may attempt to excavate solid floor substrates, which can result in trauma to the female or her eggs. Providing a suitable nesting area and substrate is critical for egg laying in captive settings. If a suitable site, temperature, and depth are not available, egg retention and eventual dystocia is likely to occur.[49,56]

Aside from covering the eggs, no further maternal care has been observed in turtles except for the Burmese mountain tortoise (*Manouria emys*).[56] In this species, the female constructs a nest of a variety of materials such as leaves and pine needles and after laying her eggs, guards the nest for several weeks.

Common behavior problems

Most of the behavioral problems encountered in captive turtles result directly from inappropriate husbandry and nutrition. It is essential to have an understanding of the natural history of the species under the clinician's care and apply that information to the captive environment. Stressors that may lead to undesirable behaviors in captive chelonians may include excessive or rough handling, inappropriate cage construction and location, lack of visual security, inadequate shelter, improper thermal range and heat sources, lack of or inappropriate substrate, inappropriate cage accessories, improper light spectrum, and photoperiod, poor nutrition, inappropriate social structure, and overcrowding.

Unless the chelonian being evaluated is a neonate, it is typically impractical to transport the entire enclosure to the veterinary clinic. It is important for the clinician to obtain a clear understanding of the patient's enclosure, nutrition, and overall husbandry. Regular site visits may be appropriate for larger facilities but in the case of the single turtle patient is usually impractical. It is helpful to instruct the client to provide photographs or digital images of the enclosure. Detailed history forms that clients can complete before appointments are also useful.

Understanding normal and abnormal behavior is critical for the chelonian veterinarian. The history should cover a variety of topics, one being the behavior of the turtle. The client should be questioned on whether the chelonian being evaluated displays the following normal behaviors: feeding, activity level, breeding and nesting behavior, ambulation or swimming, and diving. Additionally, the frequency, quantity and appearance of feces and urine are important to note. A visual examination should take place prior to handling the turtle. The clinician should focus on a number of behaviors including attitude, posture, body condition, swimming and diving capabilities, ambulation, strength, appropriate aggressive behavior, excessive basking, and respiratory rate and effort. If the chelonian is hospitalized, the clinician should pay close attention to these behaviors to get a better understanding of the patient's condition. Monitoring abnormal and normal behavior is very helpful in determining the efficacy of a particular treatment regimen.

Trauma may be a result of abnormal behaviors exhibited in captivity. Improper enclosure design may lead to excessive rubbing of the outer shell or nails. Inappropriate social structure or overcrowding may lead to bite wounds. For example, one of the authors (TMN) has observed tail and feet biting in hatchling diamondback terrapins resulting in serious wounds. Aggression may be noted in turtles that are fed in the same enclosure, especially if live prey is being offered. Some species such as snapping turtles are naturally aggressive and should be housed by themselves unless in a breeding program. Excessive breeding may cause plastron lesions and may lead to a prolapsed penis. Stereotypic pacing behavior may result in chronic rubbing and lead to abrasions and deeper wounds as described earlier in this chapter. Many of these injuries may be prevented or treated by modifying the enclosure (visual barriers, circular tanks, more space), social structure, isolating turtles during feeding, and strategic reproductive strategies (e.g., limiting time of males and females are together), and adding environmental enrichment. Chapter 5 contains more suggestions for environmental modifications that may be useful for decreasing traumatic abrasions.

Obesity is not uncommon in captive chelonians, particularly in snapping turtles and green sea turtles, and may be due to overfeeding or lack of exercise. Monitoring body weight and condition and adjusting the diet accordingly is helpful in preventing obesity. The obese chelonian may need to be provided more space and should be encouraged to move around through innovative enrichment and cage design.

Sea turtles housed in captivity and undergoing rehabilitation will eat anything in their tank including bottom substrate, heaters, and the filtration system. This may lead to fatal impactions. Bottom substrates should not be used or should be large enough that they cannot be ingested and smooth enough so that traumatic injuries do not develop from excessive rubbing.

Pain and pain management

Pain in turtles can be rather subjective and currently there is not a gold standard for evaluating pain in this group of reptiles.[64] The practitioner must be familiar with normal behavior for the species and for the patient being evaluated. Pain may manifest itself through abnormal behavior such as lethargy, anorexia, aggression, increased respiratory rate, lameness, biting at a particular area, excessive rubbing of a body part, or withdrawal and avoidance.[64] A variety of analgesics have been used for pain management in chelonians;[64] however, only recently have controlled studies been conducted to scientifically evaluate this issue.[65,66]

Enrichment and behavioral training

Behavioral training and enrichment are being used more commonly in zoological institutions and aquaria for improving the welfare of captive chelonians and other reptiles. These techniques may also be recommended by the chelonian veterinarian or behaviorist in a private practice

setting. Enrichment ideas for chelonians are included in Table 4.1.

Training has been utilized in chelonians for management and medical procedures including regular body weights, physical examination, and blood drawing. At one zoological institution, two Aldabra tortoises (*Geochelone gigantea*) were taught to extend and hold their necks for venipuncture.[67] There are extensive studies on mammals and birds correlating environmental enrichment and the reduction in stereotypical and stress-related behavior problems in captivity. A recent meta-analytic review of 54 enrichment studies on captive mammals demonstrated a 90% reduction of stereotypic behavior in those animals housed in enriched conditions when compared to control groups.[68] A few studies have been conducted in chelonians. A study involving captive eastern box turtles (*Terrapene carolina carolina*) compared enriched enclosures that had a variety of substrates and hiding places to one that had only

Table 4.1 Chelonian enrichment ideas

Enrichment pertaining to enclosures or exhibits	Provide a variety of natural substrates (i.e., leaves, rocks)
	Provide a variety of substrates (shredded paper, cardboard boxes, floating jugs, traffic cones)
	Mirrors
	Changes of light cycle
	Changes of décor
	Addition of novel items (shells, plants, rocks)
	Exercise areas
	Enrichment "playgrounds"
	Addition or removal of water features (misting, shallow pools, change water currents)
	Cover (plants, hide boxes, barrels)
	Cardboard exploration tubes or boxes
	Water and temperature changes
	Providing environment that elicits natural behaviors
	More basking/haul out places
Foraging enrichment	Add water currents during feeding time
	Insect dispensers (i.e., natural log with insects or plastic logs)
	Variety of insect prey
	Live prey
	Offer natural forage such as grass
	PVC/cardboard treat tubes (land or water)
	Spread food out to encourage foraging
	Vary the feeding times or quantities
	Drag food for scent through enclosure (banana peel)
	Vary locations of food (sunken, hidden, suspended)
Training enrichment	Change swim patterns
	Teaching targeting behavior (nose touches object)
	Stay in one place, on target
	Moving from one location to another using target
	Stretcher, scale, or crate training
	Teach to move towards people when on exhibit
	Teach to move away from open door when cleaning enclosure
Olfactory enrichment	Banana peels near enclosure
	Sunken or buried objects that are scented with food or prey
	Items scented by other animals
Social enrichment	Rotation of animals or enclosures
	Training
	Mirrors
	Touch by people, if turtle is comfortable with this

Some suggestions were taken from AAZK Forum Vol. 35 No. 2

newspaper.[69] By the end of the 30-day treatment period, the turtles in the enriched enclosures had lower heterophil to lymphocyte ratios (H/L) and spent significantly less time engaged in escape behavior. Furthermore, the turtles showed a distinct preference for the enriched environment when given free access to both enclosures. Another study was conducted to evaluate the effects of enrichment and stereotypic swimming behavior in three loggerhead sea turtles (*Caretta caretta*) and one blind green sea turtle (*Chelonia mydas*).[70] They were presented four types of enrichment: floating water cooler jugs, sunken PVC pipes with leafy greens attached, sunken jugs with holes in it so that when pushed, fish and squid floated out, and a water hose hung over the side of the tank to create a waterfall. Once enrichment was added, resting behavior decreased from 38% to 6% and stereotypic swimming decreased from 38% to 2%. Before enrichment was added, grooming and investigative type behaviors were less than 1%, but after enrichment was added those behaviors increased to 44%. This type of enrichment allows the turtles to use their olfactory, visual, and tactile senses.

More research is needed on environmental enrichment and its effects on turtles in captivity, but it is recommended to provide as much enrichment as possible for any captive animal. For turtles, this can be anything that stimulates foraging or other natural behaviors like hiding, basking, digging, and swimming. Additionally, adding items they can physically move or manipulate with their feet, mouth, or body may be enriching. Turtles have also been shown to object "play." A Nile soft-shelled turtle (*Trionyx triunguis*) showed a significant reduction in self-mutilating behavior when provided with natural and artificial objects to manipulate.[71] Once enrichment was added to this turtle's enclosure, 31% of his time was spent interacting with at least one of the objects. It is important to note that careful evaluation of new enrichment ideas needs to take place prior to implementation to ensure that it is safe for the turtle. An example would be to make sure the turtle cannot ingest an enrichment item that could possibly cause an obstruction. Providing a captive habitat that is enriching and allows turtles to express their natural behavior is likely to result in psychologically and physically healthier animals.

References

1. Bonner BB. Chelonian therapeutics. *Vet Clin North Am Exot Anim Pract* 2000;3:257–332.
2. Ernst CH, Barbour RW, Lovich JE et al. *Turtles of the United States and Canada.* Washington, DC: Smithsonian Books, 1994.
3. Norton TM. Chelonian emergency and critical care. *Semin Avian Exot Pet Med* 2005;14:106–130.
4. Moll D, Moll EO. *The Ecology, Exploitation, and Conservation of River Turtles.* New York: Oxford University Press, 2004.
5. Bonin F, Devaux B, Dupre A. *Turtles of the World.* Baltimore, MD: The Johns Hopkins University Press, 2006.
6. de Vosjoli P, Klingenberg R. *The Box Turtle Manual.* Lakeside, CA: Advanced Vivarium Systems, 1995.
7. de Vosjoli P. *General Care and Maintenance of Popular Tortoises.* Santee, CA: Advanced Vivarium Systems, 1996.
8. de Vosjoli P. Designing environments for captive amphibians and reptiles. *Veterinary Clinics of North America Exotic Animal Practice* 1999;2:43–68.
9. World Chelonian Trust. www.chelonia.org. Last accessed: July 5, 2009.
10. Chaloupka M, Musick J. Age, growth and maturation. In: Lutz ME, Musick JA, eds. *The Biology of Sea Turtles.* Boca Raton, Florida: CRC Press, 1996;233–276.
11. Cooper WE, Greenberg N. Reptilian coloration and behavior. In: Gans C, Crews D, eds. *Biology of the Reptilia Physiology E.* Chicago: The Univeristy of Chicago Press, 1992;298–422.
12. Mrosovsky N, Carr A. Preference for light of short wavelength in hatchling green sea turtles *Chelonia mydas* tested on their natural nesting beaches. *Behaviour* 1967;28:219–231.
13. Witherington BE, Bjorndal KA. Influences of artificial lighting on the seaward orientation of hatchling loggerhead turtles *Caretta caretta*. *Biol Conserv* 1991;55:139–149.
14. Witherington BE. Sea-finding behavior and the use of photic orientation cues by hatching sea turtles. PhD Thesis. Gainsville, FL: Univeristy of Florida Gainesville, 1992.
15. Lenhardt ML, Klinger RC, Musick JA. Marine turtle middle ear anatomy. *J Audit Res* 1985;25:66–72.
16. Lenhardt ML. Evidence for auditory localization ability in the turtle. *J Audit Res* 1981;21:255–262.
17. Wever EG, Vernon JA. Sound transmission in the turtles ear. *Proc Natl Acad Sci U S A* 1956;42:292–299.
18. Ridgway SH, Wever EG, Mccormic JG et al. Hearing in giant sea turtle, *Chelonia mydas. Proc Natl Acad Sci U S A* 1969;64:884.
19. Mason R, Gans C, Crews D. Reptilian pheromones. In: Gans C, Crews D, eds. *Hormones, Brain, and Behavior Biology of the Reptilia, Volume 18, Physiology E.* Chicago: University of Chicago Press, 1992;114–228.
20. Halpern M. Nasal chemical senses in reptiles: Structure and function. In: Gans C, Crews D, eds. *Biology of the Reptilia, Volume 18, Physiology E.* Chicago: University of Chicago, 1992;423–523.
21. Boiko VP. The participation of chemoreception in the organization of reproductive behavior in *Emys orbicularis* (Testudines; Emydidae). *Zool Zhurnal* 1984;63:584–589.
22. Hatanaka T, Shibuya T, Inouchi J. Induced wave responses of the accessory olfactory bulb to odorants in two species of turtle, *Pseudemys scripta* and *Geoclemys reevesii. Comp Biochem Physiol A—Physiol* 1988;91:377–385.
23. Brann JH, Fadool DA. Vomeronasal sensory neurons from *Sternotherus odoratus* (stinkpot/musk turtle) respond to chemosignals via the phospholipase C system. *J Exp Biol* 2006;209:1914–1927.
24. Grassman MA, Owens DW. Development and extinction of food preferences in the loggerhead sea turtle, *Caretta caretta. Copeia* 1982;965–969.
25. Grassman M, Owens D. Chemosensory imprinting in juvenile green sea turtles, *Chelonia mydas. Anim Behav* 1987;35:929–931.
26. Ehrenfel JG, Ehrenfel DW. Externally secreting glands of freshwater and sea turtles. *Copeia* 1973;305–314.
27. Winokur RM, Legler JM. Chelonian mental glands. *J Morphol* 1975;147:275–291.
28. Rose FL, Drotman R, Weaver WG. Electrophoresis of chin gland extracts of *Gopherus* tortoises. *Comp Biochem Physiol* 1969;29:847–851.
29. Ashton PAR. *The Gopher Tortoise: A Life History.* Sarasota, Florida: Pineapple Press, Inc, 2004.
30. Varga M. Captive maintenance and welfare. In: Girling SJ, Raiti P, eds. *BSAVA Manual of Reptiles.* 2nd ed. Quedgeley, Gloucester, England: British Small Animal Veterinary Association, 2004;6–17.
31. Boyer DM, Boyer TH. Tortoise care. *Bull Assoc Reptilian Amphibian Vet* 1994;4:16–28.
32. Jennings AH. Use of habitats and microenvironments by juvenile Florida box turtles, *Terrapene carolina bauri* on Egmont Key. *Herpetologica* 2007;63:1–10.
33. Pough FH, Andrews RM, Cadle JE et al. Temperature and water regulations. In: *Herpetology.* 3rd ed. Upper Saddle River, NJ: Pearson Prentice Hall, 2004;231–268.

34. Boyer TH. of Box Turtle Care. *Bull Assoc Reptilian Amphibian Vet* 1992;2(1):14–17.

35. Boyer TH, Boyer DM. Biology and husbandry: Turtles, tortoises, and terrapins. In: Mader DR, ed. *Reptile Medicine and Surgery*. 2nd ed. St. Louis, Missouri: Saunders Elsevier, 2006;78–99.

36. Gurley R. *Keeping and Breeding Freshwater Turtles*. Ada, Oklahoma: Living Art Publishing, 2003.

37. Licht P, Denver RJ, Pavgi S et al. Seasonality in plasma thyroxine binding in turtles. *J Exp Zool* 1991;260:59–65.

38. Pough FH, Andrews RM, Cadle JE et al. Body support and locomotion. In: *Herpetology*. 3rd ed. Upper Saddle River, NJ: Pearson Prentice Hall, 2004;353–384.

39. Walker WF. The locomotor apparatus of Testudines. In: Gans C, Parsons TS, eds. *Biology of the Reptilia, Volume 4, Morphology D*. New York: Academic Press, 1973;1–100.

40. Pough FH, Andrews RM, Cadle JE et al. Diets, foraging, and interactions with parasites and predators. In: *Herpetology*. 3rd ed. Upper Saddle River, NJ: Pearson Prentice Hall, 2004;530–566.

41. Mushinsky HR, Stilson TA, Mccoy ED. Diet and dietary preference of the juvenile gopher tortoise (*Gopherus polyphemus*). *Herpetologica* 2003;59:475–483.

42. Plotkin P. Adult migrations and habitat use. In: Lutz ME, Musick JA, Wyneken J, eds. *The Biology of Sea Turtles Volume II*. Boca Raton, Florida: CRC Press, 2003;225–233.

43. Schofield G, Katselidis KA, Pantis JD et al. Female–female aggression: Structure of interaction and outcome in loggerhead sea turtles. *Mar Ecol Prog Ser* 2007;336:267–274.

44. Pough FH, Andrews RM, Cadle JE et al. Communication. In: *Herpetology*. 3rd ed. Upper Saddle River, NJ: Pearson Prentice Hall, 2004;461–494.

45. Auffenberg W. Social behavior of *Geochelone denticulata*. *Quart J Florida Acad Sci* 1969;32:50–458.

46. Woodbury A, Hardy R. Studies of the desert tortoise, *Gopherus agassizii*. *Ecol Monogr Durham N C* 1948;18:145–200.

47. Plotkin PT, Plotkin PT. Biology and conservation of ridley sea turtles. In: Plotkin PT, ed. *Biology and Conservation of Ridley Sea Turtles*. Baltimore: Johns Hopkins University Press, 2007;68.

48. *BSAVA Manual of Reptiles*. 2nd ed. Quedgeley, Gloucester, UK: British Small Animal Veterinary Association, 2004.

49. McArthur S, Meyer J, Innis C. Anatomy and physiology. In: McArthur S, Wilkinson R, Meyer J, eds. *Medicine and Surgery of Tortoises and Turtles*. Oxford, UK: Blackwell Publishing Ltd, 2004;35–72.

50. Carr A, Carr M. Modulated reproductive periodicity in Chelonia. *Ecology* 1970;51:335.

51. Duvall D, Guillette LJ, Jones RE. Environmental control of reptilian reproductive cycles. In: Gans C, Crews D, eds. *Biology of the Reptilia Physiology D*. New York: Academic Press, Inc, 1982;201–231.

52. Krichgessner M, Mitchell MA. Chelonians. In: Mitchell MA, Tully TN, eds. *The Manual of Exotic Pet Practice*. St. Louis, MO: Saunders Elsevier, 2009;207–249.

53. Frye FL. Common pathologic lesions and disease processes. In: Frye FL, ed. *Reptile Care: An Atlas of Diseases and Treatments*. Neptune City, NJ: T.F.H. Publications, Inc., 1991;529–617.

54. Frye FL. *Reptile Care: An Atlas of Diseases and Treatments*. Neptune City, NJ: T.F.H. Publications, Inc, 1991.

55. Auffenberg W. On the courtship of *Gopherus polyphemus*. *Herpetologica* 1966;22:113–117.

56. Innis CJ, Boyer TH. Chelonian reproductive disorders. *Vet Clin North Am Exot Anim Pract* 2002;5:555–578.

57. Crowell Comuzzie D, Owens D. A quantative anaylsis of courtship behavior in captive green sea turtles (*Chelonia mydas*). *Herpetologica* 1990;46:195–202.

58. Galeotti P, Sacchi R, Pellitteri-Rosa D et al. Olfactory discrimination of species, sex, and sexual maturity by the Hermann's tortoise *Testudo hermanni*. *Copeia* 2007;980–985.

59. Auffenberg W. Sex and species discrimination in two sympatric South American tortoises. *Copeia* 1965;1965:335–342.

60. Hernandez-Divers SJ. Clinical aspects of reptile behavior. *Vet Clin North Am Exot Anim Pract* 2001;4:599–612.

61. Eisner T, Conner WE, Hicks K et al. Stink of stinkpot turtle-identified omega-phenylalkanoic acids. *Science* 1977;196:1347–1349.

62. Litzgus JD, Bolton F, Schulte-Hostedde AI. Reproductive output depends on body condition in spotted turtles (*Clemmys guttata*). *Copeia* 2008;86–92.

63. Morjan C, Valenzuela N. Is ground-nuzzling by female turtles associated with soil surface temperatures? *J Herpetol* 2001;35:668–672.

64. Hawkins MG. The use of analgesics in birds, reptiles, and small exotic mammals. *J Exot Pet Med* 2006;15:177–192.

65. Sladky KK, Kinney ME, Johnson SM. Analgesic efficacy of butorphanol and morphine in bearded dragons and corn snakes. *J Am Vet Med Assoc* 2008;233:267–273.

66. Hernandez-Divers S. Meloxicam and reptiles—A practical approach to analgesia. *Small Animal and Exotics Proceedings of the North American Veterinary Conference, Volume 20*, Orlando, Florida, USA 2006;1636–1637.

67. Weiss E, Wilson S. The use of classical and operant conditioning in training Aldabra tortoises (*Geochelone gigantea*) for venipuncture and other husbandry issues. *J Appl Anim Welf Sci* 2003;6:33–38.

68. Shyne A. Meta-analytic review of the effects of enrichment on stereotypic behavior in zoo mammals. *Zoo Biol* 2006;25:317–337.

69. Case B. Environmental enrichment for captive eastern box turtle (*Terrapene carolina carolina*). PhD Thesis. Raleigh, NC: North Carolina State University, 2003.

70. Therrien CL, Gaster L, Cunningham-Smith P et al. Experimental evaluation of environmental enrichment of sea turtles. *Zoo Biol* 2007;26:407–416.

71. Burghardt GM, Ward B, Rosscoe R. Problem of reptile play: Environmental enrichment and play behavior in a captive Nile soft-shelled turtle, *Trionyx triunguis*. *Zoo Biol* 1996;15:223–238

5

Lizards

Paul M. Gibbons and Heather Mohan-Gibbons

Introduction

Almost 5000 of the nearly 9000 reptile species in existence at the time of this writing are lizards.[1,2] Lizards can be found in almost all ecosystems and each species is uniquely suited to survive in its respective microhabitat. All-inclusive generalizations about lizards are difficult because of this diversity, and order Squamata (lizards and snakes) is generally divided into seven major phylogenetic groups (Table 5.1).[1,3] Serpentes, the snakes, are described in a separate chapter (Chapter 3) because their behavior differs considerably from other squamates. This chapter is directed toward providing clinically useful generalizations about lizard behavior, though the authors caution readers to carefully consider whether or not generalities apply among different taxonomic groups. Generalizations in this chapter may include many lizard species, a few unique lizard species, or lizard species that are commonly found in the North American pet industry.

History

Lizard behavior has been studied for over a century, and today many researchers use them to help learn about the fundamental questions of behavioral biology.[4] For example, the diverse reproduction methods of lizards provide a wealth of information about mechanisms that may influence vertebrate reproductive behavior.[5] Dissimilar patterns in closely related species are particularly interesting to researchers because other parameters are similar enough that they do not confound interpretation of the results.

Some lizards (noted by species, family, and/or subfamily) that are currently popular in the North American pet trade include green iguanas (*Iguana iguana*; Iguanidae; Iguaninae), bearded dragons (*Pogona vitticeps*; Agamidae; Agaminae), green water dragons (*Physignathus cocincinus*; Agamidae; Agaminae), Old World chameleons (e.g., panther chameleon *Furcifur pardalis*, and veiled chameleon *Chameleo calyptratus*; Chamaeleonidae), anoles (e.g., *Anolis carolinensis*; Polychrotidae), leopard geckos (*Eublepharis macularius*; Gekkonidae; Eublepharinae), day geckos (*Phelsuma* spp.; Gekkonidae; Gekkoninae), several monitors (*Varanus* spp.; Varanidae), Argentine tegus (*Tupinambis merianae*; Teiidae), and blue-tongued skinks (*Tiliqua scincoides*; Scincidae; Lygosominae). Green iguanas, leopard geckos, bearded dragons, veiled chameleons, and blue-tongued skinks have been bred in captivity for many generations, are common in the pet trade, and are frequently presented to veterinarians. Nevertheless, they are not domesticated because they are not fully adapted to life with humans and still retain the behaviors of wild conspecifics.

Each lizard species has adapted to survive in a specific ecosystem and microhabitat with complicated, unique variations and cycles of temperature, barometric pressure, altitude, vegetation, substrates, refuges, basking sites, predators, prey, lighting, humidity, rainfall, and water. Reptile caretakers must provide a captive environment that allows for expression of the behaviors exhibited in these complex environments. At least 158 stereotyped communication-related behaviors have been described in lizards.[6] These normal behaviors can be grouped into categories, of which agonistic, courtship, and mating behaviors have been best described.[6] Captive lizards will exhibit the behaviors of their wild relatives when provided with the appropriate environment. Lizard behavior is influenced by external factors, however, and individual animals do modify their behavior in response to environmental stimuli.[6,7]

Senses and communication

Most lizards have anatomical structures for sight, hearing, taste, smell, and touch that are similar to most other vertebrates. In addition, most lizards also have a chemosensory

Table 5.1 Nomenclature of the order Squamata including species cited in this chapter.

Division (Infraorder)	Family	Example cited in this chapter: Subfamily: species	Common name
Dibamia	Dibamidae		Blind lizards
Gekkota	Gekkonidae	Eublepharinae: *Eublepharis macularius*	Leopard gecko
		Eublepharinae: *Coleonyx variegatus*	Desert banded gecko
		Eublepharinae: *Hemitheconyx caudicinctus*	African fat-tailed gecko
		Gekkoninae: *Phelsuma laticauda*	Gold-dust day gecko
		Gekkoninae: *Heteronotia binoei*	Binoe's prickly gecko
		Gekkoninae: *Hemidactylus frenatus*	House gecko
	Pygopodidae	*Lialis burtonis*	Burton's legless lizard
Scincoidea	Scincidae	Lygosominae: *Tiliqua scincoides*	Blue-tongued skink
		Lygosominae: *Corucia zebrata*	Solomon Islands prehensile-tailed skink
		Scincinae: *Scincus scincus*	Sandfish
		Scincinae: *Eumeces fasciatus*	Five-lined skink
		Scincinae: *Eumeces inexpectatus*	Southeastern five-lined skink
		Scincinae: *Eumeces laticeps*	Broad-headed skink
	Cordylidae [Gerrhosauridae and Zonuridae]	Chamaesaura: *Cordylus giganteus*	Sungazer
		Gerrhosaurinae: *Gerrhosaurus major*	Sudan plated lizard
	Xantusiidae	Xantusiinae: *Xantusia vigilis*	Desert night lizard
Iguania	Iguanidae	Iguaninae: *Iguana iguana*	Green iguana
		Iguaninae: *Dipsosaurus dorsalis*	Desert iguana
		Amblyrhynchus cristatus	Galapagos marine iguana
	Polychrotidae	*Anolis carolinensis*	Green anole
		Norops (Anolis) lineatopus	Stripefoot anole
	Agamidae	Agaminae: *Pogona vitticeps*	Bearded dragon
		Agaminae: *Physignathus cocincinus*	Green water dragon
		Agaminae: *Chlamydosaurus kingii*	Frilled dragon
		Leiolepidinae: *Uromastyx spp.*	Spiny-tailed lizards
	Corytophanidae	*Basiliscus spp.*	Basilisks
	Crotaphytidae	*Crotaphytus spp.*	Collared lizards
	Phrynosomatidae	*Phrynosoma coronatum*	Coast horned lizard
		Phrynosoma platyrhinos	Desert horned lizard
		Sceloporus grammicus	Graphic spiny lizard; mesquite lizard
		Sceloporus cyanogenys	Blue spiny lizard
		Uta stansburiana	Side-blotched lizard
		Uma notata	Fringe-footed lizard
	Chamaeleonidae	*Chameleo calyptratus*	Veiled chameleon
		Furcifur pardalis	Panther chameleon
		Chameleo jacksonii	Jackson's chameleon
Serpentes	See chapter on snake behavior (Chapter 3)	See chapter on snake behavior	Snakes
Anguimorpha	Varanidae	*Varanus niloticus*	Nile monitor
		Varanus komodoensis	Komodo dragon
	Helodermatidae	*Heloderma suspectum*	Gila monster
	Anguidae	Gerrhonotinae: *Elgaria multicarinata*	Southern alligator lizard
		Anguinae: *Ophisaurus ventralis*	Eastern glass lizard
	Anniellidae		Legless lizards
	Shinisauridae	*Shinisaurus crocodilurus*	Chinese crocodile lizard
	Xenosauridae	*Xenosaurus grandis*	Knob-tailed lizard
Laterata	Teiioidea [Teiidae and Gymnophthalmidae]	*Tupinambis merianae*	Argentine tegu
		Tupinambis rufescens	Red tegu
		Aspidoscelis (Cnemidophorus) tigris	Western whiptail
	Lacertidae	Lacertinae; *Podarcis hispanica*	Iberian wall lizard
		Zootoca (Lacerta) vivipara	Viviparous lizard
	Amphisbaenia [Rhineuridae, Bipedidae, Trogonophidae, and Amphisbaenidae]	*Amphisbaena alba*	Worm lizard

vomeronasal system and some have a parietal eye. Lizards use their senses to identify food sources, avoid predation, detect diurnal patterns, thermoregulate, and communicate. Each different lizard group utilizes each of the senses according to its specifically adapted needs. Few lizards produce sounds for communication, even though most have highly sensitive, directional hearing that can be used to find prey, avoid predation, and communicate.[8–11] Unlike other lizards, chameleons lack tympana, although they probably do communicate through complex vibratory signals.[12]

Visual stimuli are important for all lizards except some worm lizards (Amphisbaenia), which have relatively small, deeply recessed, scale-covered eyes (Figure 5.1), and blind lizards (Dibamidae), which have vestigial eyes. Most lizards rely at least partially on visual cues for communication, predator avoidance, thermoregulation, feeding, and reproduction.[13] The parietal eye is closely associated with the pineal gland and has a well-developed retina, lens, and cornea; it participates not only in regulation of circadian (diurnal) and circannual (seasonal) rhythms, but also in thermoregulation and directional orientation.[14,15] Most lizards have color vision and will select certain colors over others.[16] Sensitivity to different wavelengths of light does vary among lizard species but there is no color (i.e., wavelength of the electromagnetic spectrum that is visible to humans) that is completely "invisible" to lizards, so some diurnal species will remain active under red and blue artificial lights intended for nighttime heating of reptile enclosures. Some lizards, including the desert iguana (*Dipsosaurus dorsalis*; Iguaninae), are capable not only of perceiving the spectrum of light that is visible to humans, but they also see ultraviolet wavelengths reflected by pheromone deposits.[17]

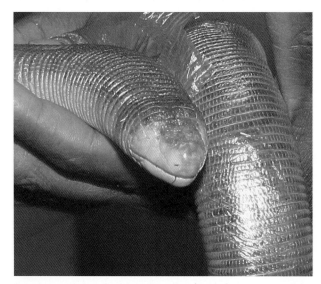

Figure 5.1 Worm lizard (*Amphisbaena alba*) at the São Paulo Zoo, Brazil. This species has adapted for a fossorial (burrowing) lifestyle and has deeply recessed, scale-covered eyes.

Male lizards are more brightly colored than females in many species, but visual cues are generally less important for communication than are chemosensory cues. In general, coloration has little or no effect on mate selection by females, but can play a role in male–male interactions.[18] In several lacertid species for example, males will attack females that have been painted to look like males but will court the painted female after licking it.[17] Male broad-headed skinks (*Eumeces laticeps*; Scincidae) have orange heads, and will normally bite and chase conspecific males. After researchers paint the heads of females orange to match the males, then males will bite the painted females before chemosensory investigation (tongue-flicking), but not after.[19]

Chemical cues are highly efficient: they work day or night, can remain after the animal has passed, and can be effective over large areas.[17] Lizards variably use licking, tongue-flicking, and biting behaviors to obtain chemical information. Secretions from the skin, femoral glands, and cloacal glands are used to mark the environment passively as a lizard moves through it, or actively when a lizard performs a specific behavior that leaves a chemical cue behind. Lizard glandular secretions can contain sterols, fatty acids, phosphatidylcholines, or hydrocarbons.[17] Lipids extracted from the skin of leopard geckos include over 40 compounds that differ between males and females and probably relay chemical signals that are important for sexual selection and mating.[17] Some male horned lizards (e.g., *Phrynosoma coronatum* and *P. platyrhinos*; Phrynosomatidae) rub their cloaca on the substrate just before breeding season, which could be a social cue that attracts females or alerts males to stay away from a breeding territory.[17] Male desert banded geckos (*Coleonyx variegates*; Eublepharinae) lick females and bite their tails to detect chemical stimuli that are necessary for breeding. A fully conscious male will lick anesthetized males and females, but will only attempt to breed with the anesthetized females.[17] When the tails of male and female desert banded geckos are detached and reattached to the opposite sex, males court females with male tails if he bites her body, but not if he bites the transplanted tail.[17] Conversely, male geckos with female tails are courted only if the tail is bitten first.[17]

Chemical communication plays an important role not only in reptile mating and social behavior, but also in predator avoidance and prey capture.[17] Different lizard species use different sensory means to locate prey depending upon the environment in which they live and their adaptations to it. Some lizards can discriminate between the odor of prey and other odors. Red tegus (*Tupinambis rufescens*; Teiidae) and Iberian wall lizards (*Podarcis hispanica*; Lacertinae) had a significantly greater number of tongue flicks and physical attacks on cotton balls scented with prey odors than on cotton balls dipped in non-food substances.[20] The five-lined skink (*Eumeces fasciatus*; Scincinae) also responds to extract of prey species over extract of non-prey species, but the closely related southeastern five-lined skink (*Eumeces inexpectatus*; Scincinae) does not discriminate prey chemicals from other odors and will respond equally to either.[20] Scent plays little or no role in prey selection for green anoles, which discriminate among prey items using taste.[21] Some lizards rely on visual or tactile cues for prey selection. For example, the stripefoot anole (*Norops* (*Anolis*) *lineatopus*; Polychrotidae) attacks four kinds of prey regardless of odor, and the sandfish (*Scincus scincus*; Scincidae), a fossorial species, is guided more by vibratory cues than any other sense when buried in the sand for hunting.[20]

Husbandry

Captive lizards require environments that are similar to the natural environment to which they are adapted, in order to allow for the most natural expression of behaviors and incur the least possible stress.[22] In order to ensure the reptile has proper welfare and husbandry, the "Five Freedoms" should be applied. The reader is encouraged to refer to Chapter 20 for more information about the "Five Freedoms." All are important in creating the right living conditions and ensuring proper welfare for the life of the captive lizard. Heat, humidity, light, water, caging, vegetation, refuges, and substrate must be considered. Temperature, light, and humidity must cycle daily and seasonally, and should vary throughout the captive environment. Nutrition must be appropriate for the species and should be based upon the best-available information about each individual species. The authors do not recommend housing multiple lizards in one enclosure except during breeding events, and multiple species should not be housed together. Not only do individuals compete for resources (heat, humidity, light, refuges, food, water, territory, and mates), but housing multiple lizards together increases disease transmission, parasites loads, and other stressors.

Construction of the enclosure

Two different categories of housing can be used to keep lizards: clinical enclosures and naturalistic enclosures. Clinical habitats have minimal cage furniture, utilize paper substrates, include a refuge to reduce stress, offer visual security on sides and back, and provide proper heat and humidity for the species.[23] These enclosures are very easy to clean and require regular maintenance to provide the level of hygiene and waste management necessary for long-term survival of the lizard.[24] Clinical habitats are ideal for the veterinary hospital, during quarantine, to isolate sick individuals, and for long-term maintenance of very large specimens.

Naturalistic habitats allow for more of the natural behaviors of the species to be exhibited and minimize stressors related to captivity. These vivaria simulate many of the elements of the environment for which the lizard is adapted, including biological processes for waste management like beneficial invertebrates, bacteria, and fungi.[24] Naturalistic habitats can facilitate gradients of light, heat, and humidity. Landscaping is based on the lizard's natural behaviors in the wild. Novice caretakers must learn about the most appropriate substrates, water sources, plants, climbing surfaces, and refuges.

Many commercial enclosures are available from retailers, though appropriate enclosures may require individualized construction. Regardless of the source, however, lizard housing must prevent escape and be non-toxic, non-porous, and easy to clean. Transparent enclosures, whether glass, plastic, or screen may stimulate repetitive behaviors (i.e., impact and rubbing) that can result in injury.

The largest cage possible should be provided for the captive lizard. A proposed minimum enclosure size recommendation for most lizards is 3 times longer and 2 times wider than the animal's body length. For arboreal lizards the minimum height is 3 times the body length.[23] For terrestrial and burrowing species the minimum height is that in which an appropriate temperature gradient can be established.

Heat

Captive heliothermic (sun-basking) lizards, such as the arboreal green iguana and the terrestrial bearded dragon, require focal radiant heat sources that mimic a natural diurnal cycle.[23] In addition, background heat must be provided to prevent the enclosure from cooling too much at night or from allowing sections of the enclosure to fall below the critical thermal minimum at any time. Species from high latitudes and montane regions, including the viviparous lizard (*Zootoca* [*Lacerta*] *vivipara*; Lacertidae) and Jackson's chameleon (*Chameleo jacksonii*) may require background cooling, such as air conditioning or misted water, to prevent overheating. Heat must be provided in horizontal and vertical gradients to allow for behavioral thermoregulation. Heat is transferred between the environment and the lizard via radiation, conduction, convection, and evaporation. Lizards maintain their core body temperature within an optimal range by shuttling among various thermal environments. Lizards generally gain heat more easily than they lose it.[25,26] Heliothermic lizards are best adapted to absorb radiant heat from above, and heart rate increases as they circulate absorbed heat from the dorsal skin to warm the internal organs.[25,26] Lizards also increase or decrease their absorption of radiant heat by varying the amount of body surface area exposed to radiant heat sources.[26] In addition, many species, including bearded dragons, horned lizards, and chameleons, will alter skin color via dermal chromatophores, because darkened skin absorbs more heat and lightened skin reflects heat.[26,27] Much heat loss occurs through the ventrum in terrestrial species when they either press their abdomen to a cool substrate in an effort to lose heat through conduction or lift their abdomen up to allow convective heat loss with the wind.[26] Heat can be lost as fluid evaporates from epithelial surfaces of the respiratory tract and oral cavity, but little or no evaporation occurs across scaled skin.[26] Most lizards cool themselves by moving air across internal membranes to lose heat through evaporation. For example, green iguanas pant, bearded dragon gape the mouth, and monitor lizards flutter the gular region.[25,28,29] Diurnal lizards may briefly utilize the ephemeral warmth of rocks and roadways to avoid heat loss for a few hours after sunset, but they avoid contact with hot surfaces during the day.[30,31] Some species jump into water or climb into trees or shrubs to lose heat and escape heat sources. Nocturnal species generally thermoregulate by shuttling among warmer and cooler areas during the day and use behavioral techniques, such as pressing the abdomen to thermoneutral substrates (e.g., leaves) or hiding in burrows, to prevent heat loss at night.

In captive environments, background warmth is provided to maintain the minimum temperature and basking sites are used to provide a small region of focal heat at the upper limit of the preferred range. Basking sites should be provided by placing radiant heat sources (e.g., tungsten filament incandescent bulbs) above the lizard. Burns are common in captive lizards when intense focal substrate heat is provided as a "basking site" because heliothermic species are better equipped to lose heat to the substrate than they are to gain it. Carefully monitored under-the-tank (external to the enclosure) heating elements can be safe, appropriate sources of background warmth, but artificially heated rocks (inside the enclosure) do not effectively warm the enclosure without serving as dangerous sources of focal heat. Lizards must be protected from direct contact with all heat sources by use of padding or caging, and the temperature must be monitored with thermometers. If background heat is provided beneath the floor of the enclosure, no more than 75% of the bottom should be covered in order to allow the lizard to move away from the heat into a cooler area. Ideally all heat sources would be controlled by a thermostat to prevent overheating. A thermometer must be placed directly in each focal hot region of the enclosure, and one thermometer should also be placed in the coolest region to monitor the entire range of temperatures.

Humidity

In the wild, lizards utilize various microhabitats within the larger ecosystem, so a captive environment should provide an array of similar microhabitats. For example, the fringe-footed lizard (*Uma notata*; Phrynosomatidae) of southern California desert regions conserves water by remaining buried under the surface (relative humidity 85%) rather than above (relative humidity <10%) for over 19 hours per day.[26] Every lizard enclosure should provide a humidity gradient so that the lizard can select a particular humidity level according to its needs at any given time. Relative humidity requirements vary among lizard species, so it should range within the various provided microhabitats from 30% to 100% depending on the species. Evaporative cooling via the buccal cavity and respiratory tract leads to water loss and potential dehydration when a lizard is kept in an environment with low humidity. Excessive cooling drives the lizard to spend more time basking to maintain body temperature, which can lead to further dehydration; so, providing the proper humidity level for each species of captive lizard is critical to its health and well-being.

Water

All lizards must be provided with clean water at all times. When offered appropriately, even desert species will soak, swim, drink, and use it as a cooling mechanism. Permanent water systems (e.g., pools or waterfalls) either need to be completely emptied and refilled several times a week or be managed to maintain a healthy biological filter by circulating the water and performing regular, partial water changes.[32] The natural behavior of each lizard must be known because some lizards, including most chameleons, arboreal geckos, and anoles, will only drink droplets of water either as condensation or while dripping from vegetation.[23] Automatic drip systems and misting systems are required for these species because free access to water must be available at all times to prevent chronic dehydration. It is not sufficient for reptile caretakers to intermittently provide manually misted water, because this coerces the lizard to select among behaviors including drinking, foraging, thermoregulating, and evading potential predators. Predator avoidance can take precedence over other important, life-sustaining behaviors.[33]

Lighting

Lizards require lighting that mimics the sun in the region and microhabitat to which they are adapted. Wavelengths of sunlight that are important to lizard health include ultraviolet A, UVB, visible (to humans), and infrared. The full array of wavelengths is important for mineral metabolism, reproduction, thermoregulation, and normal behavior. Ultraviolet B wavelengths are especially important for heliotherms such as green iguanas because they are not capable of absorbing vitamin D from the diet.[34] Crepuscular and nocturnal species including many geckos should be provided with gradients of UVB and heat during the daytime because they are adapted to bask in partial sunlight and efficiently produce vitamin D in the skin.[31,32] Lizards are particularly resistant to the damaging effects of UVB radiation[35] and no substantiated case of harm has been reported from the UVB lamps that are marketed for use with reptiles when used according to the manufacturer's specifications. The authors therefore recommend providing UVB wavelengths for all lizards regardless of the animal's lifestyle.

Light intensity decreases with distance from the source, and UVB penetrates poorly through glass, plastic, or water.[36] In one study, the UVB-attenuating properties of 14 different materials that are commonly used to cover enclosures were measured. The newly designed UV-transmitting acrylic showed adequate UVB meter irradiances, however did not allow for adequate D_3-synthesizing ability.[36] It is recommended to use air-permeable materials between the UVB source and the animal to ensure proper vitamin D_3 conversion for health and normal behavior of the lizard. Lizards should be able to move freely within 30.5 cm (12 in.) of UVB-producing fluorescent lamps to receive the beneficial effects. These fluorescent lamps should be replaced every 6–12 months because the intensity of emitted UVB decreases significantly over time. Mercury vapor lamps (e.g., PowerSun UV, Zoo Med Laboratories, San Louis Obispo, CA; or Mega-Ray, www.ReptileUV.com) can provide sufficient UVB for up to 2 years and emit visible, UVB, and infrared wavelengths (heat). The number of hours that lighting is illuminated depends upon the lizard's native latitude. Equatorial species are adapted to consistent 12 hours of daylight, and day length varies from about 8 to 16 hours of light per day throughout the year for temperate species. Lights should not be illuminated at night, regardless of the color, because many diurnal lizards will remain active, which may cause stress.

Shelters

Most terrestrial and small arboreal lizards seek shelter when not foraging or basking. Visual security is essential to reduce stress, and refuges can provide alternative locations for thermoregulation and locally high humidity. If housing more than one lizard in an enclosure, each lizard must be provided with at least one refuge in which to seek shelter. The refuge must be large enough to fit the animal comfortably but not so large that it does not provide sufficient security.[23] Ideally, several refuges should be offered to allow the lizard to select from different temperatures, humidity ranges, sizes, and shapes. Shelters can be commercial molded resin structures, cork bark sections, ceramic pots with a cutout doorway, and plastic food storage containers with a cutout entry site. Humidity can be maintained inside these enclosures with moistened paper towels, vermiculite, or long grain sphagnum moss (Figure 5.2). Areas of locally high humidity must be closely monitored for growth of fungi, which can serve as opportunistic pathogens.

Substrate

Substrates must be non-toxic, easy to clean, easy to replace, non-irritating, and non-ingestible. Unfortunately few commercially available substrates meet these criteria. Captive lizards ingest particulate substrates regardless of whether they are digestible or not.[37,38] Substrates such as wood mulch, wood shavings, wood chips, ground walnut shells, silica sand (e.g., children's play sand), gravel, and calcium sand have all been associated with serious medical problems in lizards.[38] The most notable problems include eye irritation, dermal abrasion, and gastrointestinal impaction, obstruction, irritation, ulceration, or perforation (Figure 5.3). Newsprint, unprinted newspaper, paper towels, butcher paper, and brown wrapping paper are safe, inexpensive, easily replaced, and not readily ingested.[24] Reptile cage carpet (e.g., Repti Cage Carpet, Zoo Med Labs, San Luis Obispo, CA; and Terrarium Liner, Zilla Products, Franklin, WI) is commercially available, conveniently sized, easy to clean, and safe. None of these recommended substrates allows for burrowing behaviors, however, so the authors recommend also including a shallow container with damp topsoil for species that tend to dig, a deep container of moist sand for species that must burrow (especially to lay eggs; Figure 5.4), or a shallow container with damp topsoil and leaf litter for forest floor species. A few burrowing species require particulate beddings or soil. For example, sandfish require dry, smooth-particle desert sand to pre-

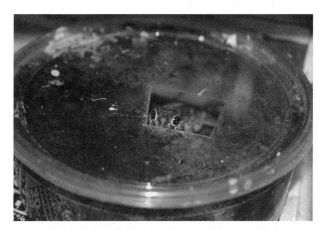

Figure 5.2   A small terrestrial gecko utilizing a humidity box that contains moistened, long-grain sphagnum moss.

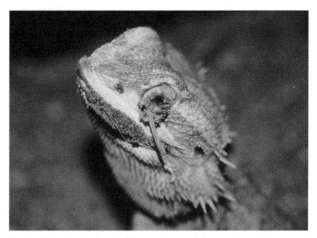

Figure 5.3   Captive bearded dragon (*Pogona vitticeps*) with sand-associated conjunctivitis and cheilitis.

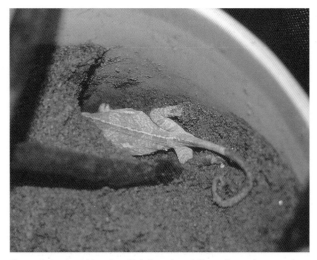

Figure 5.4 Gravid female veiled chameleon (*Chameleo calyptratus*) digging a deep burrow in moist sand to lay her eggs.

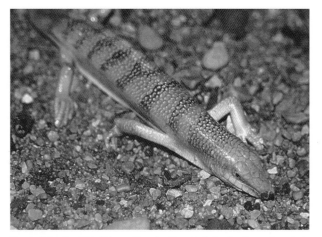

Figure 5.5 Sandfish (*Scincus scincus*) with rostral abrasion from attempts to burrow in an inappropriate gravel substrate.

vent rostral abrasions (Figure 5.5) and blue-tongue skinks do well when provided with a container of moist topsoil.[24] In order to avoid accidental ingestion of the substrate, lizards that are provided with particulate substrates should be fed either on a plate or in an area of the enclosure that does not contain the particulate bedding. Lizards that are maintained on ingestible substrates may be moved into a separate enclosure for meals, but this regular handling can be stressful; most species are not adapted to eating large infrequent meals and some lizards simply will not eat under these circumstances. Whenever possible, it is better to provide a substrate that is unlikely to be ingested.

Locomotion

Lizards use different locomotor patterns at different speeds and in different media (e.g., sand, water, air, horizontal surfaces, and vertical surfaces). Lateral footfall patterns that provide maximum stability are used at slow speeds on the ground. The movement of the forefoot on each side follows movement of the hind foot on the same side in the following order: right hind, right front, left hind, and left front.[39] At a trot, diagonal limbs move in synchrony and the body may be supported only by two diagonal limbs for much of the gait cycle. Stride length is increased in many lizards by a unique joint between the pectoral girdle and sternum. Most lizard hind limbs are much longer and more muscular than the forelimbs and provide most of the propulsive force. Tarsal joint anatomy and function differs significantly from that of mammals.[39]

Speed is generally correlated with hind limb length in lizards, and the Komodo dragon (*Varanus komodoensis*; Varanidae) can briefly achieve speeds of up to 18.5 km/h (11.5 mph) with sustained speeds of about 14 km/h (8.7 mph) for more than 0.5 km.[39] Dynamic bipedal lizards can support themselves on their hind legs while running. Species that exhibit this behavior include basilisks (*Basiliscus* spp.; Corytophanidae), collared lizards (*Crotaphytus* spp.; Crotaphytidae), the frilled dragon (*Chlamydosaurus kingii*; Agaminae), and juvenile green iguanas.[39] Basilisks exhibit the behavior while running across the surface of water and are aided by fringed scales on the caudal surfaces of their digits that provide resistance as they strike the surface of the water. A video clip of this behavior can be seen at http://www.people.fas.harvard.edu/~glauder/videos/13_lizard/lizard.mov. Bipedal locomotion requires few unique anatomical differences from other lizards, but the species that use it do tend to have a caudally shifted center of gravity resulting from relatively long hind limbs, short forelimbs, a short presacral vertebral column, and a relatively long tail.[39]

During locomotion, lizards that have legs will lift the entire torso off the substrate. Most lizards usually do not, however, remain standing for long periods of time while motionless. Instead, they allow their body to rest on the substrate, minimizing the energy required for postural support.[39] It is not normal for a terrestrial lizard with legs to use undulatory, sliding movements to propel the body along a solid surface like a snake, even on very smooth surfaces such as a clinical examination table. Veterinarians should consider musculoskeletal, neurological, nutritional, or metabolic (e.g., hypocalcemia) disease etiologies for lizards that exhibit undulatory, sliding locomotive behavior in the examination room. Some members of a few families of lizards have partial or complete reduction of limbs. These include Pygopodidae (flap-foots), Scincidae (skinks), Anguidae (glass lizards), Amphisbanidae (worm lizards), Cordylidae (grass lizards), and Dibamidae (legless lizards).[40] The locomotion of these species combines that of other lizard families with many features of snake locomotion. Quite a few of these species use the reduction in limb size, along with a few other anatomical adaptations to live a fossorial (burrowing) lifestyle.[40,41]

Aquatic locomotion (swimming) can be undulatory or oscillatory. Undulatory propulsion results from waves of movement along the body and oscillatory propulsion results from back and forth movement of limbs. Many lizards flatten their limbs against the sides of the body and tail and utilize undulatory movement to move through the water. The Galápagos marine iguana (*Amblyrhynchus cristatus*; Iguanidae) is one notable example that also utilizes sculling (lateral undulation) with its laterally compressed tail.[40]

Many lizards are scansorial (climbing); they dwell on rocks (saxicolous) or in trees (arboreal). Adaptations for climbing include prehensile tails (in tree skinks [e.g., *Corucia zebrata*; Lygosominae], some geckos, and Old World chameleons) and specialized feet. The zygodactyl, syndactyl feet of Chameleonidae are especially well adapted to life on tree branches. Other lizard toe adaptations include sturdy claws and transversely expanded platelike scales termed "scansors." Scansors use a dry adhesive system that depends upon van der Walls forces (molecular attraction between closely associated surfaces due to transient changes in electrons) and are found in many geckos, some anoles, and the green tree skink (*Prasinohaema virens*; Scincidae).[39]

A few species of lizards use aerial locomotion. Two adaptations are used to slow the rate of descent to a glide (angle of descent less than 45°), either webbed digits (e.g., in *Ptychozoon* spp.; Gekkoninae) or broad flaps of lateral skin termed patagia (e.g., in *Ptychozoon* spp. and the flying dragon, *Draco volans*; Agamidae).

Social behavior

Lizards communicate through an array of complex visual, acoustic, and chemical signals that vary with each species.[13] Iguania and Laterata primarily utilize visual cues, whereas other Squamata primarily use chemical cues. Gekkota and a few lacertid species also use acoustic signals.[13] Communication signals may be associated with territoriality, aggression, courtship, mating, submission, or simply to indicate presence to conspecifics; a single behavior can communicate different information depending upon the circumstances.[42–44]

Aggression

Aggression directed toward conspecifics is normal lizard behavior that increases with age and sexual maturity; it frequently results in severe injury.[22] Incubation temperature can affect expression of aggressive behaviors during the life of lizards. Both male and female leopard geckos are more likely to show conspecific aggressive behavior as adults if they hatched from incubation at higher temperatures in their incubation range.[4] Other potential causes of aggression in lizards include hormonal changes, breeding behaviors, defensive response when threatened, lack of choices for escape

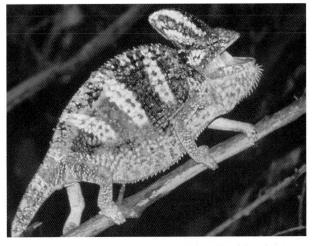

Figure 5.6 Recently wild-caught male veiled chameleon (*Chameleo calyptratus*) demonstrating aggressive behaviors immediately after being released from a shipping container. Note the contrasting skin coloration, flattened body, and open mouth.

in environment, and pain. Offensive aggression is related to breeding and territory, whereas defensive aggression is associated with fear or threats.[45] Body language used to display aggression includes: lateral posturing, body flattening, mouth-gaping (Figure 5.6), body raising, back arching, dewlap extension, throat enlargement, head-bobbing, push-ups, head-shaking, biting, tail raising, striking with head or tail, and tail-whipping.[44,45] Submissive behaviors during aggressive events can include head lowering, arm-waving (circumduction), and pressing the body against the substrate.[42,45,46] Head-bobbing and arm-waving can also occur in the absence of conspecifics; these behaviors may indicate territorial status or notification of presence.[42,45] It is interesting that, although most lizards live solitary lives, some will aggregate without aggressive behavior in large groups that include both sexes. For example, desert-banded geckos (*Coleonyx variegatus*; Eublepharinae) aggregate without agonistic behavior throughout the year to conserve moisture.[47] Broad-headed skinks (*Eumeces laticeps*; Scincinae), however, aggregate without aggression during winter hibernation, but exhibit courtship and agonistic behaviors in late spring after most individuals have emerged for the breeding season (concurrent with increasing testosterone).[17]

Predator defense

Defensive mechanisms against predators generally include crypsis, locomotor escape, struggling, defecating, hissing, and biting.[48] Many tropical lizards bask in branches that overhang water so they can either swim away or dive into deep water when approached by a predator. Some lizards also exhibit ritualized displays, expose startling color patterns, or release noxious secretions. Horned lizards squirt blood from their eyes when threatened by carnivores, but not when attacked by birds or rodents.[48] Australian

Diplodactylus spp. geckos squirt a liquid from their tail that attaches to potential predators and becomes a sticky thread.[49] Many lizards use the tail to distract predators. Tail autotomy is common among many species, and the dropped tail will often continue to move involuntarily for several minutes, which distracts predators.

Reproductive behavior

Male lizards of many species display colorful patches or patterns during combat or courtship. Bright coloration is presumed to be used for social communication and is kept hidden most of the time. Flashing of bright colors may be linked to dominance.[16] Colors are exposed by changes in dermal chromatophores (e.g., Old World chameleons) or exposure of normally hidden skin (e.g., anole dewlap). Soon after hatching, male green anoles exhibit displays that are associated with mating in adults.[50]

Female sexual behaviors are grouped into three patterns, associated, dissociated, and constant.[5] Associated reproduction describes that in which sex hormone secretion and gonadogenesis stimulate copulation, egg formation, and fetal development. It is most common in subtropical and temperate lizards and typically requires hibernation before breeding. Bearded dragons, blue-tongued skinks, leopard geckos, and green anoles all have associated reproduction patterns. Female green anoles oviposit one egg every 5–14 days and females are then receptive to courtship by males for about 1 week as the upcoming follicle grows from about 3.5 mm to 8 mm diameter. A female green anole will usually copulate when receptive even though a single mating is all that is required for her to produce fertile eggs for an entire breeding season.[51] Similarly, in lizards with dissociated cycles, insemination occurs prior to the active season. Dissociated reproduction is characterized by mating that occurs when the testes and ovaries are small and sex hormone levels are low. Sperm is stored in the vas deferens before copulation or in the female reproductive tract until ovulation. It is more characteristic of viviparous species, but does occur in several oviparous skinks, a gecko, and a spiny lizard (Phrynosomatidae).[5,51] Continuous reproduction occurs in some lizards from tropical regions where temperature and rainfall remain relatively constant throughout the year; it does not occur in any species that is commonly kept in captivity.

Some lizards are oviparous (producing shelled eggs that are incubated outside the body before hatching), whereas others are viviparous (embryo retained in the oviduct during development, live birth). Both gestation methods can occur within the same subfamily. Some chameleons, for example, lay eggs (e.g., veiled chameleon) whereas others give birth to live young (e.g., Jackson's chameleon). Parthenogenic reproduction (offspring from a single parent) occurs in a few lizards species including several whiptails (*Aspidoscelis* [*Cnemidophorus*] spp.; Teiioidea),

some rock lizards (*Lacerta* spp.; Lacertidae), a few geckos (*Heteronotia* spp.; Gekkoninae), and a skink (*Menetia greyii*; Scincidae).[52–55] Parthenogenic female lizards can exhibit mounting (male-associated), receptive (female-associated), and copulatory behaviors.[4] No parthenogenic species is common in the North American pet trade.

Proper husbandry, good physical condition, freedom from disease, and appropriate nutrition are essential for reproductive success in captive lizards. Breeding reptiles in captivity can be challenging, and requires detailed knowledge of the environment to which each species has adapted. Parameters including temperature, photoperiod, humidity, rainfall, nutrition, and social factors may all require manipulation for breeding success.[56] Several species are, however, commonly bred in captivity in sufficient numbers to supply the pet trade. These include bearded dragons, leopard geckos, Argentine tegus, blue-tongued skinks, veiled chameleons, panther chameleons, and a few species of monitor lizards.

Mate selection is crucial for reproductive success in any reptile. Simply placing members of the opposite sex together is not likely to result in viable breeding, even if the two were each successful with a different mate during previous breeding. Clients who are interested in breeding should be advised to either purchase pairs that have already produced offspring together, or at least purchase individuals that have already been housed together to improve the probability of success. Wild reptiles have many potential mates among which to select and it can be difficult to match a breeding pair in captivity. In addition, a few species are monogamous.[57,58] Problems can arise when the male has not had contact with the female prior to introducing them for courtship and mating. Certain social interactions can also inhibit breeding. For example, males that lose in combat with another male or females that are frequently exposed to aggressive males can stop mating for a period of time.[56]

In general, though, mating behavior occurs because females release pheromones that signal the male they are sexually receptive. These pheromones are released from glands such as the precloacal or femoral pores of geckos and iguanas, and the mental, axillary, and inguinal glands of chameleons.[56] In many cases, specific behaviors must occur for lizards to become receptive to copulation (Figure 5.7). Females of some species can store sperm for years, however, so the association between sexually receptive behavior, copulation, and fertilization is not always clearly defined.[5] Desert-banded gecko males, for example, begin courtship by waving the tail while holding the head and body near to the ground. The male will then lick the female's body and bite her tail during courtship. Mounting and copulation begin after these behaviors have been repeated several times.[17] Male blue spiny lizards (*Sceloporus cyanogenys*; Phrynosomatidae) scrape their pelvis (i.e., drag the vent) on the ground when approaching females from a distance, but

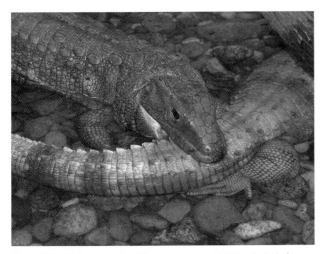

Figure 5.7 Male caiman lizard (*Dracaena guianensis*) biting the tail of a female during courtship in an exhibit at the San Diego Zoo.

not when approaching other males.[17] Males of several other species in the Phrynosomatidae family approach females and lick the area surrounding the pelvis and vent before and after mating. Tongue flicking behavior is also a common prelude to mating in many lizards.[17] When a group of female leopard geckos is introduced to a resident male, he will lick them all and then respond aggressively to females that are nearing ecdysis (i.e., cloudy skin) and court those that are not.[17] Given this, female geckos, and possibly all lizards, should not be introduced to each other when shedding is imminent. Female leopard geckos that hatched from incubation at a relatively high temperature grow into adults with relatively high androgen levels, relatively low estrogens, and physical characteristics that are much like males. These females should not be included in breeding colonies because they do not become sexually receptive and have not been observed to mate, ovulate, or lay eggs.[4]

Maternal behavior and neonatal development

Some families of lizards are entirely oviparous (e.g., Dibamidae, Helodermatidae, Pygopodidae, Teiidae, and Varanidae), whereas others are entirely viviparous (e.g., Shinisauridae, Xantusiidae, and Xenosauridae).[51] The remaining lizard families include some oviparous and some viviparous species. In general, viviparity is associated with high altitudes or cool climates and closely related species will utilize the reproductive mode that is most suitable for the local conditions to which they are adapted.[51] Viviparous lizards usually produce a single clutch per season, but the number of clutches per season varies among the different oviparous species. Overall fecundity is, however, associated with numerous environmental and species-specific factors.[51] Many gravid viviparous females require additional energy and nutrients to nourish the developing fetuses, though this ranges among viviparous species

from nearly complete dependence upon maternal nutrition to total dependence upon nutrients stored within the yolk.[51]

Many female lizards develop brighter colorations when gravid. In addition, many become highly aggressive toward males after being fertilized; they may roll onto their back or gape their mouth if a male approaches.[16] Gravid lizards often spend more time basking, may spend more time digging, and can become more secretive or aggressive before delivery. Oviparous species generally require a specific substrate in which to build a nest, and some species (e.g., many arboreal chameleon species) will dig deep burrows into moist sand to lay their eggs. Dystocia results in many cases when adequate nesting substrate is not provided. Although many lizards will tolerate being removed from their normal enclosure to a site with adequate nesting substrate during late gestation, it is best to avoid disturbing them during the nest-building process because this may lead to abandonment of the nest and failure to lay the eggs.[56] Some viviparous species require a brood box during late gestation to avoid dystocia. The box must be large enough for the female to move around easily, and several boxes at different temperatures and humidity levels should be provided to allow the gravid female to select the most appropriate environment.[56] Some arboreal lizards, including many geckos, lay sticky eggs that attach directly onto vertical surfaces such as leaves, branches, rocks, or glass. These eggs harden within hours and cannot be removed without causing damage to the shell. It is notable that house gecko (*Hemidactylus frenatus*; Gekkoninae) eggs are sticky when laid on vertical surfaces, but are not sticky when laid on horizontal surfaces.[40]

Females of most oviparous species will not produce shelled eggs unless they have been exposed to a reproductively mature and sexually active male.[56] Conversely some species, including green water dragons and green iguanas, commonly form shelled eggs in the absence of a male, which can lead to dystocia, especially when appropriate nesting substrate is not provided. The sex of fetal lizards is determined either by sex chromosomes or by the temperature of gestation and incubation. Chromosomes probably determine the sex of developing fetuses in most viviparous lizards, though temperature can also be involved when gestating females select body temperature via basking behavior.[59] The sex of many oviparous lizards is determined by post-fertilization temperature, but the temperature ranges vary among different species. For example, mostly female leopard geckos are hatched at low incubation temperatures, whereas mostly males are produced at high temperatures.[4]

A few lizard species exhibit brooding and maternal behaviors; most of these are members of the Scincidae and Anguidae.[17,60,61] Researchers have observed two species of skinks in the genus *Eumeces* that continually turn the eggs in their nests. These skinks use their head to roll eggs back into the nest if removed and placed near the nest.

They will also brood eggs of other skinks when they are about the same size, but not eggs of other lizards.[17] The skinks use chemical cues to locate and recognize their eggs, and will flick the tongue to the eggs a single time when returning to the nest.

Even when maternal care is not evident, the proximity of neonates to mature adults can be critical for survival of some species. Many neonatal herbivorous reptiles must ingest feces of older animals to obtain gut flora necessary to digest cellulose.[51] Some young reptiles raised in isolation from conspecifics may not learn the social cues needed for successful mating as an adult.[56] When monitor lizards are raised singly, the first interactions with others are very aggressive and can result in severe injuries, but normal breeding behavior will be exhibited if raised in groups.[56] Hatchling green iguanas separate into sibling groups within 24 hours after they have been mixed with others from different parents. This grouping occurs in response to chemical cues received from licking one another.[17] Overcrowding of neonates can, however, result in aggression. To reduce injuries and stress, offer the largest possible enclosure with a variety of hiding places, visual barriers, thermal and moisture gradients, feeding and water stations, and excess food.[56] Most lizard species should be raised singly after a brief period of exposure to their siblings because they compete for resources, fight, and may attempt to eat one another.

Ingestive behavior

Lizards may be herbivores, carnivores, or omnivores, and can be specialized or opportunistic. Less than 1% of all lizard species are herbivorous, and only about 11% are omnivorous.[48] Some carnivorous lizards thrive on a single type of invertebrate prey (e.g., ants), while others eat an array of different vertebrates and invertebrates. Active foragers are often specialists and more sedentary reptiles often eat a greater variety of food items.[62] Some "sit-and-wait" predators use parts of their body to lure prey; for example the legless lizard, *Lialis burtonis* (Pygopodidae), attracts small frogs and lizards by waving or twitching its tail.[48] Foraging style is associated with many traits including movement rate, movement frequency, sensory mode, types of prey, body form, crypsis, skin toxins, predators, daily energy expenditure, endurance, and fecundity.[48]

Common captive herbivores include green iguanas, spiny lizards (*Uromastyx* spp.), and Solomon Islands prehensile-tailed skinks. Almost all monitor lizards eat a diet of vertebrate animals, though chameleons, leopard geckos, day geckos, collared lizards, and water dragons are mainly insectivorous. In addition to insects, many geckos also eat nectar and soft fruit, and water dragons will eat fish, newborn rodents, and hatchling birds. Many carnivores scavenge for carrion in addition to capturing live prey.[48] Common captive omnivores include bearded dragons, blue-tongued skinks, plated lizards, and tegus. Omnivorous lizards may vary their diet with the season of the year and availability of feed, though they sometimes preferentially select certain items (e.g., flowers) over others (e.g., insects) even when all are abundant.[48] Dietary preference of omnivores can change with age as well. For example, the diet of juvenile basilisks is almost exclusively composed of insect and small vertebrate prey, whereas that of adults is largely omnivorous.[48] Each individual of one *Anolis* species has a specific preference for insect species as a hatchling that becomes expanded to a greater diversity of prey types in adulthood.

Captive lizard diets would ideally be based upon items that are eaten in their naturally adapted habitat.[62–64] Reports of the stomach contents of wild-caught individuals and observations of ingestive behavior are available for many species, but the most readily available sources of feed for captive lizards rarely match the plant and animal prey eaten by wild conspecifics. Studies that use information about the nutrient composition of the diet in the wild and the nutrients found in convenient items from grocery stores and pet shops must be employed to make reasonable husbandry decisions.[62,64] Unfortunately, no prospective study has been reported that proves any commercial diet is capable of meeting nutritional requirements throughout all life stages for many generations. Many commercially formulated diets are available for reptiles and claim to be nutritionally complete, but such claims remain unsubstantiated without published reports of lifetime feeding trials. Therefore, broad generalizations of nutrient requirements are the best information available, and these exist for only a few lizard species.[62] Many herpetoculturists have noted that herbivorous lizards are often attracted to red items, and will eat red fruits or vegetables preferentially. It is important, however, to ensure that herbivores eat a variety of food items, because reliance on one or two items is likely to lead to deficiencies of some nutrients and excesses of others. Gut transit time for lizards varies with the species and ranges from 1 to 8 days.[62] Herbivorous lizards have gastrointestinal adaptations that are similar to hindgut fermenting mammals and digestive efficiency that compares closely to ruminants.[48] Few lizards exhibit parental care of their young and gastrointestinal symbiont flora are not passed directly from parents to offspring. Instead, hatchling green iguanas ingest soil from the nest cavity and then enter the forest canopy where they seek out and eat the feces of adults.[48] Little is known about the strategies other juvenile herbivorous lizards use to inoculate their gut with the proper gastrointestinal flora.

Energy requirements of reptiles are much lower than those of similarly sized mammals, and lizards do not need to eat as frequently or spend as much time eating as mammals.[62] Green iguanas, for example, spend an average of only 9 minutes a day feeding.[62] Lizards select food items through a variety of sensory cues. Most species rely primarily on one sensory modality, however. Iguania rely primarily on visual cues, whereas geckos, dibamids, and skinks rely primarily on chemosensory cues.[48] Sit-and-wait foragers tend to rely on vision to detect moving prey. Chameleons use acute stereoscopic vision to track insects and precisely target them in three-dimensional space before launching the tongue to capture the prey item and retrieve it by retracting the tongue back onto the enteroglossal bone inside the mouth.

All aspects of nutrition must be considered in feeding captive lizards, this includes trophic level, species of feed offered, prey size, time of day for feeding, nutritional composition of diet, and presentation of feed. Nutrition-related problems are common in captive lizards and include rickets, nutritional secondary hyperparathyroidism, hepatic lipidosis, xanthomatosis, obesity, anorexia, and chronic renal failure. Many of these problems can be solved by considering ingestive behaviors of wild conspecifics. Environmental temperature has a profound effect on digestion. Suboptimal temperature can lead to maldigestion, bloat, constipation, and death.[62] Green iguanas kept at 28°C (82°F) will eat voluntarily, but can have maldigestion.[62] Monitor lizards cannot assimilate nutrients properly when housed in temperatures below the optimal range.[62] Diurnal lizards should be fed during the late morning, after they have had an opportunity to warm up and in time to allow digestion to begin before the temperature drops in the evening.

Common behavior problems: Diagnosis and treatment

Most of the undesirable or problem behaviors exhibited by lizards result directly from inappropriate husbandry, so clinical management is closely linked to providing appropriate nutrition and environmental conditions. The first steps in solving behavior problems in lizards include learning about the natural history of the species and how to apply that information to the captive environment. Environmental stressors that may lead to undesirable behaviors include excessive or rough handling, inappropriate cage construction, inappropriate cage location (lack of visual security), inadequate shelter, improper thermal range, inappropriate heat sources, improper substrate, inappropriate cage accessories, improper light spectrum, improper diurnal and seasonal cycles, inappropriate prey or feed, multiple individuals in a single enclosure, and overcrowding.

When the reptile's enclosure is too large to bring into the exam room, it is essential to gather a thorough history and to view photos of the reptile's environment. A form can be used that includes all the pertinent questions about all of the various husbandry parameters. It is useful, for example, to know at what locations the lizard spends its time relative to heat, light, humidity, and shelter. Clients may then be counseled about the best cage setup including ranges and cycles of temperature, lighting,

and moisture. Normal lizards will take advantage of a complex array of appropriately configured microenvironments throughout the day, so a captive environment must be redesigned if a lizard spends nearly all of its time in just one or two locations within the enclosure.

Aggression

The most common undesirable behavior category is aggression, either toward people or toward other lizards in the same enclosure. Behaviors associated with aggression and several of its causes are described in a previous section of this chapter; it is usually a normal response to environmental stimuli. In general, lizards should be housed singly and with visual barriers between individuals in separate cages to reduce aggression that is related to territory and competition for resources.

While green iguanas remain with siblings after hatching and do not show aggression to them, they will aggress to unrelated conspecifics of a similar age. Adult green iguanas may be kept in groups (no more than one male per group) in extremely large outdoor enclosures with excess resources, but constant behavioral evaluation and removal of aggressive individuals is required.[22] Iguana groups are most compatible if all are a similar size and were raised together. Juvenile bearded dragons will tolerate siblings in large groups immediately after hatching, but within a few months some individuals become larger than others and aggressive individuals begin to inflict severe bite wounds upon cage mates. Adult chameleons exhibit aggressive behaviors in response to their own image reflected by glass-walled enclosures, so screening and other non-reflective materials are recommended for cage construction instead of glass to reduce the stress associated with territorial defense against reflected images. Adult chameleons should never be housed together because of the stress involved with constant territorial aggression.

Defensive aggression directed toward humans can result from repeated aversive events, such as forced displacement from basking site or refuge, removal of resources (food), and excessive force during handling. Ideally this is prevented through gentle handling that starts from a very young age, but might be manageable with desensitization and counterconditioning. In addition, several interventions have been suggested to reduce aggressive behaviors in captive lizards:[23,45,65–67]

- house individual lizards alone;
- eliminate contact with other reptiles;
- increase the number of resource locations (e.g., hiding places, feeding stations, water stations, and basking sites);
- reduce the number of daylight hours (<10 h/day);
- provide a surrogate mate (e.g., stuffed animal);
- increase the complexity of the environment;
- increase the visual barriers between individuals;
- castration.

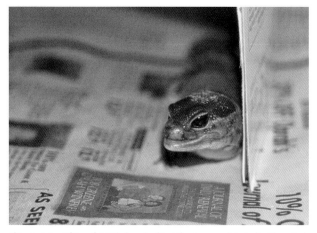

Figure 5.8 African fat-tailed gecko (*Hemitheconyx caudicinctus*) with rostral abrasion as a result of trauma from impact against solid surfaces during normal prey capture behavior.

Castration may reduce territorial or breeding aggression, but is not likely to have an effect on aggression that is based on defense or fear. Pain-induced aggression is not likely to respond to behavioral therapy and must be managed medically.

Abnormal repetitive behaviors

Saltatorial (jumping) species, such as water dragons and frilled dragons, will leap powerfully into translucent barriers (e.g., glass or Plexiglas) in response to certain visual stimuli, and fat-tailed geckos (*Hemitheconyx caudicinctus*; Eublepharidae) will forcefully impact solid surfaces with the rostrum while prehending insect prey (Figure 5.8). Many terrestrial species will press the rostrum into a translucent barrier as they move from one side of the enclosure to the other. These behaviors can result in captivity-associated disease including rostral abrasions, soft-tissue necrosis, and osteomyelitis. Possible solutions include:

- reduce glare and reflection by moving the light
- provide additional cage plantings or refuges
- place a physical obstruction inside the cage to prevent access to the region where the injury is occurring
- attach an opaque visual barrier, such as masking tape or paper, to the transparent surface in the location where the lizard is rubbing
- provide a much larger, more complex environment

Burrowing species, such as the sandfish (*Scincus scincus*; Scincidae), require soft sand because they will attempt to burrow into the substrate and will abrade the rostrum on substrates to which they are not adapted. Fine desert sand should be provided instead of abrasive children's play sand or commercially available reptile calcium sand.

Treatment for behavioral problems in lizards should be adapted from techniques used in other animals. Lizards do learn new behaviors in response to antecedents and consequences (see Chapter 18). Komodo dragons at Disney's Animal Kingdom were taught to enter a stanchion for physical examination and blood collection (http://www.animaltraining.org). The following website includes numerous videos that demonstrate lizards trained to perform an array of different behaviors—http://reptilebehavior.com/lizard_training.htm.

More research is needed on environmental enrichment and its effects on lizards in captivity, but biologically relevant enrichment should be available to all captive animals. For lizards, this can be anything that stimulates foraging or other natural behaviors such as hiding, sunbathing, digging, foraging, or swimming. Also, any item that they can physically move or manipulate with their feet, mouth, or body may be enriching. Refer to the "Behavior problem" section in Chapter 4 for supportive research on reptile enrichment and to view a table on enrichment ideas that could also be used for lizards. Providing a captive habitat that is enriching and allows the lizard to express its natural behavior is likely to result in psychologically and physically healthier animals.

Pain and pain management

Clinical signs that indicate pain have not been well documented in lizards, and currently there is no gold standard for evaluating pain in any non-human patient.[68] The practitioner must be familiar with normal behavior for the species and what the owner reports for that individual. Pain in lizards may manifest itself through abnormal behavior such as changes in attitude, appetite, activity, and posture; muscle contraction during palpation; withdrawal from a stimulus; aggression in a normally non-aggressive animal; color changes of skin; rapid respiration; polydipsia; repeated swallowing; aerophagia; scratching or flicking a foot at the affected area; elevated extended head; abnormal posture; lameness; ataxia; avoidance; partially or fully closed eyes; escape behaviors; biting or licking at affected areas; and changes in usual daily routine.[69–71] A variety of analgesics have been used on lizards for pain relief;[68] however, only recently have controlled studies been conducted to scientifically evaluate this issue.[70–73]

Acknowledgments

All photos in this chapter courtesy of Paul Gibbons.

References

1. Vidal N, Hedges SB. The molecular evolutionary tree of lizards, snakes, and amphisbaenians. *Comptes Rendus Biologies* 2009;332:129–139.
2. Uetz P. The TIGR reptile database. Available at: http://www.reptile-database.org/, J. Craig Venter Institute. Last accessed Nov 17, 2008.
3. Fry BG, Vidal N, Norman JA et al. Early evolution of the venom system in lizards and snakes. Nature 2006;439:584–588.

4. Crews D, Gans C. The interaction of hormones, brain, and behavior: An emerging discipline in herpetology. In: Gans C, Crews D, eds. *Biology of the Reptilia: Hormones, Brain, and Behavior*. Chicago: The University of Chicago Press, 1992;1–23.

5. Whittier J, Tokarz R. Physiological regulation of sexual behavior in female reptiles. In: Gans C, Crews D, eds. *Biology of the Reptilia: Hormones, Brain, and Behavior*. Chicago: University of Chicago Press, 1992;25–69.

6. Carpenter CC, Ferguson GW. Variation and evolution of stereotyped behavior in reptiles. In: Gans C, Tinkle EW, eds. *Biology of the Reptilia: Ecology and Behaviour A*. New York: Academic Press, 1977;335–554.

7. Garrick LD. Lizard thermoregulation: Operant responses for heat at different thermal intensities. *Copeia* 1979;258–266.

8. Manley GA. Spontaneous otoacoustic emissions in monitor lizards. *Hear Res* 2004;89:41–57.

9. Labra A, Sufan-Catalan J, Solis R et al. Hissing sounds by the lizard *Pristidactylus volcanensis*. *Copeia* 2007;1019–1023.

10. Christensen-Dalsgaard J, Manley GA. Acoustical coupling of lizard eardrums. *J Assoc Res Otolaryngol* 2008;9:407–416.

11. Manley GA, Koppl C. What have lizard ears taught us about auditory physiology? *Hear Res* 2008;238:3–11.

12. Barnett KE, Cocroft RB, Fleishman LJ. Possible communication by substrate vibration in a chameleon. *Copeia* 1999;225–228.

13. Pianka ER, Vitt LJ. Social behavior. In: *Lizards: Windows to the Evolution of Diversity*. Berkeley: University of California Press, 2003;85–106.

14. Pough FH, Andrews RM, Cadle JE et al. Movements and orientation. In: *Herpetology*, 3rd ed. Upper Saddle River: Pearson Prentice Hall, 2004;431–460.

15. Ellis DJ, Firth BT, Belan I. Circadian rhythm of behavioral thermoregulation in the sleepy lizard (*Tiliqua rugosa*). *Herpetologica* 2006;62:259–265.

16. Cooper WE, Greenberg N. Reptilian coloration and behavior. In: Gans C, Crews D, eds. *Biology of the Reptilia: Hormones, Brain, and Behavior: Physiology E*. Chicago: The University of Chicago Press, 1992;298–422.

17. Mason RT. Reptilian pheromones. In: Gans C, Crews D, eds. *Biology of the Reptilia: Hormones, Brain, and Behavior: Physiology E*. Chicago: The University of Chicago Press 1992;114–228.

18. Pough FH, Andrews RM, Cadle JE et al. Communication. In: *Herpetology*. 3rd ed. Upper Saddle River: Pearson Prentice Hall, 2004;461–494.

19. Copper W, Vitt LJ. Orange head coloration of the male broad headed skink (*Eumeces laticeps*); a sexually selected social cue. *Copeia* 1988; Issue 1 (Feb. 5) 1–6.

20. Halpern M. Nasal chemical senses in reptiles: Structure and function. In: Gans C, Crews D, eds. *Hormones, Brain, and Behavior: Physiology E*. Chicago: The University of Chicago Press, 1992;423–523.

21. Stanger-Hall KF, Zelmer DA, Bergren C et al. Taste discrimination in a lizard (*Anolis carolinensis*, Polychrotidae). *Copeia* 2001;490–498.

22. Schumacher J, Kohler G, Maxwell LK et al. Husbandry and management. In: Jacobson ER, ed. *Biology, Husbandry, and Medicine of the Green Iguana*. Malabar: Krieger Publishing Co, 2003;75–95.

23. Varga M. Captive maintenance and welfare. In: Girling SJ, Raiti P, eds. *BSAVA Manual of Reptiles*. 2nd ed. Gloucester: British Small Animal Veterinary Association, 2004;6–17.

24. de Vosjoli P. Designing environments for captive amphibians and reptiles. *Vet Clin North Am Exotic Anim Prac* 1999;2:43–68.

25. Bartholomew GA. Physiological control of body temperature. In: Gans C, Pough FH, eds. *Biology of the Reptilia Volume 12 Physiology C*. London: Academic Press, 1982;167–204.

26. Pough FH, Andrews RM, Cadle JE et al. Temperature and water regulations. In: *Herpetology*. 3rd ed. Upper Saddle River: Pearson Prentice Hall, 2004;231–268.

27. de Velasco JB, Tattersall GJ. The influence of hypoxia on the thermal sensitivity of skin colouration in the bearded dragon, *Pogona vitticeps*. *J Comp Physiol B* 2008;178:867–875.

28. Tattersall GJ, Cadena V, Skinner MC. Respiratory cooling and thermoregulatory coupling in reptiles. *Respir Physiol Neurobiol* 2006;154:302–318.

29. Cadena V, Tattersall GJ. The effect of thermal quality on the thermoregulatory behavior of the bearded dragon *Pogona vitticeps*: Influences of methodological assessment. *Physiol Biochem Zool* 2009;82:203–217.

30. Belliure J, Carrascal LM. Influence of heat transmission mode on heating rates and on the selection of patches for heating in a Mediterranean lizard. *Physiol Zool* 2002;75:369–376.

31. Hitchcock MA, McBrayer LD. Thermoregulation in nocturnal ectotherms: Seasonal and intraspecific variation in the Mediterranean gecko (*Hemidactylus turcicus*). *J Herpetol* 2006;40:185–195.

32. Carman EN, Ferguson GW, Gehrmann WH et al. Photobiosynthetic opportunity and ability for UV-B generated vitamin D synthesis in free-living house geckos (*Hemidactylus turcicus*) and Texas spiny lizards (*Sceloporus olivaceous*). *Copeia* 2000;245–250.

33. Robert KA, Thompson MB. Is basking opportunity in the viviparous lizard, *Eulamprus tympanum*, compromised by the presence of a predator scent? *J Herpetol* 2007;41:287–293.

34. Allen ME, Oftedal OT. Nutrition in captivity. In: Jacobson ER, ed. *Biology, Husbandry, and Medicine of the Green Iguana*. Malabar: Krieger Publishing Company, 2003;47–74.

35. Cope RB, Fabacher DL, Lieske C et al. Resistance of a lizard (the Green Anole, *Anolis carolinensis*; Polychridae) to ultraviolet radiation-induced immunosuppression. *Photochem Photobiol* 2001;74:46–54.

36. Burger RM, Gehrmann WH, Ferguson GW. Evaluation of UVB reduction by materials commonly used in reptile husbandry. *Zoo Biol* 2007;26:417–423.

37. Gibbons PM. What's your diagnosis: Pica in a bearded dragon (*Pogona vitticeps*). *Bull Assoc Reptilian Amphibian Vet* 1999;9:34–36.

38. Bradley T. Coelomitis secondary to intestinal impaction of calcisand in a leopard gecko, *Eublepharis macularius*, in *Proceedings of the Seventh Annual Conference of the Association of Reptilian and Amphibian Veterinarians* 2000;27–28.

39. Pough FH, Andrews RM, Cadle JE et al. Body support and locomotion. In: *Herpetology*. 3rd ed. Upper Saddle River: Pearson Prentice Hall, 2004;353–384.

40. Pianka ER, Vitt LJ. From geckos to blind lizards. In: *Lizards: Windows to the Evolution of Diversity*. Berkeley: University of California Press, 2003;171–192.

41. Pianka ER, Vitt LJ. Getting around in a complex world. In: *Lizards: Windows to the Evolution of Diversity*. Berkeley: University of California Press, 2003;19–40.

42. Watt MJ, Joss JMP. Structure and function of visual displays produced by male jacky dragons, *Amphibolurus muricatus*, during social interactions. *Brain Behav Evol* 2003;61:172–183.

43. Radder RS, Saidapur SK, Shine R et al. The language of lizards: Interpreting the function of visual displays of the Indian rock lizard, *Psammophilus dorsalis* (Agamidae). *J Ethol* 2006;24:275–283.

44. Ord TJ, Blumstein DT. Size constraints and the evolution of display complexity: Why do large lizards have simple displays? *Biol J Linn Soc Lond* 2002;76:145–161.

45. Lock BA. Behavioral and morphologic adaptations. In: Mader DR, ed. *Reptile Medicine and Surgery*. 2nd ed. St. Louis: Saunders Elsevier, 2006;163–179.

46. Labra A, Carazo P, Desfilis E et al. Agonistic interactions in a *Liolaemus* lizard: Structure of head bob displays. *Herpetologica* 2007;63:11–18.

47. Lancaster JR, Wilson P, Espinoza RE. Physiological benefits as precursors of sociality: Why banded geckos band. *Anim Behav* 2006; 72:199–207.

48. Pough FH, Andrews RM, Cadle JE et al. Diets, foraging, and interactions with parasites and predators. In: Herpetology. 3rd ed. Upper Saddle River: Pearson Prentice Hall, 2004;530–566.

49. Weldon PJ, Flachsbarth B, Schulz S. Natural products from the integument of nonavian reptiles. *Nat Prod Rep* 2008;25:738–756.

50. Moore MC, Lindzey J. The physiological basis of sexual behavior in male reptiles. In: Gans C, Crews D, eds. *Biology of the Reptilia: Hormones, Brain, and Behavior. Physiology E.* Chicago: The University of Chicago Press, 1992;70–113.

51. Pough FH, Andrews RM, Cadle JE et al. Reproduction and life histories of reptiles. In: Herpetology. 3rd ed. Upper Saddle River: Pearson Prentice Hall, 2004;331–352.

52. Fu J, Murphy RW, Darevsky IS et al. Divergence of the cytochrome b gene in the *Lacerta raddei* complex and its parthenogenetic daughter species: Evidence for recent multiple origins. *Copeia* 2000; 432–440.

53. Adams M, Foster R, Hutchinson MN et al. The Australian scincid lizard *Menetia greyii*: A new instance of widespread vertebrate parthenogenesis. *Evolution* 2003;57:2619–2627.

54. Walker JM, Cordes JE, Carpenter GC. Can parthenogenic *Cnemidophorus tesselatus* (Sauria: Teiidae) occasionally produce offspring markedly different from the mother? *Southwest Nat* 2003;48:126–129.

55. Kearney M, Shine R, Wiens J. Developmental success, stability, and plasticity in closely related parthenogenic and sexual lizards (Heteronotia, Gekkonidae). *Evolution* 2004;58:1560–1572.

56. Wright KM. Breeding and neonatal care. In: Girling SJ, Raiti P, eds. *BSAVA Manual of Reptiles.* 2nd ed. Gloucester: British Small Animal Veterinary Association, 2004;40–50.

57. Chapple DG, Keogh JS. Complex mating system and dispersal patterns in a social lizard, *Egernia whitii. Mol Ecol* 2005;14:1215–1227.

58. Bull CM. Monogamy in lizards. *Behav Process* 2000;51:7–20.

59. Robert KA, Thompson MB. Viviparous lizard selects sex of embryos. *Nature* 2001;412:698–699.

60. Greene HW, Rodriguez J, Powell BJ. Parental behavior in anguid lizards. *South Am J Herpetol* 2006;1:9–19.

61. deFraipont M, Clobert J, Barbault R. The evolution of oviparity with egg guarding and viviparity in lizards and snakes: A phylogenetic analysis. *Evolution* 1996;50:391–400.

62. Calvert, I. Nutrition. In: Girling SJ, Raiti P, eds. *BSAVA Manual of Reptiles.* 2nd ed. Gloucester: British Small Animal Veterinary Association, 2004;18–39.

63. Baer DJ. Nutrition in the wild. In: Jacobson ER, ed. *Biology, Husbandry, and Medicine of the Green Iguana.* Malabar: Krieger Publishing Company, 2003;38–46.

64. Donoghue S. Nutrition. In: Mader DR, ed. *Reptile Medicine and Surgery.* 2nd ed. St. Louis: Saunders Elsevier, 2006;251–298.

65. Moore MC. Testosterone control of territorial behavior: Tonic-release implants fully restore seasonal and short-term aggressive responses in free-living castrated lizards. *Gen Comp Endocrinol* 1998;70:450–459.

66. Sakata JT, Gupta A, Chuang CP et al. Social experience affects territorial and reproductive behaviours in male leopard geckos, *Eublepharis macularius. Anim Behav* 2002;63:487–493.

67. Weiss SL, Moore MC. Activation of aggressive behavior by progesterone and testosterone in male tree lizards, *Urosaurus ornatus. Gen Comp Endocrino,* 2004;136:282–288.

68. Hawkins MG. The use of analgesics in birds, reptiles, and small exotic mammals. *J Exotic Pet Med* 2006;15:177–192.

69. Read MR. Evaluation of the use of anesthesia and analgesia in reptiles. *J Am Vet Med Assoc* 2004;224:547–552.

70. Mosley CAE. Anesthesia and analgesia in reptiles. *Sem Avian and Exotic Pet Med* 2005;14:243–262.

71. Sladky KK, Kinney ME, Johnson SM. Analgesic efficacy of butorphanol and morphine in bearded dragons and corn snakes. *J Am Vet Med Assoc* 2008;233:267–273.

72. Mosley CAE, Dyson D, Smith DA. Minimum alveolar concentration of isoflurane in green iguanas and the effect of butorphanol on minimum alveolar concentration. *J Am Vet Med Assoc* 2003;222:1559–1564.

73. Mosley CA, Dyson D, Smith DA. The cardiovascular dose-response effects of isoflurane alone and combined with butorphanol in the green iguana (*Iguana iguana*). *Vet Anaesth Analg* 2004;31:64–72.

6

Ferrets

Megan J. Bulloch and Valarie V. Tynes

Natural history

It is generally believed that the ferret was first domesticated 2000–3000 years ago but there is some debate as to where domestication actually began. Some believe ferrets originated in Northwest Africa and Iberia where they were used primarily for hunting rabbits. Eventually, the species was spread by humans, along with the rabbit, throughout Europe.[1] Other researchers argue that Europe is the more probable place of origin.[2] The most likely ancestor of the domesticated ferret (*Mustela putorius furo*) is the European polecat (*Mustela putorius*).[1,2] However, the close phylogenetic relationship of the polecats and a long history of hybridization makes this difficult to confirm. The steppe polecat (*Mustela eversmanni*) and the black-footed ferret of North America (*Mustela nigripes*) are all very similar genetically, as well as in appearance and behavior.[2,3,4] Studies of the social behavior of the polecat, ferret, and F1 hybrids of the two have found their behavior to be virtually identical[5,6,7] and several authors appear to use the term polecat and ferret interchangeably.[8,9,10] The primary differences are those that would be expected to occur with domestication; ferrets are less alert, less fearful of humans, more tolerant of changes in their environment and generally less neophobic (fearful of novel things and places) than the polecat.[11]

The term "ferret" comes from the Latin *furonem*, or little thief. Indeed, if the scientific name, *Mustela putorius furo*, is taken literally, domesticated ferrets are thieving, smelly weasels. These members of the Mustelidae family, like the stoat, weasel, badger, skunk, otter, and mink, have retained a diversity of primitive characteristics, such as their small size, stocky legs, elongated brain case, and short rostrum. Although they were originally domesticated for hunting and pest control, they are currently used as animal models in biomedical research programs and are popular companion animals.[2]

Ferrets reach mature size at about 1 year of age. Males, or hobs, and females, or jills, are sexually dimorphic: hobs weigh between 0.68 and 2.7 kg (1.5 and 5 lbs), whereas jills are 2–3 times smaller, at 0.2–0.9 kg (0.5–2 lbs). Additionally, hobs typically measure 38–46 cm (15–18 in.) long, whereas jills measure 33–36 cm (13–14 in.), not including the tail. Neutered hobs are slightly smaller than intact hobs.[12] Ferrets have been bred for a large variety of different coat colors including, butterscotch, chocolate point, cinnamon, lilac, sable point, Siamese, and silver, to name but a few.[12,13]

Sensory systems

Visual system

Ferrets' visual system is similar to cats'. Indeed, recent research has identified 12 cortical areas in the ferret visual system that are homologous to those in the cat.[14] Ferrets have a retina rich in cones and ganglion cells. They can distinguish the color red but not blue, yellow, or green, and they are more sensitive to light intensity than color.[15,16] It appears that ferrets see best at dawn and dusk, when there is muted light. Their low visual acuity and reliance on olfactory and aural cues is typical of a nocturnal species.

Ferrets will preferentially follow and attack targets moving at 25–45 cm/sec (10–17in./sec), approximately the same speed as an escaping mouse.[17] This visual ability supports the hunting efficiency of this species.

Auditory system

The auditory system of the ferret is similar to that of the cats' as well.[18,19] However, the startle response to loud noises is not present until 32 days after birth, much later than this behavior is seen in cats. Ferrets' hearing is most sensitive to frequencies in the range of 4–15 kHz.[19] Ferrets are capable of localizing sounds very accurately and react quickly to the slightest of noises such as rustling grass.[20]

Interestingly, the ferret brain is organized tonotopically, with neurons responding to low frequencies located dorsally, and neurons responding to high frequencies located ventrally.[21] There is evidence that cells in the superior colliculus fire preferentially to sounds from specific directions.[22,23] Thus, the superior colliculi might provide the animal with a spatial map derived from sound, and an efficient means of locating prey within the environment.

Olfactory system

While the visual and auditory systems are both important, the role of the olfactory system in hunting and mating for ferrets cannot be overstated. Ferrets, like many other mammals, use odors to identify individuals, and distinguish gender and reproductive status.[24] Researchers have demonstrated that the glomerular activation of the main olfactory bulb in both male and female ferrets is different, depending on whether the ferrets smell odors from a male or female anal scent gland.[25,26]

Ferrets possess a variety of different secretory glands that play a role in mediating their social behavior. These include anal sacs, proctodeal glands that open into the rectum, and preputial glands that release secretions into the preputial skin, as well as sebaceous glands all over the body.[27]

Different behaviors are used to spread the chemical messages contained in these secretions. The anal drag, performed equally by both males and females, is a behavior in which the anus is lowered to the ground while the animal walks forward wriggling its hindquarters. Anal drags are performed most often around latrine sites and do not appear to change in frequency with the season.[27] Anal gland secretions appear to carry much of the information that allows individuals to recognize other individuals.[24] Urine contains compounds unique from anal secretions and urine marking may provide another method by which ferrets can recognize individuals and their gender.[28]

Wiping behaviors include the belly crawl, where the chest is lowered to the ground and the body pushed forward by the back legs, and another behavior where the urogenital region is wiped over an object with the tail raised. Sometimes one leg is raised during the urogenital wiping and urination may also occur. Males wipe significantly more often than females and perform wiping behaviors more often in the Spring than in other seasons. Dominant males wipe more often than subordinate males, and the wiping occurs equally throughout the territory.[27]

Both sexes rub their neck, flanks or sides on the ground. This body rubbing behavior is often followed by rolling on the ground. Males are more likely to perform this rubbing behavior when meeting other males and at the boundary of their territory (or what they perceive to be their territory). The differing forms of marking behavior allow different messages to be dispersed throughout the territory. These messages allow for mutual recognition of individuals as well as allowing for the overlap of territories such that ferrets can use a system of mutual avoidance while traveling about their territories.[27]

Ferrets also rub their chin backward and forward over substrates. This behavior is expressed equally by males and females and frequently occurs at feeding sites. It has been hypothesized that, because ferrets typically cache their food, these marks may allow them to rapidly identify locations where they have stored food. Conversely, the behavior might also serve as a threat to other individuals that approach the stored food.[27]

Ferrets do have a vomeronasal organ (VNO) but it is rudimentary and morphologically different from that of most other animals. Unlike changes in plasma testosterone, testes and brain size, the VNO does not change in size or structure during the mating season. This suggests that the VNO plays a limited role, if any, in mediating reproductive behavior in the ferret.[29]

Additionally, researchers have found that the olfactory system is particularly important in food imprinting. For instance, there appears to be a critical period, between 2 and 4 months of age, in which ferrets establish food preferences and the odors associated with these preferred foods. This critical period occurs concomitantly with morphological changes in the granules of the olfactory bulb.[30,31]

Body care

Much like cats, ferrets will groom themselves and each other by licking. However, the motor patterns and sequences of behavior associated with grooming have not been well studied or documented as in the cat.

One reason why ferrets have become such popular pets is because they are relatively easy to care for, involving little grooming work on the part of their owners. In one author's experience (MJB) ferret baths should be limited to once a month because although it seems counterintuitive, excessive bathing actually appears to increase their natural odor by stripping the natural body oils from their coats and causing them to produce more oils to compensate for the dryness.

Locomotion

Ferrets engage in forms of locomotion typical of most four-legged mammals. Ferrets will crawl, walk, and run. Their walk can best be described as an ambling gait, where the body is fully stretched out and the head held close to the ground. When running the ferret's back is repeatedly arched, giving the appearance of a hopping scamper.[20] They can pivot, run backward, jump, and can right themselves when falling from a height, a useful trait given their adeptness at climbing.[4,32] Ferrets will slither or slink, sliding along the ground on their bellies. This behavior has also been referred to by Poole as belly crawling. In his studies of play and social behavior, belly crawling was often seen to occur after a brief period of rest where the ferret lay flat on its belly with is back legs splayed[6] (see Figure 6.1). Clapperton, however, mentions belly crawling in the context of marking behavior, where the ferret lowers its chest to the ground and pushes its body forward until the ventral surface is flat on the ground and the rear legs splayed out behind.[27] This action also presses the urogenital region to the ground.

Ferrets also hop and "dance," a behavior performed by springing into the air from all four feet (see Figure 6.2). They can dance either forward, backward or in place and often do so with their mouth open while weaving their head back and forth.[7] Dancing is most often performed when the ferret is excited and/or soliciting play. It has also been referred to as the "happy dance," "dance of joy," "the war dance," or any number of other names devised by ferret owners.

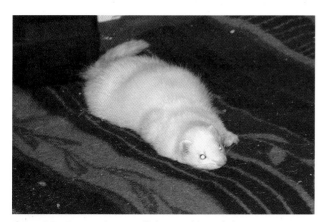

Figure 6.1   Ferret resting sternally between bouts of play.

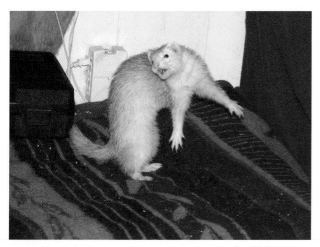

Figure 6.2   Ferret dancing and demonstrating the "open mouthed play face."

Social behavior

The ancestor of the domestic ferret, the European polecat, is a solitary, nocturnal species and both males and females define their territories using scent marks.[24,27,33,34] These marks appear to allow individuals to avoid interactions with other territory holders except during the mating season.[35] When two individuals do meet at other times, male–male encounters are likely to be more aggressive than female–female ones and aggressive interactions do appear to increase with age.[35] Aggression between adult males is likely to be most severe during the breeding season.

Vocalizations

Ferrets have a variety of entertaining and fascinating vocalizations that have not been well studied or clearly documented. The most commonly heard vocalization of the ferret is the chattering, chuckling, or clucking sounds[5] that have been referred to by pet owners as the "dook." When excited and when playing, ferrets will "dook." When two unfamiliar animals meet, they will begin clucking after they have examined and sniffed the other. The clucking becomes more rapid and staccato as they begin interacting.[6] High-pitched chattering (very much like monkeys) is an alarm call. Extreme agitation or fear induces hissing[6,36] but hissing may also be a part of an offensive threat.[6] Additionally, females will make a whimpering noise to encourage young to follow.[36] One author (MJB) has noted that most ferret noises are made "under their breath" in a sort of muttering hoot as they climb or explore or play. Finally, ferrets will scream when they are in pain or very afraid. According to one researcher, the hiss and the scream are most likely to be produced in a defensive context and are commonly produced by the ferret that is being attacked and losing in a contest with another individual.[6] Female ferrets may also squeal or scream during copulation.[6]

Play

Like most young mammals, ferrets engage in play behavior. Play is at its maximum level between 6 and 14 weeks although it may be seen in animals as young as 4 weeks of age, even before their eyes are open.[5] Males tend to be more playful than females and there is some suggestion that this sex difference is linked to testosterone.[37,38]

Ferret play is very aggressive and active, consisting of several adult patterns of behavior which are stereotyped and do not appear to change significantly with experience.[5] Social play consists of locomotor play, and rough-and-tumble play (wrestling, biting, rolling, and mouthing). Rough-and-tumble play often consists of one individual jumping onto the back of another and attempting to bite its neck but all biting during play is inhibited compared to the uninhibited biting of genuine aggression[5] (see Figure 6.3).

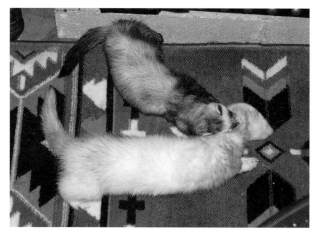

Figure 6.3 Neck biting during play.

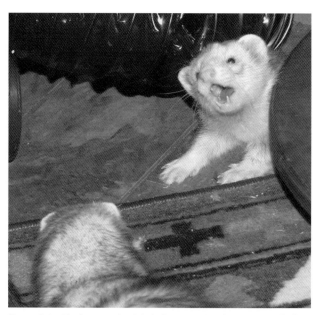

Figure 6.4 The ferret on the right is demonstrating the "open mouthed play face" while trying to initiate play with the ferret on the left.

Locomotor play can be differentiated from genuine aggression by the loose, bouncy, and jerky galloping movements displayed by the ferret during play. Ferrets will alternate the role of aggressor and defender with the defender attempting to push the aggressor away with its forepaws, while directing bites at the neck and muzzle. Individual ferrets have been noted to more consistently take the role of either aggressor or defender, while reversing roles less often than is commonly seen in other young mammals.[39] Uninhibited play bites are rarely directed at limbs or tails. As the level of excitement rises, the aggressor may shake the opponent by the neck and attempt to drag it around by the neck. If an individual tires of the rough play, they may whine or hiss and attempt to flee. This usually results in the attacker stopping its attack.[5]

Another feature common to play and not seen in genuine aggression is referred to as the "open mouthed play face" (see Figure 6.4). This consists of the ferret holding its mouth wide open without retracting its lips to display teeth (as may be seen in genuine aggression). Frequently a ferret will turn and orient the open-mouthed play face toward its attacker while wagging its head back and forth, as it flees an encounter. This frequently leads to a chase suggesting that the behavior is an invitation to play.[39]

Ferrets will engage in object play but the presence of another ferret is the best stimulus for play. If an individual is playing with an inanimate object and another ferret is introduced to its pen, the ferret is likely to stop playing with the object in order to engage the introduced ferret in play. If a strange juvenile ferret is introduced to a group of juvenile ferrets that have not previously been playing, the presence of the stranger is likely to lead to play in much the same way that an adult ferret introduced to a group of adult ferrets will lead to aggression. The introduction of a novel object is also likely to lead to play behavior.[5]

Certain situations will predictably inhibit play in the ferret: the presence of a fear-inducing stimulus, the presence of prey, and being placed in a strange environment.[5] When placed in a novel environment, the ferret's behavior will immediately be focused on exploration, whereas when exposed to a fear-inducing stimulus, the animal will become defensive or try to escape or hide. The presence of prey will usually lead to the chasing and killing of the prey, if possible.

After 18 weeks, polecat play decreases dramatically, coinciding with the time that they would be leaving their nest and setting out on their own.[37] This decrease, though present, is less notable in the domestic ferret and may be due to early gonadectomy that is common in pet ferrets, or it may be a sign of the juvenilization of behavior that is commonly associated with domestication or, possibly, even a combination of the two.

Play behavior in ferrets, as in other young mammals, may provide the opportunity for honing the hunting and fighting skills needed by adults in the wild. Adult, domestic ferrets retain these behavioral traits, and owners need to remember that although the wrestling may seem to be vicious, ferrets rarely hurt each other in this type of play. The extremely thick skin over the thick muscular neck usually serves to prevent actual injury.[6] Owners should still use caution if attempting to intervene, as they might be accidentally injured by the ferret's sharp canines.

Aggression

Aggression between ferrets can be a problem, especially if attempting to introduce two adult ferrets. Aggression is less likely when animals are familiar with each other[40] and familiarization is more important than kinship.[35] Aggression between familiar ferrets may be inhibited and yet sustained.[41] Aggression between unfamiliar ferrets is uninhibited and is intended to result in the formation of a rank order. Ferrets that are removed from a group of familiars for as little as 2 days may be viewed as a stranger when returned and uninhibited fighting may occur.[41] Animals that have been raised together demonstrated less aggressive interactions but one researcher determined that aggressive interactions do appear to increase with age.[35] Whereas it is not impossible to introduce two unfamiliar adult ferrets, one cannot be certain that the two chosen ferrets will ultimately be able to cohabitate and little is known about what makes any two particular ferrets compatible. If plenty of space and slow introduction time is not provided when introducing unacquainted ferrets, serious fights can ensue. This fighting can be very vigorous and persistent but it is rare for serious injury or death to occur.[41] Pet owners desiring to keep more than one ferret together should be encouraged to acquire both ferrets when young so that they can mature together rather than attempting to add a new ferret after the first ferret is grown. While it is generally recommended that gonadally intact males should not be housed together due to the potential for aggression, current research suggests that there is little to no difference in aggression when introducing intact male or female ferrets and gonadectomized male or female ferrets. In one study, levels of aggression were found to be similar when any combination of the above was paired.[40]

Staton et al. also looked at the effects of pre-familiarization to determine if it could decrease aggression between previously unacquainted ferrets. Ferrets were housed in cages side by side for a period of 2 weeks and then introduced into a test pen. While this period of familiarization was not enough to decrease fighting significantly in most ferrets,[40] a longer period of pre-familiarization might be effective and warrants further study.

While genuine aggression can be difficult to differentiate from play, there are four patterns of behavior that occur during adult aggression that have not been documented during play: the sustained neck bite, sideways attack, the defensive threat, and screaming.[5] During the breeding season, the aggression between gonadally intact adult males can be especially fierce and prolonged.

During genuine aggression, the attacker uses uninhibited bites to its opponent's neck and holds on. The opponent may attempt to fight back and gain its own hold on the attacker's neck but if intimidated and afraid it may attempt to escape, often while screaming. If the attacker is highly motivated to continue attacking it is likely to use a sideways attack, where the attacker approaches the victim while walking sideways with its head turned away from the victim, threatening in an attempt to prolong the interaction. This persistent attack often leads to the victim performing a defensive threat where it stands with an arched back and raised head facing its aggressor with bared teeth while hissing and/or screaming.[5] If the attacker continues to attack, he will usually do so with the sideways

attack while running sideways at the victim in an attempt to roll over him and grasp his neck. The defensive animal will attempt to back away from this offensive tactic or he may attempt to flee. However, fleeing opens his neck to attack from the aggressor, who may attempt to leap upon him and grasp his neck.[6] When adult ferrets fight, the larger, stronger animals usually win the battle, achieving a dominant status to the smaller, weaker opponent.[5]

A recent study that looked at the effects of surgical and chemical castration on male ferrets found that ferrets with a deslorelin implant had lower rates of aggression between male ferrets both when a receptive female was present and when she was absent.[42] In addition, both chemically and surgically castrated ferrets had reduced sexually motivated behaviors, and increased play behavior (slightly higher in the chemically castrated animals).[42] Chemical castration appears to be more effective at promoting "pet appropriate" behavior than surgical castration. Due to the fact that early surgical castration is correlated with onset of hyperadrenocorticism, exploring the use of chemical castration to reduce aggressive interactions seems particularly promising.[42,43,44]

The juvenilization of behavior that accompanies domestication may be the cause of the domestic ferrets appearing to be much more sociable than their solitary living ancestors. Nevertheless, other than occasional allo-grooming and the fact that many ferrets appear to prefer sleeping in groups, ferrets show little of the cohesive behaviors typical of most social animals.[41] Therefore, it cannot be overstated that ferrets, like other animals, have individual personalities. In general, some ferrets are better off with companions, whereas some, like some cats and dogs, prefer to be an "only child."

Interspecific interactions

Ferrets are curious creatures and will interact with other animals, such as cats, dogs, other pets, and people; however, ferrets are predators, so common sense should be used when introducing them to other animals. For example, ferrets and rodents, birds, or other small animals might not be a safe pairing. Additionally, ferrets themselves might trigger predatory behavior in some dogs or cats so caution should be used especially during initial introduction until it can be determined how the other animal will respond to the ferret.

Housing

In the wild, polecat home ranges average from 12.4 ha (30 acres) for females to 31.3 ha (77 acres) for males[4] and they have been known to travel significant distances when foraging (up to 7.5 km or 4.6 mi) according to one author.[45] Thus, caretakers are encouraged to provide ferrets with as large a cage as possible, and lots of playtime outside of the enclosure. Commercial ferret cages are commonly made of wire. Wire should be 0.75 × 0.75 in.

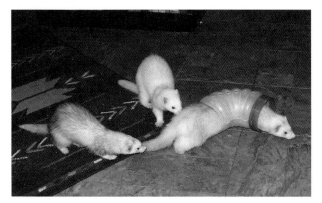

Figure 6.5 A group of ferrets playing in plastic tubing.

(2 × 2 cm) and a heavy gauge, to ensure that ferrets do not stray. Wire on the flooring of the shelter should be covered by smaller gauge wire to protect feet and nails from becoming caught. Most commercial ferret cages are two or three stories, hence, the wire ladder might pose a problem for ferret feet; a wooden ramp with tacked on "steps" is a better alternative, or else a single story ferret warren might provide a safer environment.

In the wild, polecats and ferrets dig and spend much of their time in underground tunnels.[4,46] Providing ferrets with plastic pipes or other similar objects for them to crawl in and around, and to rest in, allows them to perform more of their normal behaviors and may be inherently enriching (see Figure 6.5). Ferrets appear to prefer a smaller enclosure within their cage for nesting. Including plenty of soft bedding under which they can burrow also appears to be appreciated. Hammocks, when available, are also often the chosen sleeping site for ferrets and hammocks designed specifically for ferret cages are available commercially. When familiar ferrets are housed together, they will generally sleep together and it is important to provide sleeping space so that they can snuggle together, as well as separate sleeping arrangements to accommodate the times when the animals seek solitude.

Ferrets should be kept within a temperature range of 15–21°C (59–70°F).[47] Ferrets are very sensitive to high temperatures and may suffer from heat prostration if the temperature exceeds 29°C (85°F).[48]

Reproductive behavior

Ferrets engage in a polygynous mating system.[49] Hobs will attempt to mate as many jills as possible. Ferrets reach sexual maturity at 8–12 months of age.[50] In hobs, puberty is characterized by an increase in testicular size and male sexual behaviors. These behaviors include neck gripping, an interest in estrus jills and pelvic thrusting. If these sexual behaviors appear in an adult gonadectomized ferret, a diagnosis of hyperadrenocorticism should be considered.[43]

In jills, the onset of first estrus indicates sexual maturity. Estrus in jills is seasonal, linked to changes in day length, and characterized by a swollen vulva, due to increases of estrogen in her system.[51] Jills will remain in estrus indefinitely unless they are bred or given hormones to induce ovulations.[50]

Ferret copulation is noisy and aggressive. The hob will grasp the jill by the nape of the neck and sometimes drag her about. The jill's response is dependent upon her stage of estrus. When in estrus, the jill will remain in close proximity to the hob, often crawling under and over him and repeatedly presenting her genital area to his head. Copulation takes place with the jill's belly flat on the ground and her neck stretched forward. The hob's pelvic region is brought forward and his back arched. Multiple pelvic thrusts are used to achieve intromission.[7,52] Intromission can last for minutes to hours.[50] Fox and Bell report a mean length of 1 hour for mating sessions.[51]

Although ferret breeding can be manipulated through changes in length of daylight, typically hobs will mate from December to July.[4] Interestingly, jill breeding season is from March to August.[50] During mating season hobs should not be kept together, given heightened conspecific aggression. Estrous females should not be housed together nor should females who have been mated. Such a situation risks pseudopregnancy and eliciting of ovulation.[51]

As noted earlier, the VNO does not appear to play a role in sexual behavior of male ferrets. It appears that male ferrets rely on smell using the olfactory bulbs in mate choice rather than the VNO as other mammals. That said, there is evidence that an olfactory circuit in female ferrets, terminating on the ventromedial hypothalamus, does contribute to facilitation of female sexual receptivity and the seeking out of male partners.[53]

Maternal behavior

Healthy domestic ferrets can have up to three successful litters per year, although one to two is most common. Gestation length is about 42 days. Ferrets have on average, 8 kits in a litter (with a range of 1–18).[50] Although pregnant jills will likely not act aggressively toward each other, it is worthwhile to house them individually 2 weeks prior to birth of the litter. This will minimize disturbances and conspecific stress. Excessive or unusual noises, temperature extremes, strange people, or animals should all be kept away from the pregnant and birthing jill. Normal birthing occurs very swiftly, and is generally over in 2–3 hours. Mother and kits should be left alone for several days after birth to ensure that she does not cannibalize the kits.[51] It has been reported that jills will accept the kits of other jills so cross-fostering can be a solution when a jill dies or fails to care for her litter.[48] If the litter is small (less than 5 kits), jills may experience a lactational estrus.[51]

Newborn kits weigh about 6–12 g (0.21–0.42 oz.) (about 1% or less of the adult ferret's weight).[51] Kits begin nursing almost immediately after birth, and remain attached to the jill's nipples almost all the time.[51] Their eyes and ear canals are closed at birth and they are covered by fine white hair. They are able to pull themselves about using their front legs and can initiate suckling on their own.[8] The kits' eyes and ears open by 4–5 weeks of age.[8]

Lactating females preferentially orient themselves to frequencies greater than 16 kHz. Neonate distress calls typically have frequency components up to 100 kHz.[51] Females who are not lactating do not orient to these stimuli. During the first few weeks of life, the dam must lick the newborns' anogenital region to stimulate defecation and urination. The young ferrets are able to defecate without stimulation at about the same time as they begin eating solid food.[8]

Weaning of the kits begins at approximately 3 weeks of age, when the mother begins to bring food to the nest. By 4–5 weeks they are eating solid food and weaning is generally completed by 5–6 weeks. By the seventh week of life the differences in male and female body weight begin to show and by the ninth week, differences in length are obvious. While the males are ultimately larger in size, the female reach mature body size sooner.[8]

Ingestive behavior

Eating

The polecat is primarily a nocturnal predator with its activity patterns coinciding with the activity patterns of its prey. Polecats will feed upon a variety of vertebrate and invertebrate prey including rodents, small birds, reptiles, amphibians, spiders, beetles, slugs, snails, and earthworms.[4] Ferrets and polecats will stalk and then leap upon their prey, seizing it by the neck with its large canine teeth and holding firmly.[20,46] Numbers of different types of prey taken varies with the season in polecats, as do their activity patterns. In the wild, polecats are more active when their primary prey is most active.[54,55] This ability to adapt to prey availability can be useful to the pet owner desiring to increase their pet's activity levels during the daytime hours when the pet owner is most active. Feeding and allowing the ferret out of its cage for exercise and interaction can all be done during the day to encourage the ferret to be active during the day and sleep during the night.

The ferret, though an obligate carnivore, has a stomach similar in shape to those of dogs. When fed a mostly carnivorous diet, ferrets have a short transit time, 148–219 minutes.[56] To maintain body weight, ferrets must eat approximately 90–140 kcal per pound of body weight per day[12] and one study of two adult hobs demonstrated that, given free access to food, they ate 9–10 small meals per day.[57] The amount of food needed will differ for individual ferrets depending on his/her gender and activity levels; growing kits and pregnant jills will require significantly more nutritious food.

Ferrets require diets high in protein and fat. They have a limited capacity to digest fiber, and carbohydrates do not play an important role in their nutrition.[58] In general, however, a good ferret food or kitten food will provide adequate nutrition. Ideally, the majority of the protein should come from an animal source rather than corn or other plant source.[48]

Ferret owners must remain vigilant for decomposing food. Ferrets are well known for their caching behavior.[59] They are likely to hide away food, favorite treats, toys, and in one author's experience (MJB), cell phones, keys, and computer wires. While hiding objects is a behavior that many find endearing, rotting food can lead to bacterial growth that may be harmful to the health of the ferret and their human caretaker, so the ferret's environment should be monitored closely for hidden foods. In addition, many items can lead to illness and even death if chewed on or eaten, so ferrets should be monitored closely when out of their cages and their environment carefully "ferret-proofed."

Drinking

A healthy adult ferret will drink approximately half a cup of water per day[12] so fresh water should be available all day. Ferrets will dig in and tip over all but the sturdiest of water bowls. To ensure that fresh water is available, use heavy-bottomed, small water bowls. There are varieties of bowls that can be clamped to the sides of cages and rodent water bottles may also be used. No evidence exists that one form of providing water is superior to the other; however, in one author's experience (MJB), some ferrets may refuse to drink out of a rodent water bottle, so close attention should be paid to the ferret to confirm that it is drinking from the provided water source.

Elimination

Ferrets in the wild use multiple different latrine sites within their territories and may use the same sites for several months at a time. These sites are often located near their den and will usually be visited at the beginning and/or end of activity periods.[27] Ferrets do not bury their feces like cats but due to their tendency to use one or two locations for elimination they can be litter trained as easily. Ferrets in captivity have demonstrated a preference for defecating in corners, where they will scuttle backward until their hindquarters touch. Generally a ferret will choose a preferred corner of their cage, or the room when they are allowed out. Corner-shaped litter boxes with low openings are ideal for the ferret and pelleted type litters are the safest to use. Clumping litter and clay litters are not recommended.

Common behavior problems

Biting or nipping

Many ferrets will bite until they are trained otherwise. Just like dogs, different responses will work for different ferrets.

Caretakers must try to figure out what works for each individual ferret. Smacking, flicking, shaking, or any other violent behavior will not work. It will simply scare the ferret, possibly teaching it to fear humans or human hands, and thus lead to more biting.

The best way to deal with biting behavior is to try to determine the cause. A common way for ferrets to try to get attention or initiate play is to sneak up and bite. Whereas this is normal and acceptable among ferrets, it can be painful and annoying when directed at a person's ankles or hands. If picked up and removed from a toy or treat, some ferrets may turn and bite, probably in an attempt to get the person to let them return to what they were doing. Although no controlled studies have been done comparing the different ways in which to prevent nipping or biting, basic learning principles apply to ferrets as well as to other mammals. The most important thing for owners or caretakers to remember is that corrections must happen immediately in order for them to be effective. If delayed for more than a second or two, the ferret will not understand what it is being corrected for and may simply become fearful of the person administering the correction. Positively reinforcing non-biting behavior (by food reward or attention) will likely work better than any training regimen dominated by punishment. See Chapter 18 for more detailed information about the proper use of punishment and reinforcement for correcting behavior problems.

Destructive behaviors

Digging is a normal exploratory behavior for ferrets. When carpeting is present in the home, ferrets are likely to dig and claw the edges. Clearly, this behavior can very quickly lead to expensive damage to a home and an unhappy ferret owner. In one author's experience (MJB), the best course of action is to vigilantly "ferret proof" the home, or at least a few rooms, where the ferret can safely spend some time outside of its cage. This may include replacing all carpeting with tile, linoleum, or wood floors or covering corners of carpeting with metal plates. Alternatively, heavy, solid pieces of furniture can be placed on the corners or edges of carpeting. Owners not willing to try any of these solutions may find that a ferret is not the best pet for them. All dirt and plants must be well out of ferret reach (which is surprisingly high), but putting foil around the bottoms of plants may keep the ferret from digging in them.

One of the best ways to prevent ferrets from chewing on unacceptable items is to provide them with plenty of acceptable items for them to chew. These can include hard rubber toys (Kong makes a very small version that many ferrets like [*pers. ob.*, MJB]), hard rubber disks attached to the inside of the ferret enclosure, stuffed animals, and other similar toys. Any toy containing small parts that can be torn off by the ferret or soft foam rubber must be avoided as these can be a common cause of gastrointestinal blockage. To prevent chewing on furniture, stairs, carpeting, etc., a bite deterrent such as bitter apple or a hot sauce may be applied to the area but prevention is the best insurance (close supervision or denying access to that area).

Litter training

Ferret litter training is surprisingly easy. Consistency is the key. Ferrets prefer to back into a corner, thus the typical litter pans designed for ferrets work very well. Use very little litter; ferrets do not cover their scat, and this may lessen litter digging by bored ferrets. To begin with, placing a litter pan in each corner of the enclosure will assist in keeping the enclosure clean and in helping the ferret to succeed. Once the ferret picks a favorite spot, that litter pan can remain while the others are removed.

When the ferrets are out of their enclosures for daily play sessions, put the other litter pans in the corners of the room. This will provide the ferret with plenty of opportunities to eliminate in a location acceptable to the owner. Due to their short gastrointestinal transit time, ferrets eliminate frequently. They are likely to eliminate immediately after waking, after eating and 2–3 more times during the course of a day. Picking the ferret up when first removed from the enclosure and placing him or her in the litter pan is helpful, especially if they have just woken up.

It is also important to be attentive to the ferrets' choices when eliminating. If the ferret shows a preferred corner, the box should be placed in that corner. Once the ferret is using the box reliably, the owner may attempt to move the box, slowly (over a period of several days) to the location the owner prefers. If the owner is reluctant to follow these instructions, and they remain observant, they can physically place the ferret in the corner they prefer every time they see the animal posturing to eliminate. Eventually the ferret might choose to use this location exclusively.

Younger ferrets may be inclined to play in a litter box, as they love to dig, but are tidy animals and this behavior usually ceases as they learn what the litter box is for. Nevertheless, wiring litter boxes to the side of the cage will prevent them from being turned over if the ferret does spend some time digging and playing in the litter.

Rubbing a ferret's nose in his elimination when he has eliminated outside of the litter pan will never teach the ferret to use the litter pan successfully. Instead, this is confusing and heightens the likelihood that the ferret will bite.

Lost ferrets

Teaching the ferret to come to a particular sound (shaking a treat can, squeaking a favorite toy) is highly recommended. The easiest way to do this is to make a noise and provide a treat. The ferret will associate the sound with the treat and eventually come running when it hears the sound.

Conclusion

A recent study found that 91% of the ferrets that were adopted from veterinary surgery teaching hospitals were rated as good pets (total $N = 43$ adult ferrets, responses cover 53% of the ferrets). Only 4.5% were rated as poor pets. The most common problems, found in 36% of the ferrets, were behavioral issues such as nipping and failure to litter train.[60] This underscores the trainability of ferrets regardless of their early rearing histories, and the importance of addressing behavioral issues as soon as they appear, before the human–pet bond becomes irreparably damaged.

Acknowledgments

All photos in this chapter courtesy of M. C. Tynes, copyright 2010.

References

1. Owen C. Ferret. In: Mason IL, ed. *The Evolution of Domesticated Animals.* England: Longman Group Limited, 1984; 225–228.

2. Church B. Ferret polecat domestication: Genetic, taxonomic and phylogenetic relationships. In: Lewington JH, ed. *Ferret Husbandry, Medicine, and Surgery.* New York: Elsevier Saunders 2007;122–150.

3. Miller BJ, Anderson SH. Comparison of black-footed ferret (*Mustela nigripes*) and domestic ferret (*M. Putorius furo*) courtship activity. *Zoo Biol* 1990;9:201–210.

4. Blandford PRS. Biology of the polecat, *Mustela putorius*: A literature review. *Mammal Rev* 1987;17:155–198.

5. Poole TB. Aggressive play in polecats. *Symp Zool Soc Lond* 1966;18:23–44.

6. Poole TB. Aspects of aggressive behaviour in polecats. *Z Tierpsychol* 1967;24:351–369.

7. Poole TB. Diadic interactions between pairs of male polecats (*Mustela furo* and *Mustela furo* × *Mustela putorius* hybrids) under standardized environmental conditions during the breeding season. *Z Tierpsychol* 1972;30:45–58.

8. Shump AU, Shump KA. Growth and development of the European ferret (*Mustela putorius*). *Lab Anim Sci* 1978;28:89–91.

9. Norbury GL, Norbury DC, Heyward RP. Space use and denning behaviour of wild ferrets (*Mustela furo*) and cats (*Felis catus*). *N Z J Ecol* 1998;22(2):149–159.

10. Poole TB. Detailed analysis of fighting in polecats (Mustelidae) using ciné film. *J Zool Lond* 1974;173:369–393.

11. Poole TB. Some behavioral differences between the European polecat, *Mustela putorius*, the ferret, *Mustela furo* and their hybrids. *J Zool* 1972;166(1):25–35.

12. Fox, J. *Biology and Diseases of the Ferret.* Philadelphia: Williams & Wilkins, 1998.

13. Lewington J. *Ferret Husbandry, Medicine, and Surgery.* Philadelphia, PA: Butterworth Heinemann, 2002.

14. Manger P, Nakamura H. Visual areas in the lateral temporal cortex of the ferret (*Mustela putorius*). *Cereb Cortex* 2004;14:676–689.

15. Neumann F, Schmidt HD. Optische Differenzierungsleistungen von Musteliden. Verusche an Frettchen und Iltisfrettchen. *Z für Vergleichende Physiologie* 1959;42:199–205. (Cited in Blandford PRS. Biology of the polecat, *Mustela putorius*: A literature review. *Mammal Rev* 1987;17:155–198.)

16. Gewalt W. Beiträge zur Kenntnis des optischen Differnzierungsvermögens eineger Musteliden besonderer Berücksichtigung des Farbensehens. *Zoologische Beiträge* 1959;5:117–175. (Cited in Blandford PRS. Biology of the polecat, *Mustela putorius*: A literature review. *Mammal Rev* 1987;17:155–198.)

17. Apfelbach R, Wester U. The quantitative effect of visual and tactile stimuli on the prey-catching behavior of ferrets. *Behav Process* 1977;2:187–200.

18. Bizley J, Nodal F, Nelken, I et al. Functional organization of ferret auditory cortex. *Cereb Cortex* 2005;15:1637–1653.

19. Moore DR, Semple MN, Addison PD. Some acoustic properties of the neurons in the ferret inferior colliculus. *Brain Res* 1983; 269:69–82.

20. Poole TB. Polecats. *Forestry Commision Forest Record No. 76.* HMSO: London 1970. (Cited in Blandford PRS. Biology of the polecat, *Mustela putorius*: A literature review. *Mammal Rev* 1987; 17:155–198.)

21. Mrsic-Flogel T, King A, Schnupp J. Encoding of virtual acoustic space stimuli by neurons in ferret primary auditory cortex. *J Neurophysiol* 2005;93:3489–3503.

22. Mrsic-Flogel TD, Versnel H, King A. Development of contralateral and ipsilateral frequency representations in the ferret primary auditory cortex. *Eur J Neurosci* 2006;23:780–792.

23. Bajo V, Nodal F, Bizley J, Moore, D. The ferret auditory cortex descending projections to the inferior colliculus. *Cereb Cortex* 2007;17:475–491.

24. Clapperton BK. An olfactory recognition system in the ferret *Mustela furo* L. (Carnivora: Mustelidae). *Anim Behav* 1988;36:541–553.

25. Rehn B, Breipohl W, Mendoza AS et al. Changes in granule cells of the ferret olfactory bulb associated with imprinting on prey odours. *Brain Res* 1986;373:114–125.

26. Woodley SK, Baum MJ. Differential activation of glomeruli in the ferret's main olfactory bulb by anal scent gland odours from males and females: An early step in mate identification. *Eur J Neurosci* 2005;20:1025–1032.

27. Clapperton BK. Scent-marking behavior of the ferret (*Mustela furo*). *Anim Behav* 1989;38:436–446.

28. Zhang JX, Soini HA, Bruce KE. Putative chemosignals of the ferret (*Mustela furo*) associated with individual and gender recognition. *Chem Senses* 2005;30:727–737.

29. Weiler E, Apfelbach R, Farbman AI. The vomeronasal organ of the male ferret. *Chem Senses* 1999;24:127–136.

30. Apfelbach R, Weiler E, Rehn B. Is there a neural basis for olfactory food imprinting in ferrets? *Naturwissenschaften* 1985;72: 106–107.

31. Apfelbach R. Imprinting on prey odors in ferrets (*Mustela putorius furo*) and its neural correlates. *Behav Process* 1986;12:363–381.

32. Christensson M, Garwicz M. Time course of postnatal motor development in ferrets: Ontogenetic and comparative perspectives. *Behav Brain Res* 2005;158:231–242.

33. Powell, RA. Mustelid spacing patterns: Variations on a theme by *Mustela. Z Tierpsychol* 1979;50:153–165.

34. Moors PJ, Laver RB. Movements and home range of ferrets (*Mustela furo*) at Pukepuke Lagoon, New Zealand. *N Z J Zool* 1981;8:413–424.

35. Lode T. Kin recognition versus familiarity in a solitary mustelid, the Europena polecat *Mustela putorius. C R Biol* 2008;331:248–254.

36. Hillman CN, Clark TW. *Mustela nigripes. Mammal species* 1980;126:1–3.

37. Biden M. Sex differences in the play of young ferrets. *Biol Behav* 1982;7:303–308.

38. Stockman ER, Callaghan RS, Gallagher CA et al. Sexual differentiation of play behavior in the ferret. *Behav Neurosci* 1986; 100: 563–568.

39. Poole, TB. An analysis of social play in polecats (Mustelidae) with comments on the form and evolutionary history of the open mouth play face. *Anim Behav* 1978;26:36–49.

40. Staton VW, Crowell-Davis SL. Factors associated with aggression between pairs of domestic ferrets. *J Am Vet Med Assoc* 2003;222: 1709–1712.

41. Poole TB. The aggressive behavior of individual male polecats (*Mustela putorius, M. furo* and hybrids) towards familiar and unfamiliar opponents. *J Zool Lond* 1973;170:395–414.

42. Vinke CM, van Deijk R, Houx BB, Shoemaker NJ. The effects of surgical and chemical castration on intermale aggression, sexual behaviour and play behaviour in the male ferret (*Mustela putorius furo*). *Appl Anim Behav Sci* 2008;115:104–121.

43. Schoemaker NJ, Schuurmans M, Moorman H, Lumeij JT. Correlation between age at neutering and age at onset of hyperadrenocorticism in ferrets. *J Am Vet Med Assoc* 2000;216:195–197.

44. Schoemaker NJ, Teerds JK, Mol JA et al. The role of luteinizing hormone in the pathogenesis of hyperadrenocorticism in neutered ferrets. *Mol Cell Endocrinol* 2002;197:117–125.

45. Rusakof OS. Some data on the nutrition of the European polecat in Leningrad, Pskov, and Novgorod oblasts. *Sbornik Nauchnykh Statei Zapadnogo Otdela Vsesoyuznogo Nauchno-Issledovatel' skogo Instituta Zhivotnogo Syr'ya Pushniny* 1963;2:195–199. (Cited in Blandford PRS. Biology of the polecat, *Mustela putorius*: A literature review. *Mammal Rev* 1987;17:155–198.)

46. Progulske DR. Observations of a penned, wild-captured black-footed ferret. *J Mammal* 1969;50:619–621.

47. Andrews PLR, Illman O. The ferret. In: Poole TB, Robinson R, eds. *The UFAW Handbook on the Care and Management of Labo-ratory Animals*. 6th ed. New York: Churchill Livingstone, 1986; 436–445.

48. Ball RS. Husbandry and management of the domestic ferret. *Lab Anim* 2002;31:37–42.

49. Lode T. Mating system and genetic variance in a polygynous mustelid, the European polecat. *Genes Genet Syst* 2001;76:221–227.

50. Lindeberg H. Reproduction of the female ferret. *Reprod Dom Anim* 2008;43(Suppl 2):150–156.

51. Fox JG, Bell JA. Growth, reproduction and breeding. In: Fox JG, ed. *Biology and Diseases of the Ferret*. Philadelphia: Williams & Wilkins, 1998;211–230.

52. Miller BJ, Anderson SH. Courtship patterns in induced oestrous and natural oestrous domestic ferrets, *Mustela putorius furo*. *J Ethol* 1989;7:65–74.

53. Robarts DW, Baum MJ. Ventromedial hypothalamic nucleus lesions disrupt olfactory mate recognition and receptivity in female ferrets. *Horm Behav* 2007;51:104–113.

54. Lode T. Activity pattern of polecats *Mustela putorius L.* in relation to food habits and prey activity. *Ethology* 1995;100:295–308.

55. Lode T. Time budget as related to feeding tactics of European polecat *Mustela putorius*. *Behav Proc* 1999;47:11–18.

56. Bell JA. Ferret nutrition. *Vet Clin North Am Exotic Anim Pract* 1999;2:169–192.

57. Kaufman LW. Foraging costs and meal patterns in ferrets. *Physiol Behav* 1980;25:139–141.

58. Fekete SGY, Fodor K, Proháczik A et al. Comparison of feed preference and digestion of three different commercial diets for cats and ferrets. *J Anim Physiol Anim Nutr* 2005;89:199–202.

59. Raber H. Versuche zur Ermittlung des Beuteschemas an einem Hausmarder (Martes foina und einem Iltis (*Putorius putorius*). *Revue Suisse de Zoologie* 1944;51:293–332. (Cited in Blandford PRS. Biology of the polecat, *Mustela putorius*: A literature review. *Mammal Rev* 1987;17:155–198.)

60. Harms CA, Stoskopf MK. Outcomes of adoption of adult laboratory ferrets after gonadectomy during a veterinary student teaching exercise. *J Am Assoc Lab Anim Sci* 2007;46:50–54.

7

Rabbits

Sharon L. Crowell-Davis

The modern domestic rabbit originated in southwestern Europe, specifically the Iberian peninsula or modern day Spain and Portugal. The wild European rabbit, *Oryctolagus cuniculus*, whose name roughly translates as "hare-like digger of underground passages," was kept in cages approximately 3000 years ago, when the Phoenicians reached Spain. They were subsequently carried by the Romans across much of Europe and to the British Isles, where escaped or released rabbits established wild populations, greatly expanding their range.[1] Eventually, human migrations caused their spread to all continents except Antarctica. *O. cuniculus* is the sole remaining member of the genus *Oryctolagus*. Taxonomically, *Oryctolagus* is a member of the order Lagomorpha, which includes two families, the Leporidae, or hares and rabbits, and the Ochotonidae, or pikas. The most common native wild rabbits of the Americas are in the order Sylvilagus, of which there are 16 species. The smallest member of the Leporidae, the pygmy rabbit *Brachylagus idahoensis* which weights 375–500 g (13.2–17.6 oz.), also resides in North America.

Hares, comprising three genuses, *Lepus*, *Caprolagus*, and *Pronolagus* live most of their lives above ground. Their young are precocial, born fully furred, and with their eyes and ears open. In contrast, rabbit species, except for the cottontail rabbit *Sylvilagus*, spend much of their life underground, with *Oryctolagus cuniculus* being a rabbit species that builds extensive underground warrens. Rabbit young are altricial, born hairless, blind and deaf, although they subsequently mature very rapidly. Female rabbits (called does) prepare underground nests for their altricial young. This may be a shallow nest hole in the case of *Sylvilagus* spp., but can be very deep within a warren in the case of *O. cuniculus*.

When rabbits were first kept in cages, they were portable sources of fresh meat rather than pets. The fact that they were already adapted to living in social groups and confined spaces probably made them pre-adapted to surviving what was doubtless a very harsh living environment, with little concern for the rabbits' welfare.

In about the 6th century AD, monks began breeding rabbits of various sizes and colors. Subsequently, during the industrial revolution, people who had moved from the country to the crowded cities still desired some contact with animals and nature. While the keeping of cattle and flocks of sheep was quite impossible in the cities, the keeping of small livestock, such as rabbits and pigeons, was often feasible, which led to the development of the rabbit fancy and a broader variety of shapes and colors.

In the modern day, domestic rabbits are kept for a variety of purposes, including personal and commercial meat production, laboratory research, wool production, showing, and breeding for the pet market. There is no single source that keeps population data on all rabbit populations. The USDA reports that there are approximately 5 million pet rabbits owned by 2.2 million US households. This makes rabbits the most popular mammalian house pet after dogs and cats. Rabbits make good house pets for multiple reasons. They are generally small, ranging in size from 1 to 8 kg (2.2–17.6 lbs.), depending on breed. They can be trained to use a litterbox and, raised appropriately, make friendly and playful pets. Altogether, the entire rabbit industry in the United States consists of approximately 9 million rabbits.[2]

Social organization of wild rabbits

Wild *O. cuniculi* live in social groups that number up to 300 or 400 rabbits, although most groups are smaller. Individual rabbits and groups of rabbits typically leave the warren to graze at dawn and at dusk, that is they are crepuscular. When multiple rabbits are out together, they take turns checking for predators, which they do by discontinuing feeding, standing up on their hind limbs, and raising their ears.[3] The more rabbits that are out at one time, the less time any one rabbit spends checking for predators. Thus, one advantage of group living is the ability to spend more time eating when in the vulnerable position of being outside the warren. If a rabbit sights a predator it will rapidly strike the ground with its hind limb, making the distinctive sound of the "alarm thump," which will result in all of the rabbits running into the warren. Outside housing for rabbits should allow them to be psychologically safe, as well as physically safe, from predators. For example, if the rabbit is kept in a hutch that primarily has wire sides, floor, and roof, it should have an enclosed box, not only to protect it from the elements, but to allow it to retreat into the safety of a pseudo warren if it hears or sees things that alarm it.

Within the colony, there are typically multiple subgroups, each consisting of 2–8 individuals.[4–6] Females within the group are usually related, while males (referred to as bucks) within the group maintain a rigid dominance hierarchy that is maintained primarily through ritualized signaling. As males mature, they may remain with the subgroup with which they grew up, migrate to another subgroup, or even migrate to another warren.[7] Rabbits grazing in groups also show subtle vigilance when a conspecific that is a potential competitor is nearby. Among groups of wild, sexually intact rabbits, subtle vigilance is primarily exhibited by males when another male is close, and by females whose social status is unstable when either females or males are close.[3] Keeping in mind the natural social organization of wild rabbits, it is generally best to keep pet rabbits in similar, small social groups.[8–11]

Warrens

When they are not eating, wild rabbits live in underground warrens.[12–14] A large warren may have 50 entrances or more (Figure 7.1). Some exits are very obvious from the outside, with an opening that is free of brush with earth mounded up around it, and latrines filled with feces nearby. Others, called bolt holes, are dug from within the warren so that no dirt around the opening marks the opening. Bolt holes can be vertical, allowing a rabbit to enter or exit quickly but making passage by a number of predators quite difficult. In addition, bolt holes usually come out under dense brush or within tall, dense grasses. While most tunnels are narrow, about 15 cm (5.9 in.) in diameter, wider sections of 40 cm (15.7 in.) diameter allow rabbits to pass each other in the tunnels. Various dead-end tunnels within the warren end in a side gallery, a small "room" where rabbits rest, groom, and consume their caecotrophs. In the keeping of pet rabbits, it is best to allow

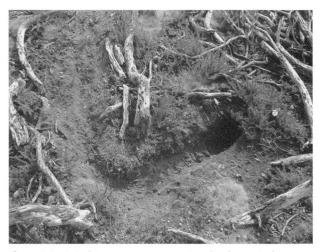

Figure 7.1 A single entrance to a warren. Note that the approach turns at a sharp angle, allowing a rabbit that is running away from a predator appear to be escaping in one direction, then abruptly turn and escape down a hole.

for their natural behavior, and make sure that they have a secure, cave-like area where they can also rest undisturbed (Figure 7.2a–c).

Sensory abilities and communication

Rabbits' sensory abilities are adapted to spending much of their lives underground in lightless tunnels. They have an excellent sense of smell and can hear very low volume sounds that a human would not hear. Their long ears can be rotated independently, facilitating their ability to identify the direction from which a predator is approaching. Their eyes are prominently located on the side of their head and their total field of vision is close to 360°. Rabbits can also have a wide field of vision upward, above their head, allowing them to spot approaching raptors. There is a small blind spot directly in front of their nose. Rods are the predominant photoreceptor cells, giving the rabbit excellent vision in dim light.[15]

While people who are not familiar with rabbits tend to think of them as being silent animals, they have a number of auditory communications, most of which are low volume. Purring, clicking, and quiet tooth grinding can generally be interpreted as indicating contentment, as these are sounds that humans can hear when a rabbit that is well habituated to humans is in a secure, comfortable situation. Loud tooth grinding, grunting, or growling are threat behaviors. Their growl sounds similar to that of a dog but, as with all of their vocalizations, is generally of such a low volume that the inattentive handler may miss it. Likewise, the purr sounds similar to that of the cat, but is very low volume. Rabbits in pain may also grind their teeth loudly, and it is important to pay attention to this when caring for a rabbit that is sick or injured. One sound that humans readily recognize is the thump, a distinct and fairly loud sound

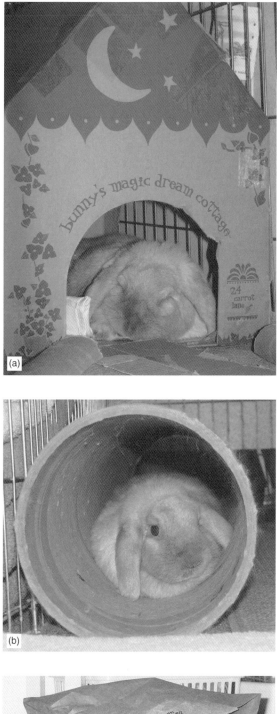

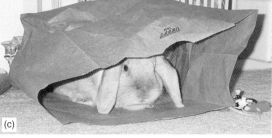

Figure 7.2(a–c) Even in the security of a household, pet rabbits prefer to have access to shelters reminiscent of the warren. These can be tubes, houses, or other devices produced specifically for pet rabbits, or something as simple as a paper bag. (Photos courtesy of Angela Curtis.)

produced by rapidly striking a hind foot against the ground. It is as an alarm signal. Frequent thumping by pet rabbits indicates that their environment is excessively threatening and stressful. In cases of extreme distress or fright, rabbits also scream, a sound that is very similar to the sound of a young child's scream.

Having a good sense of smell, rabbits also communicate via scent-marking that is sometimes sufficiently strong for humans to detect. Most notably, males scent mark by urine spraying. They will spray lower ranking males and will also spray females in estrus as part of courtship behavior.[7,16] If a male rabbit has a strong social bond with a human, they may spray the human. This is accomplished by running past the doe or human, lifting the hindquarters and directing them toward the object of spraying, and sending a spray of urine backward as the buck rapidly moves on. While not 100% effective, neutering male rabbits decreases the likelihood of this behavior. Rabbits often mark both their environment and each other with glands located on the chin. In my own household, that has both cats and rabbits, the two species may get into a kind of marking competition, with the cats rubbing various objects in the house which the rabbits overmark. Then the cats overmark the rabbits, etc. In the wild, latrines serve as both visual and scent markers. Rabbits housed side-by-side in cages are likely to eliminate in the corner or side of the cage nearest the neighboring rabbit. The characteristic odor of rabbit feces comes from the anal glands.[17]

The rabbit's posture gives further information about its emotional state. A relaxed rabbit will lie on its side with its hind limbs stretched out. Alternatively, it may squat with its limbs tucked under it. The eyes will be partially or fully closed and the ears will be relaxed, often hanging down from the upright posture of an alert rabbit. Rabbits showing submission to another rabbit, or fear of a human or something else in the environment, will crouch low to the ground and lay their ears flat against their neck and body.[18] In intraspecies interactions, the submissive or fearful rabbit will avoid eye contact. In contrast the alert rabbit will not only hold its ears up, it will rotate them as it listens to various sounds in the environment. The alert rabbit will also sit up on its hind limbs and turn its head, scanning the environment around it.

Locomotor behavior

The lack of activity by rabbits confined to small hutches is profoundly misleading. Wild rabbits and domestic rabbits that have adequate space are very active. There is only one gait, the hop, in which the powerful hind limbs push the rabbit forward and the forelimbs function to hold the front part of the rabbit off the ground when it is standing on all four limbs. The hop can be done slowly, for example when a rabbit is grazing, it will take a bite of grass, make one slow hop, take another bite, and so forth. At the other extreme, the rabbit can hop very rapidly, for example to escape predators. Pet rabbits will hop on and off of various objects, such as furniture. They will also stand up on their hind limbs, balancing easily while they scan their surroundings. Rabbits kept in cages that have too low a ceiling to allow them to stand like this do not have the opportunity to properly develop the extensor muscles of their back. I adopted one laboratory rabbit that had been kept in housing where she could not stand up. When she was first moved into a situation where she could stand, she would try to but could only elevate her torso to about 60°, at which point her forequarters would fall. Within a few weeks, her back muscles had strengthened and she was able to sit up perpendicular to the ground for extended periods of time.

Intraspecies affiliative behavior

The most common affiliative behavior between rabbits with amicable relationships is "cuddling up," that is lying side-by-side in direct contact with each other. Rabbits with amicable relationships will also allogroom each other by licking, although this is less frequent than lying side by side.[18]

Reproduction and care and rearing of kittens

Rabbits are induced ovulators, that is the doe only ovulates upon copulation. Gestation lasts approximately 31 days. As parturition, called kindling in rabbits, approaches, the doe will build a nest from a mixture of grasses and fur that she pulls from her own body. In the wild, some side galleries are used as nesting rooms, or nest stops. Higher ranking does will control access to the nest stops that are positioned most deeply in the warren, making access to her young by predators difficult. Lower ranking does will have to use nest stops located more superficially in the warren or may even have to dig a short tunnel with a nest stop at the end a short distance away from the warren. This situation obviously places the kits at high risk of predation. Because access to the best nesting sites can be critical to the survival of a doe's young, aggression between intact does can be quite severe, a behavior that can transfer to the domestic situation and is one of several reasons that does being kept as pets should be neutered.[5,6,8]

The kits are born blind, deaf, and hairless. The doe will return to the nest once or twice a day to nurse the kits. It is important to understand that this is normal, as pet owners who are accustomed to the much more frequent nursing of dogs, cats, and many other mammals, may think that the doe is being a poor mother. The kits identify and localize nipples in response to a mammary pheromone that is present in rabbit's milk.[19] The kits will spend the time between nursings inside the warmth of the nest. They will exit to nurse, urinate on the outside of the nest, then burrow within the warmth of the nest again. At about 8–12 days of age the kits will begin eating the grass that forms part of the nest, as well as fecal pellets left by the mother. When bottle raising baby rabbits, their natural cycle for nursing should be followed, that is they should not be overfed by attempting to get them to suckle from the bottle too frequently. Also, the caregiver of bottle-fed kits should be prepared for the kits to eliminate on their hand at the end of bottle feeding.

In about 18 days, the kits will have fur and can see and hear. At this time they will begin venturing outside the nest. When they are about 24 days, or 3½ weeks old, the mother ceases returning to the nest to nurse them. At 4 months of age they will have become sexually mature, but they will not reach full adult size until they are about 9 months of age. Females will typically breed as soon as they are sexually mature. Bucks, that must compete with other bucks, will usually not be able to breed until they have attained full adult size, enabling them to successfully compete.

If the warren is crowded, does may kill kits, particularly of other does. This can also occur in a domestic environment in which does are group-housed in an overcrowded environment, for example if a hobby rabbit owner keeps bucks and does together in a single enclosure, allowing them to breed freely and reproduce past the point of the individual rabbits being able to have adequate personal space and nesting areas.

Ingestive behavior

Rabbits are strict herbivores whose normal diet consists primarily of various grasses, herbs, and clovers. Their digestive system is designed for a high fiber diet.[20] While it can be very tempting to the owners of pet rabbits to give their rabbits lots of treats that are high in calories and low in fiber, this type of feeding should be avoided in order to avoid obesity and detrimental health sequelae. Hay should form the bulk of a pet rabbit's diet, with treats being used in small quantities for training and facilitation of the human–pet bond.

Coprophagy

Rabbits have two kinds of feces: most feces are eliminated as small, rounded, firm balls, approximately 1 cm in diameter. If a rabbit is litterbox trained, most or all of them will be deposited in the box. If the rabbit gets excited, or has its schedule disturbed so that it does not go to the litterbox, these feces may be deposited elsewhere, but are easily picked up with a tissue. The other kind of feces is the caecotroph. A healthy rabbit will consume their caecotrophs as they come out of the anus, and the owner or caregiver will never see the caecotroph. Among pet rabbits, caecotrophs are often erroneously referred to as "night feces," because of the tendency of pet rabbits to produce and eat their caecotrophs at night. What is actually happening is that rabbits produce and eat their caecotrophs when their environment is quiet and they are unlikely to be disturbed. Among pet and laboratory rabbits, this is often at night. However, wild rabbits will consume their feces during the day, when they are underground, as well.

Litterbox training and litterbox problems

Rabbits are usually easy to train to use a litterbox because of their natural habit of eliminating in specific latrines, also called scrapes, rather than randomly, when living in the wild (Figure 7.3).[6,13,21] We train cats to use litterboxes because of their predisposition to dig and subsequently bury their excrement. Rabbits do not dig and bury their excrement, and this is not the instinctive mechanism by which we facilitate their using a designated litterbox. Before a new rabbit owner brings their rabbit home, they should consider the question of where they want the litterbox to be. If they want it to be in some section of a particular room, they should initially confine the rabbit to that area with temporary fencing or other structural constraints. As soon as the rabbit has selected the area where it is going to eliminate, a litterbox should be placed at that site. If the owners want the litterbox to be in a cage, they should initially confine the rabbit to the cage, observe which corner of the cage the rabbit eliminates in, and then place the litterbox there. For this situation, triangular litterboxes designed to fit in the corner of a cage often work best. In both cases, the rabbit selects the latrine within the options it initially has. Once the rabbit's use of the box has been established, the owner can begin gradually allowing it more freedom, both in terms of time that it is able to leave the immediate vicinity of the litterbox, and the distance from the litterbox it has access to.

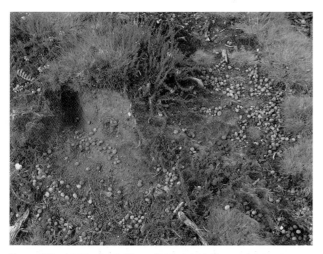

Figure 7.3 A latrine located immediately outside the opening to a warren. The quantity of pellets indicates that this is a toileting area, and warns rabbits that are not members of the warren to stay away.

If the rabbit is allowed to wander over an extensive area of the house, it may be necessary to add one or more boxes in other locations. If the rabbit is going to be allowed in a large area of the house, this situation can be anticipated by moving a litterbox that already has some of the rabbit's excrement to a new location in the house where the owner considers it acceptable for the rabbit to eliminate, and placing a new box in the location where the rabbit is already eliminating. The scent of its own excrement can facilitate the rabbit using the box that is in a new location.

Cats typically jump into their box, eliminate, bury their excrement, and exit the box. Rabbits, in contrast, may spend long periods of time in their box, just sitting or lying and resting there. This is normal. Sometimes a rabbit will backup to the edge of the box and urinate over the side. One technique for dealing with this is to place a washable mat under the box. Otherwise, a box with higher sides may have to be used. Some rabbits, having identified the box as their latrine and, apparently, wanting a new location, may move their box, either pushing it with their paws or head, or grabbing the edge with their teeth and pulling it. In this situation, it is generally best to allow the rabbit to move the box to the location it desires. If this change is totally unacceptable, it may be necessary to tie or clamp the box in place.

Rabbits will commonly eat the contents of their litterbox. Therefore, it is essential that toxic litters and litters that could potentially clump in the rabbit's gut not be used. One example of these types of unsafe litter are the clumping litters offered to cats that are designed to facilitate removing urine from the box. Pine or cedar shavings, and litters with deodorizing crystals are also unsuitable for rabbits. Aspen bark, compressed sawdust, straw, hay, peat moss, litter made from oats or alfalfa, and litter made from paper products are usually suitable, although the ingredients list should be carefully studied, especially if the litter is not labeled as safe for rabbits. Ground corn cobs can also work well, although there have been cases of rabbits developing impactions consisting of this substrate. A number of litters have now been developed specifically for rabbits, taking into consideration their behavior. Litters marketed for cats are generally not safe or appropriate for rabbits, although a non-clumping, unscented clay litter with very low dust may be acceptable in some circumstances.

Rabbit litterboxes are cleaned by dumping out all litter and excrement at once. Scooping, as is usually done with cat litter, does not work for several reasons. First, since clumping litter is dangerous for rabbits, the urine simply percolates to the bottom of the litter and collects there. Second, the rabbit deposits numerous small, firm balls of feces in a layer on the top of the litter. These are not readily scooped, as are the larger feces of the cat. As with cats, rabbits that have historically consistently used their box may develop an elimination behavior problem in which they urinate and/or defecate outside the box. Occasional dropping of the small, firm fecal balls outside of the box is normal, especially if the box not cleaned frequently enough or the rabbit is startled. In this case, simply picking up the occasional "accident" with a tissue and ensuring that the excrement and litter are dumped and changed frequently enough, (about every 1–2 days) is the best solution. Stress, changes in schedule, changes in the household, such as the addition of new pets or rearranging the furniture, can all cause the rabbit to respond by seeking a new location for its latrine. An examination of the environmental changes and retraining the rabbit to using a specific site may be necessary. For example, if the rabbit is accustomed to using a litterbox in a particular bedroom, and a rabbit-friendly dog that gives the rabbit unwanted attention when it is trying to spend time in its box is added to the household, the rabbit may seek a quiet area away from the dog for a new latrine. In this case, blocking the dog's access to the litterbox, either at the original site or a new site may be necessary.

Introducing unfamiliar rabbits

Rabbits recognize other rabbits, and know if another rabbit is a member of their social group, and therefore familiar, or if the rabbit is not a member of their social group, and a stranger. Ideally, rabbits that are going to be kept as housemates should be introduced when young.[22] If there are already one or more rabbits in a household and a new adult rabbit is brought home, the new rabbit is likely to be chased and attacked.

Introductions must be done gradually and under supervision. When a new rabbit is brought home, it should be kept totally separate from the existing household rabbits at first for medical quarantine. Once the medical quarantine is complete, rabbits should be kept separate by one or more barriers, such as baby gates or cages, so that they can become familiar with each other via scent, vision, and sound. Having double barriers, such as is provided by having the rabbits in separate cages that are positioned about 1.3–2.54 cm (0.5–1.0 in.) apart will make it impossible for them to injure each other by reaching through the barrier. At first, they may charge at each other, thump and/or urinate, and defecate in the section of the cage closest to the other rabbit, as a means of providing threats and marking barriers. With time, as they become familiar, hostility will generally decrease. Once this happens, housing arrangements can be changed so that there is only a single barrier between the rabbits. For example, one rabbit can be loose while one is in a cage, two cages can be placed in contact with each other, or the rabbits can be separated by a baby gate. Once they are not aggressive through this barrier, more direct introductions can be initiated.

Ideally, both rabbits should be familiarized with a harness and leash before being introduced with no barrier between them. There are harnesses designed specifically for rabbits, and many cat harnesses also work well on rabbits. While rabbits initially respond to a harness being placed on them in a fashion similar to cats, i.e., they are very inhibited in their movement, familiarity with the harness will gradually lead to ignoring its presence and moving normally. Encouraging movement while wearing the harness can be facilitated by placing the rabbit in a location where it must move a little in order to reach some tasty food, such as on a lawn, a few hops away from blooming clover. If there are more than two rabbits to be introduced, it is best to limit actual first introductions to pairs, to minimize the level of general arousal. Each rabbit should be leashed and have a separate handler. Take them both to neutral territory, that is do not do introductions in an area that one rabbit spends a lot of time in. Ideally, take them to an area where neither rabbit has been. A slightly slippery floor can be of benefit because the insecure footing discourages leaping on another rabbit to attack it. The rabbits should be allowed to approach and sniff each other. Curious mutual exploration and ritualized dominance signaling without aggression, such as one rabbit placing its head over the other rabbit, should be allowed. Some rabbits will mount. This is particularly likely if a male and female are being introduced, even if they are neutered. In most cases, mounting should be ignored, unless it escalates to fighting. Sometimes a rabbit will be particularly persistent in mounting, which can eventually lead to aggression by the rabbit being mounted, even if it was initially totally tolerant of the mounting. If one rabbit becomes aggressive, it should be gently but quickly pulled back. Some rabbit pairs will be friendly or at least neutral in their interactions quite rapidly, while others require multiple introductions before aggression ends. Occasionally, two rabbits do not ever get along, in spite of substantial effort and time spent trying to introduce them.

Once the rabbits proceed to the stage of getting along well with harnesses on, they can be allowed loose together with no harnesses, but under supervision in case a fight breaks out. Placing the rabbits in an empty bathtub can be useful in this step as, again, the insecure footing can inhibit attack behavior. Sometimes introduction cannot be readily accomplished by owners because personal attachment and/ or lack of experience make it difficult for them to remain calm if minor aggression occurs during initial interactions. In this case, introductions may best be accomplished by a veterinary technician or other person experienced with rabbits, in a location away from the home where the rabbits live.

If they engage in serious fighting, rabbits can cause substantial injury and even kill each other. During transitional stages of introduction, it is useful to have a heavy towel or blanket available. If a serious fight starts, it can most safely be disrupted by throwing the towel over the rabbits and then pushing them apart with the towel as protection for human hands from the biting and scratching that the rabbits are engaging in.

Human-directed aggression

Human-directed aggression that is not caused by a medical problem is primarily due to fear. If a rabbit has not been properly socialized and/or is mishandled so that it associates humans with frightening, painful experiences, it will be afraid of humans. Conversely, association of humans with pleasant experiences, such as being fed pieces of apple, are likely to produce rabbits that approach humans without fear.[23] Fear of humans can be decreased by even brief handling both when the rabbits are very young[24] and when they are adults (Swennes, unpublished data). While rabbits are not known for being highly dangerous animals, in good part due to their small size, their long claws can cause serious scratches, while their incisor teeth are capable of causing painful bites. If a rabbit is presented for human-directed aggression it is essential to start with a thorough physical evaluation. As with other species, discomfort and pain can lead to aggressive behavior. For example, a rabbit that has historically been friendly might start biting people whenever they attempt to rub its ears if it has ear mites. Also, as prey animals, rabbits may hide even significant injuries, so that behaviors that one might expect to change as a consequence of injury do not occur. For example, a rabbit with a broken limb bone may have a totally normal gait, but alter its reaction to humans who attempt to pick it up.

There is not a significant difference in the prevalence of human-directed aggression between intact versus neutered males or intact versus neutered females. However, if an aggressive intact rabbit of either sex is neutered or spayed, there is a significant decrease in the incidence of aggression. Neutering or spaying does not, however, eliminate all human-directed aggression, which is consistent with much human-directed aggression being caused by fear, rather than being motivated by sex hormones (Reinisch, Bergman, unpublished data).

Prevention of fear-induced aggression is accomplished by the combination of regular handling of a rabbit from a young age, so that it habituates to smells, sights, and sounds of humans, and to the sensations it will experience as it is picked up, held, touched, and petted. Equally important, the handling should not be frightening or harmful. The limbs and weight of the body should be supported at all times This is particularly important regarding the handling of rabbits by young children as, through lack of skill, co-ordination, naiveté, or other problems, they may inadvertently pick the rabbit up and carry it in an uncomfortable or frightening manner, or even drop it. If this happens, the rabbit will become classically conditioned to be frightened of humans and may begin defending itself by use of aggression. If the aggression results in people leaving it alone, the behavior will be negatively reinforced.

Treatment of the rabbit that has developed fear aggression is best done by someone who is familiar with rabbits and is comfortable interacting with them even when they are aggressive. Treatment is best begun by someone being near the rabbit with a protective barrier, such as a baby gate or a cage between the rabbit and the person. Rabbits with severe aggression may attempt to attack through the barrier, but will eventually stop reacting. Once this happens, the person can offer small treats through the barrier, beginning the process of associating the presence of humans with pleasant experiences. If, at this point, the rabbit is housed in a cage, it should not be forcefully removed unless absolutely necessary. Caregivers should wear protective leather gloves or gauntlets when they need to place their hands in the cage to change litter, etc. Once the rabbit has become non-aggressive to someone sitting immediately outside the cage, progress to direct interaction can proceed.

Protective clothing such as sturdy denim pants, shoes that cover the feet entirely, and leather gauntlets are usually adequate protection. Ideally, the rabbit should be outside of its cage, either because it has been kept in a room with a baby gate up to this point, or because the door to the cage is left open until the rabbit exits, after which the door is closed. The person carrying out the treatment should calmly sit or stand near the rabbit and not respond to attempts by the rabbit to drive them off. Once the rabbit ceases responding in an aggressive fashion, the handler can begin offering the rabbit treats and/or gently petting it. Eventually, proceed to gentle restraint, lifting, and holding. If a rabbit has had a very traumatic experience at the hands of a human, this process can take weeks or even months. Rabbits that have been successfully treated can be susceptible to relapse. The best way to prevent a relapse is to ensure that anyone who interacts with the rabbit is physically capable of handling it appropriately and knows how to do so.

Chewing and digging

Rabbits have long, strong front claws for digging into dirt and creating a warren. In the wild, rabbits also chew a lot of herbage in their environment, some of it very tough. In the domestic environment, these behaviors remain as natural, normal behaviors for this species. If the pet rabbit is not provided with ways to dig and chew that are acceptable and safe, it is likely to engage in digging and chewing behaviors that are dangerous and/or destructive. For example, the rabbit may chew electric cords, and dig holes in furniture cushions. Therefore, household areas where rabbits will be allowed to run loose need to rabbit-proofed, particularly in terms of safety issues. Electrical and other cords should be wrapped with duct tape, run through PVC pipe, or otherwise made inaccessible to rabbits. Valuable items should be placed up high, out of the rabbit's reach.

Various toys that are designed for rabbits can provide suitable substrates for chewing. Parrot toys are also mostly safe for rabbits. While most people provide objects for the rabbit to chew on the floor, hanging an object, such as from the roof of the rabbit's housing or some other object, will sometimes stimulate the rabbit to rear up to interact with the toy. Rabbits that do not have toys available will chew in the interior of their cage, feed bins, and other structures. Rabbits that have toys available to chew on spend significantly more time chewing than do rabbits that do not have toys (Poggiagliolmi, unpublished data). Since the rabbit's teeth grow continuously throughout life, facilitating chewing by offering appropriate toys may help prevent dental problems. A basket or box filled with hay can provide the rabbit with an area to dig in. Given sufficient hay, domestic rabbit's will even dig and arrange the hay so as to form a kind of warren, complete with tunnels and resting rooms.

Environmental enrichment

Small cages, such as are often available in pet stores, are not suitable for continuous housing of the pet rabbit. They are derived from keeping rabbits as meat animals, and fail to address a number of requirements for optimizing the rabbit's welfare, including the provision of adequate space for a rabbit to move and explore its environment, as well as objects to chew, manipulate, and explore.[9,25–27] Suitably large rabbit housing is now available through many providers of pet rabbit equipment. Small cages can be suitable as areas for resting and retreating from the activity of the household, at night, and when no one is home to ensure supervision, especially in a mixed species household. If the rabbit is allowed access to a sufficiently large area of the house, it can self-exercise by hopping around. Rabbits can also be trained to hop on a harness and leash and taken outside for "walks" or, more precisely, hops (Figure 7.4a and b). It is important to make sure that they are walked only on lawns that are free of herbicides and pesticides. Providing a rabbit with substrates that they can safely dig in and chew on is also important.

Large outdoor enclosures have advantages and disadvantages. An outdoor enclosure can be used to provide the rabbit with the space and resources to engage in vigorous activities such as digging, which may not be possible even if the rabbit is allowed access to a large house. However, care must be taken to make sure the play space is predator proof, or else the rabbit must be continuously supervised when it is outside. Do not leave a rabbit outside in extremely hot or cold temperatures, or other severe weather. In addition, being outside potentially exposes the rabbit to insect attack, including flies, fleas, and mosquitoes. Rabbits that are in a location where they may be exposed to flies, whether it is inside or outside, should be checked frequently, at least twice a day, for signs of maggots. Checking the skin and hair for any sign of other parasites is also important. In areas where mosquitoes are a problem, covering the outdoor housing with mosquito netting can be useful, and the mosquito netting can block access by flies as well. Using citronella around the housing may be useful, but citronella should not be used within the housing or on the rabbit, as the rabbit's grooming can lead to ingestion.

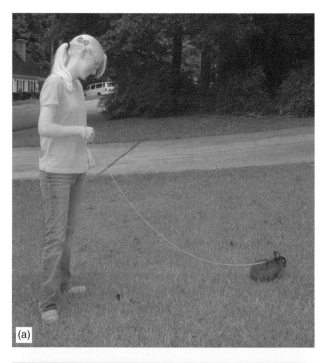

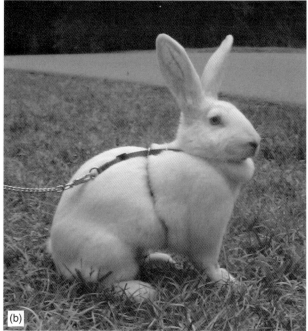

Figure 7.4(a and b) Rabbits can be trained to go on "hops," using a harness and leash.

Ways to maintain a behaviorally healthy pet rabbit:

1. Socialize it to humans and other rabbits when it is young.
2. Always pick up and carry a rabbit in a way that provides adequate support for its limbs and its body.
3. Have more than one rabbit. Wild rabbits socialize in small groups. Having other, familiar rabbits in the household gives the pet rabbit a playmate and grooming companion.

4. Provide environmental enrichment via toys to play with and acceptable digging sites.
5. Make sure the rabbit has frequent, preferably daily, opportunities to exercise and explore its environment.
   (a) Provide your rabbit with access to one or more rooms of the house for at least part of the day.
   (b) Take the rabbit on walks, but make sure it is not exposed to pesticides or herbicides.
   (c) Provide a large outdoor enclosure, making sure to protect the rabbit from predators, insects, and severe weather.
6. Neuter male rabbits to decrease the likelihood of urine spraying.

Acknowledgments

Except where otherwise noted, all photos in this chapter are courtesy of the author.

References

1. Sandford JC. Notes on the history of the rabbit. *J Appl Rabbit Res* 1992;15:1–28.
2. United States Department of Agriculture. U.S. Rabbit Industry Profile;2002.
3. Monclús R, Rödel HG. Different forms of vigilance in response to the presence of predators and conspecifics in a group-living mammal, the European rabbit. *Ethology* 2008;114:287–297.
4. Cowan DP. Group living in the European rabbit (*Oryctolagus cuniculus*): Mutual benefit or resource localization? *J Anim Ecol* 1987;56:779–795.
5. Lockley RM. *The Private Life of the Rabbit.* New York, NY: Macmillan Publishing Co, 1903;27–70.
6. Mykytowycz R. Territorial marking by rabbits. *Sci Am* 1968;218:116–126.
7. Mykytowycz R, Fullagar PJ. Effect of social environment on reproduction in the rabbit, *Oryctolagus cuniculus. J Reprod Fertil Suppl* 1973;19:503–522.
8. Crowell-Davis SL. Behavior problems in pet rabbits *J Ex Pet Med* 2007;16:38–44.
9. Hulls WL, Brooks DL, Beans-Knudsen D. Response of adult New Zealand white rabbits to enrichment objects and paired housing. *Lab Anim Sci* 1991;41:609–612.
10. Love JA. Group housing: Meeting the physical and social needs of the laboratory rabbit. *Lab Anim Sci* 1994;44:5–11.
11. Whary M, Peper R, Borkowski G et al. The effects of group housing on the research use of the laboratory rabbit. *Lab Anim* 1993;27:330–341.
12. Nelissen M. On the diurnal rhythm of activity of *Oryctolagus cuniculus* (Linne, 1758). *Acta Zool Pathol Antverp* 1975;61:3–18.
13. Southern HN. The ecology and population dynamics of the wild rabbit (*Oryctolagus cuniculus*). *Ann Appl Biol* 1940;27:509–526.
14. Stodart E, Myers K. A comparison of behavior, reproduction, and mortality of wild and domestic rabbits in confined populations. *CSIRO Wildl Res* 1964;9:144–159.
15. Bagley LH, Lavach D. Ophthalmic diseases of rabbits. *Calif Vet* 1995;49:7–9.
16. Mykytowycz R. Reproduction of mammals in relation to environmental odours. *J Reprod Fertil Suppl* 1973;19:443–446.
17. Fennessy BV, Mykytowycz R. Rabbit behavior research in Australia and its relevance in control operations. In: Fennessy BV, ed. *Proceedings 6th Vertebrate Pest Conference: Rabbit Behavior Research in Australia and its Relevance in Control Operations.* University of Nebraska-Lincoln, 1974;184–187.
18. Lehmann M. Social behavior in young domestic rabbits under seminatural conditions. *Appl Anim Behav Sci* 1991;32:269–292.
19. Coureaud G, Rödel HG, Kurz CA et al. The responsiveness of young rabbits to the mammary pheromone: Developmental course in domestic and wild pups. *Chemoecol* 2008;18:53–59.
20. Harcourt-Brown F. Diet and husbandry. In: *Textbook of Rabbit Medicine.* Edinburgh: Butterworth Heinemann, 2002;19–51.
21. Lockley RM. Social structure and stress in the rabbit warren. *J Anim Ecol* 1961;30:385–423.
22. Bigler L, Oester H. Paarhaltung nichtreproduzieren-der Hauskaninchen-Zibben im Käfig [Raising pairs of young non-reproductive female rabbits in cages]. *Berl Munch tierarztl* Wochenschr 1994;10:202–205.
23. Davis H, Gibson JA. Can rabbits tell humans apart? Discrimination of individual humans and its implications for animal research. *Comp Med* 2000;5:483–485.
24. Csatádi K, Kustos K, Eiben Cs. et al. Even minimal human contact linked to nursing reduces fear responses toward humans in rabbits. *Appl Anim Behav Sci* 1995;205:123–128.
25. Baumans V. Environmental enrichment for laboratory rodents and rabbits: Requirements of rodents, rabbits, and research. *ILAR J* 2005;46:162–170.
26. Hansen LT, Berthelsen H. The effect of environmental enrichment on the behavior of caged rabbits (*Oryctolagus cuniculus*). *Appl Anim Behav Sci* 2000;68:163–178.
27. Maertens L, De Groote G. Influence of the number of fryer rabbits per cage on their performance. *J Appl Rabbit Res* 1984;7:151–155.

8

Guinea pigs

YeunShin Lee

History

Phylogenetic information on the evolutionary history of the subfamily Caviinae is limited due to an incomplete fossil record. Thus comparisons between extant wild caviomorph rodents (spp. *Microcavia*, *Galea*, and *Cavia*) and the domesticated guinea pig (*Cavia porcellus*) yield inferential results at best. With this in mind, evidence suggests that although the guinea pig is larger than its putative wild ancestor, the cavy (*Cavia aperea*),[1] it retains the same range of behavior patterns, with differences appearing in the frequencies and thresholds for expression of the behaviors. For instance, captive-housed wild cavies tend to be more aggressive and explore more than domestic guinea pigs housed under identical conditions. On the other hand, domestic guinea pigs will engage in more sociopositive behaviors (grooming and nudging) and courtship than wild cavies.[2–4] Less reactive stress axes in the domestic guinea pig when compared to wild cavies have been proposed as the mechanism behind these differences in behavior.[3]

Natural history of wild cavies (*Cavia aperea*)

Cavies are medium-sized, agouti-colored rodents with either a short tail or lacking one altogether and bilateral secretory anal glands. Broadly distributed across Venezuela, Colombia, and northern Argentina, they are the most abundant mammal species found in Argentina and are conferred "pest" status in some regions.[4] Thus, the IUCN (International Union for Conservation of Nature) Red List continues to list cavies as species of "lower risk/least concern."[5]

Cavies observe predominantly diurnal behavior patterns with crepuscular bouts of activity. In the wild, this pattern may be due to the animals' aversion to intense sun exposure. Cavies forage largely on short grasses, but will also consume forbs, leaves, and bark. Though cavies occupy semi-arid habitats, they do not avoid water and have been observed wading in puddles and even swimming several kilometers after floods.[4]

Cavies are socially tolerant and spend a significant proportion of their day foraging in mixed-sex, mixed-age groups (see Figure 8.1). Aggression, when it does occur, tends to arise between same-sex adults, typically males, and between adult females and dispersal-aged adolescents.[4] Cavies frequently interrupt feeding bouts to dash toward cover. Once near shelter they will freeze, seeking refuge only if the potential predator approaches to within a few meters. Cover-seeking occurs in response to both visual and auditory cues, is often contagious, and can be elicited by heterospecific cues such as avian alarm calls. Cavies travel through home ranges over paths trampled in

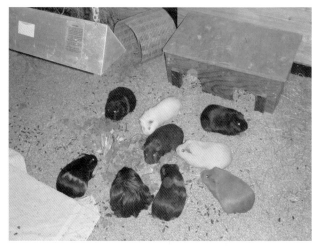

Figure 8.1 In captivity, given enough space guinea pigs will live together peacefully. (Photo courtesy of Lisa Nelson, VMD.)

the grass with latrines at intervals along the paths.[6] Cavies tend not to occupy exclusive home ranges, with most of the overlap occurring at resources such as food and water.[4] However, a single male will often control a territory that encompasses those of several females.[7,8] Social hierarchies, once established, are fairly stable, as are home ranges which are relatively large for such a small mammal, ranging from 1575 m^2 (5167 ft^2) for females to 2475 m^2 (8120 ft^2) for males.[6]

The domestic guinea pig

The guinea pig, or "cuy" as it is called by Native Americans from the Central Andes, has existed in close association with humans for approximately 3000 years. Initial contact between humans and the guinea pig's wild ancestor is hypothesized to have occurred inadvertently through guinea pigs opportunistically scavenging on human garbage. Humans subsequently domesticated the guinea pig as a food source and/or pet, functions which guinea pigs serve to this day[9] (Figure 8.2).

The guinea pig currently fills a wide variety of roles, ranging from pet to animal model for human disease. Because the guinea pig is such an appealing laboratory animal, it has been used extensively as an experimental subject. This versatility in function can be attributed, in part, to their relatively low maintenance, space requirements, and tractability.

Senses and communication

Vision

Early histological and behavioral studies of guinea pig vision described guinea pigs as possessing "pure rod-eyes,"[10,11] leading to the assumption that guinea pigs lacked color vision. Later histological examinations of guinea pig retinas confirmed the presence of both rods and cones in the

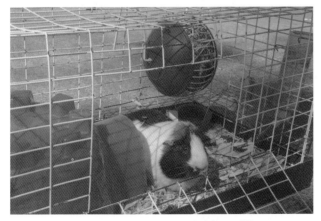

Figure 8.2 A pet guinea pig in a cage typical of those sold by pet stores for housing large pet rodents. (Photo courtesy of M. C. Tynes, copyright 2010.)

guinea pig eye, though rods outnumbered cones by a 4:1 ratio.[12] A recently developed technique that specifically labeled the outer segments of green- and blue-sensitive cones in mammals[13] led to the identification of both types of cones in the guinea pig retina.[14] Further physiological and behavioral studies provided supporting evidence that guinea pigs do indeed possess dichromatic color vision.[15]

Collectively, these and subsequent studies have revealed that guinea pigs possess retinas with rods (peak sensitivity: 494–500 nm),[15–17] S cones (peak sensitivity: 400–420 nm), and M cones (peak sensitivity: 520–540 nm).[15,17] Since guinea pig vision is limited to the visible spectrum, they do not require any special lighting conditions when housed indoors. Thus, standard housing practices for guinea pigs recommend that guinea pigs be housed under a 12–14:12–10 L:D illumination cycle of 325 lux at 1 m above the floor.[18,19]

Olfaction

Guinea pigs utilize olfactory cues for individual recognition. Typically they initiate social encounters with a brief nose–nose investigation, often followed by nuzzling around the muzzle area, also known as a kiss. Depending upon the information gathered and conveyed during this greeting ritual, the encounter can either escalate into aggression or settle into an affiliative interaction.[4] Beauchamp demonstrated that olfactory bulbectomy in group-housed male guinea pigs resulted in disruption of sexual activity, failure to form species-typical dominance hierarchies, almost complete elimination of male-on-male aggression, and a reduction in scent-marking.[20] In a discrimination learning study, male and female guinea pigs successfully discriminated among odors of colony-mates from swabbings of the ano-genital region and control non-specific odors. Both sexes also demonstrated they could learn to distinguish between swabbings collected from females in and out of estrus.[21]

The guinea pig vomeronasal organ has been implicated in the maintenance of behavioral responses to repeatedly presented olfactory stimuli. Male guinea pigs with their vomeronasal organ removed were less likely to investigate conspecific urine than males subjected to a sham surgery. With repeated exposure over 6.3 months postoperatively, males without vomeronasal organs eventually investigated water as much as conspecific urine. Interestingly the males who had undergone vomeronasal organ removal continued to express a preference for female over male urine. They also did not exhibit any change in social or sexual behaviors, unlike the differences in behavior described earlier when guinea pigs underwent bulbectomy.[22] Apparently, the change in responsiveness over time observed in the males who had undergone vomeronasal organ removal is an example of behavioral extinction. Male guinea pigs presented with female guinea pig urine for the first time 15 weeks postoperatively investigated the urine at levels similar to males who had just undergone the surgery and for longer durations than other males 15 weeks after surgery who had first been exposed to female urine immediately afterward.[23] The influence on behavior of the vomeronasal organ is age dependent. Male guinea pigs who had their vomeronasal organs removed at 4–7 days of age did not exhibit differences in behavioral responses to olfactory stimuli when compared to males who underwent sham surgery (also at 4–7 days of age) until after they became sexually mature.[24]

Olfactory cues in urine provide information about the individual's gender and reproductive condition. Sexually experienced males prefer non-receptive female urine over intact male urine.[25] Gonadal hormones appear to play a role in the recognition process. When the same sexually experienced males were presented with urine from castrated males or ovariectomized females, their responses began to change 14 days postoperatively. The males preferred the urine of ovariectomized females up to 14 days after surgery over intact male urine, but the preference was extinguished beyond this point. With urine from castrated males, the subject males did not distinguish between castrated male urine and sham castrated male urine until 14 days postoperatively.[25] This author suggests that urinary gonadal metabolites, both ovarian and testicular, may continue to exert a residual olfactory effect up to 14 days postoperatively, contra Beauchamp.[25] Although these effects may operate as potent signals, the signals produced by females tend to be fleeting. When presented with urine that had dried for 3 hours, males could no longer discriminate between a sample collected from a familiar female versus one collected from an unfamiliar female. However, the same males demonstrated that they could distinguish their own urine from other male urine that had dried for up to 8 days.[26]

Olfactory cues contribute to the formation and maintenance of the mother–offspring and filial bonds. Guinea pig pups demonstrated preferences for stimulus guinea pigs anointed with the synthetic odor with which they had been reared over stimulus guinea pigs with either natural or an unfamiliar synthetic odor.[27] Urinary olfactory cues also play a role in offspring recognition of their mothers. Beginning at 5 days of age and definitely by 10 days, pups preferred their own mother's urine over urine from a lactating, unfamiliar, unrelated female, a lactating unfamiliar, related female, and a familiar unrelated female, but not urine from a familiar, related female. By the age of 1 month, roughly the age at which guinea pigs become independent from their mothers, the ability to discriminate among females waned.[28]

Perineal gland secretions may convey even more information than urine. Male guinea pigs distinguished between urine of two individuals when primed with the sebum from the perineal gland of those two individuals first. However, they failed to distinguish between the sebum from two individuals when presented with those individuals' urine first. Thus, male guinea pigs appear to generalize information about individual identity obtained from perineal gland secretions to urine, but not vice versa.[29] However, the cues appear to be short-lived, as males ceased to discriminate their own sebum from that of an unfamiliar male after 72 hours.[30]

Another role of perineal gland secretions may be to communicate information about and help maintain stable dominance hierarchies. Beauchamp found that although sebum production from perineal glands prior to social group formation did not predict social rank, after group formation, the amount of sebum secreted positively correlated with social rank, as did the frequency of scent-marking/perineal gland drag. Changes in the amount of sebum production subsequent to disruption in the social hierarchy also mirrored the direction of rank change.[31] Apparently, social rank also affects the quality of perineal gland sebum produced by an individual. Males responded with more aggressive behaviors when presented with the sebum of higher than lower ranking males.[32]

Guinea pig responses to olfactory stimuli may serve as an excellent environmental enrichment opportunity. The aforementioned studies demonstrate that guinea pigs investigate and scent-mark when presented with conspecific olfactory stimuli. These types of behavioral responses imply that guinea pigs become aroused when presented with such stimuli. Therefore, an interesting experiment may be to determine a regimen for the presentation of conspecific olfactory stimuli, the frequency of which would challenge the guinea pigs without actually causing them distress.

Audition

The hearing range, auditory anatomy, and sensitivities of guinea pigs have been well documented. Some variability in the reported values of the guinea pig peak acoustic sensitivity range exists, though the majority of the sources overlapped around 4–8 kHz.[33–41] In addition, because they are capable of detecting sounds up to 30–46.5 kHz,[35,39] guinea pigs are capable of hearing and possibly communicating well into ultrasound (>20 kHz). The large range in values reflects the large range of methodologies used to obtain this information.[33,34,36,42]

The response of several rodent species, including guinea pigs, to high intensity noise has been extensively studied.[43,44] Although all three species responded with increased HPA (hypothalamic–pituitary–adrenal)-axis activity, guinea pigs tended to be more sensitive to the acoustic stimuli than rats or mice, as indicated by a greater latency to resume normal behaviors after noise exposure.[43] One study demonstrated that male guinea pigs exposed to high intensity noises for 6 weeks tended to have smaller adrenal and thymus glands and more gastric pitting than controls.[44]

The preceding studies raise an issue regarding housing conditions for guinea pigs. Although most facilities have eliminated or at least attempt to minimize the opportunities for guinea pigs to receive chronic exposure to high intensity noises, managed environments immerse the animals in an evolutionarily novel acoustic milieu. Thus, captive guinea

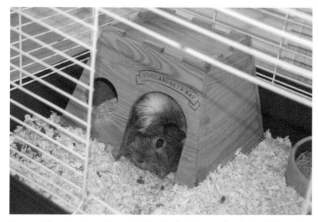

Figure 8.3   A guinea pig, startled by loud noises, seeks shelter. (Photo courtesy of M. C. Tynes, copyright 2010.)

pigs are continuously bombarded by anthropogenic noise from which they cannot escape (see Figure 8.3). Loss of control from not being able to escape such stimuli could compound an already potentially stressful experience and compromise their well-being. Although progress has been made to improve conditions for animals in captivity, for example References [45,46–57], the effect of ambient anthropogenic noises on guinea pigs has yet to be examined and further study is needed.

Vocalizations

The guinea pig vocal repertoire consists of 11 vocalizations: chut, purr, chutter, whine, low whistle, squeal, scream, tweet, drrr, and chirrup. These fall loosely into five functional categories as proposed by Berryman: increase proximity, greeting/maintain proximity, regain proximity, pain/distress, and alarm.[58] While some vocalizations clearly fit into a single category, such as a scream which is issued only by the loser of an aggressive encounter or when the individual is in pain, others, such as the purr or drrr, are emitted under a broader range of contexts spanning from sexual encounters to mother–offspring interactions and can often be contagious.[58] In addition, some vocalizations can convey information about the social status of the individual. For instance, the purr is issued only by the subordinate individual in paired fights.[59]

Much of the research on guinea pig vocalizations has concentrated on either brain mapping or behavioral reactions to vocalizations, predominantly pup isolation calls. Brain mapping studies have identified regions responsible for the production of specific calls: the dorsomedial thalamus elicited pup-like isolation calls from adult guinea pigs, the mesencephalic region surrounding the periventricular gray caused subjects to scream,[60] and the periaqueductal gray triggered low whistles and purrs.[61]

Playback experiments comparing the responses of pups, virgin females, and lactating females reveal that age and reproductive state determine the level of responsiveness to conspecific vocalizations. Pups responded similarly to conspecific vocalizations and single frequency tones. In all instances, pups tended to freeze whenever a playback was heard. Although they were more responsive to conspecific adult vocalizations, virgin females were also likely to freeze in response to both conspecific vocalizations and single tone frequencies. Most significantly, they did not exhibit any discernable behavioral changes when played pup vocalizations. Lactating females, on the other hand, discriminated among the stimuli, with infant vocalizations eliciting the most pronounced responses.[62]

As with olfactory cues, vocalizations appear to influence the formation and maintenance of the mother–offspring bond. Female guinea pigs need to learn to recognize their own pups' isolation calls. Lactating mothers consistently respond to pup isolation calls and do so preferentially to calls from their own pups over all other vocalizations, including calls of unfamiliar pups.[63] In contrast, neither fathers[64] nor pregnant guinea pigs[63] exhibited responses to pup isolation calls. This heightened sensitivity to pup isolation calls in lactating females is temporary and begins to wane after the first week postpartum.[64] The ability of lactating females to differentiate between vocalizations of their own pups from unfamiliar pups seems to imply that pup isolation calls carry information about the identity of the individual. In fact, individual differences in pup isolation calls have been identified by acoustic analysis.[65] For guinea pig pups, pairing a moving fuzzy model with conspecific vocalizations increased the likelihood that pups isolated immediately after birth would initiate and maintain contact with the model.[66] Thus for pups, conspecific vocalizations appear to increase the salience of mother-like visual and tactile stimuli.

In addition to providing information about individual identity, pup isolation calls may convey information about the pup's condition. For instance, the call rate emitted by isolated pups is influenced by social context and separation duration. Solitary pups placed in a novel enclosure with a mesh top called at the highest rate.[67–70] Presence of their mother,[67,68,70] even when unconscious,[68] or when physical contact was prevented,[70] and presence of littermates[69] resulted in a slower call rate. Duration of separation has an interesting effect on call rate. After 15 minutes of isolation in a wooden box, pups reduced the length of their calls, thus increasing their call rate.[71] However, beginning at 30 minutes post-isolation in a clear-sided, uncovered novel cage pups began to reduce their call rate and locomotion.[72] By 90 minutes they had dramatically reduced their call rate.[73] Hennessy and colleagues noted that this reduction in call rate was accompanied by behaviors associated with the "despair" phase of the maternal separation response[74] and hypothesized that it may be indicative of a complex known as "stress-induced sickness behaviors."[75] They also demonstrated that the reduction in rate reflects, in part, the high concentration of HPA-axis hormones circulation in the pups' bloodstream by this time. When they injected CRH (corticotropin-releasing hormone) peripherally to 20-day old pups 1 hour prior to separation, the pups issued isolation calls immediately upon separation at a rate usually not seen until after 60–90 minutes of isolation.[76] Some sex differences in response do exist. When isolated in a novel enclosure, males tend to vocalize more while females exhibit a higher cortisol response.[68] However, female pups vocalized more than males while in their home cages with their mothers removed.[77]

In their study, Hennessy and Ritchie observed an unusual response from guinea pig pups. They noticed that despite the novelty of the environment, pups placed alone in an enclosure with solid walls and top, as opposed to a mesh top, neither vocalized nor exhibited a rise in plasma cortisol levels.[68] Perhaps the mesh top lent to the perception of exposure whereas the solid top provided the pups with a sense of security similar to a shelter. Thus, it appears as if the maternal separation response can be modified by the physical characteristics of the surroundings in which the isolated pups find themselves and that separation from their mother alone may not necessarily be sufficient to trigger a full-blown response.

The body of research conducted on pup isolation calls has yielded information that can be applied toward preserving the welfare of guinea pig pups. Since isolated pups appear to be affected by their perception of exposure, when pups need to be removed from their mothers, it is recommended that they are placed in enclosures or cages with solid tops. Additionally, because pups find maternal separations that exceed 1 hour to be distressing, separations greater than 1 hour should be avoided if possible. However, waiting until the 1 hour point may already have subjected the pups to a state of compromised welfare, as indicated by their elevated HPA-axis hormones and expression of the "stress-induced sickness behavior" complex. Thus, since call rate is likely to fall off gradually, the appropriate time to intervene and terminate a maternal separation may be as soon as a change in call rate is detected.

Locomotion

Guinea pigs are strictly fossorial so their primary means of locomotion are walking and running. Young guinea pigs during play and sexually aroused adults will perform frisky hops as well.[4] When startled, guinea pigs may leap and then dash away from the startling stimulus.[78] Although not noted for their climbing abilities, if provided with shelters in their cages, guinea pigs will occasionally climb onto them (*pers. obs.*).

Social behavior

Studies on colony-housed guinea pigs revealed that they can express intraspecific variation in social systems (IVSS)[79]

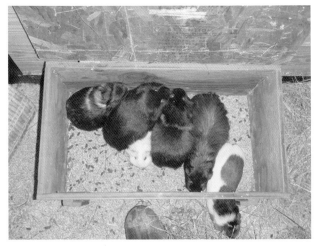

Figure 8.4   Group-housed guinea pigs sharing a shelter. (Photo courtesy of Lisa Nelson, VMD.)

in response to different population densities (Figure 8.4). Thus at lower population densities, male guinea pigs organize themselves into linear[58,59,80,81] and occasionally despotic[82] dominance hierarchies while females form loose, flexible dominance hierarchies.[80] Under this social organization, adults will engage in sociopositive behaviors opportunistically. For instance, King reported that his guinea pigs would huddle together only when they were exposed to the elements or follow one another when frightened and that they did not exhibit any particular social preferences among colony members.[80] When males establish themselves in this kind of hierarchy, they pursue a polygynous mating system, with the alpha male obtaining the greatest numbers of copulations.[58,59,80–82] In contrast, at higher densities, males become territorial,[81,83] forming strong attachments to only a few females and almost completely disregarding other females; even ones in estrus.[81,84,85]

A considerable amount of research has been conducted on guinea pig social behavior. Studies have examined the formation of social attachments, the effects of long-term isolation on social responses, the influence of adult males on the development of pup social behavior, the impact of social buffering on responses to novel environments, and the effect of pre-natal stress on later social tendencies. Most of this research has been conducted on males,[81] perhaps because the process of male hierarchy formation and the outcomes of that process are so conspicuous whereas females tend to be more subtle. Thus, we know that males take approximately 1 month to form a stable linear dominance hierarchy,[80] dominant males are more likely to scent-mark,[86] males who form attachments to females in response to high population densities are more likely to acquire territories and that nomadic, but bonded males rank below bonded territory holders but above non-bonded males.[81,83] In contrast, throughout most of these studies, females are described as passive recipients of male attention[81,83,85] and, in some cases, are defined as "owned" by males.[81,83]

Pup social attachment

Pups can readily discriminate between their mothers and unrelated adults. Although they will interact with unrelated adults when provided the opportunity, the quality of these interactions differs substantially from interactions with their mothers.[86] And, given a choice, guinea pig pups raised with their mother will consistently prefer her over other social alternatives[66,87,88] with the exception of their littermates.[88] This preference manifests physiologically as well: prior to weaning, presence of the mother can attenuate the stress response in pups exposed to a novel environment.[89] However, this response is context-specific: plasma cortisol does not rise in response to removal of the mother from the home cage.[73] The strength of the maternal attachment can be varied depending upon rearing condition and age of pups. Pups will imprint upon an inanimate, fuzzy object when removed from their mothers and isolated immediately after birth.[66,90] Furthermore, pups who had imprinted upon the inanimate object remained responsive to it even after exposure to and experience nursing on their mothers.[66] The age effects on social preferences begin to manifest around weaning. Despite their preference for their mother, as pups begin to approach weaning age, they will gradually spend more time with an unrelated female stimulus.[88]

Isolation effects

It appears as if isolation from birth does not profoundly affect either social or reproductive behavior. Generally speaking, both male and female guinea pigs isolated from birth demonstrated competence at interacting with other guinea pigs as adults and eventually reproduced.[91] However, unlike with females, the *quality* of social interactions isolate males are capable of engaging in does appear to suffer from long-term isolation (see later for impact on sexual behavior). Nagy observed that isolation-reared pups were more hesitant at approaching like-aged congeners than either communal- or mother-reared pups.[92] Also, in contrast with either colony-reared or older, socially experienced males, 7–8 month old isolate males failed to integrate themselves when introduced to either a colony[93] or a small group of 1 adult male and 2 adult females.[94] Additionally, in these experiments, the isolation-reared males lost significant amounts of weight, had higher plasma glucocorticoids levels,[93] and decreased complement system activity[94] when compared to both the colony-reared and socially experienced older males.

Adult male effect studies

Although adult males do not actively participate in rearing offspring, nor are they a preferred social partner, it appears as if they play a vital role in the development of normal social behaviors of guinea pig pups. Pups raised in a colony without adult males did not initiate aggressive and sexual behaviors until puberty[95] in contrast to pups raised in colonies with males, who began to express aggressive and sexual behaviors at weaning.[96] Adult males appear to exert their greatest influence during the period between weaning and puberty.[97] One group of studies found that male guinea pig pups, isolated from all adult males from 30 days to 6–7 months of age, demonstrated markedly higher levels of male–male aggression later in life.[98,99] The endocrine profiles of the male pups not exposed to adult males between weaning and puberty rose more quickly and remained at higher levels than the male pups who remained in the colony beyond puberty.[98,99]

The most significant behavioral differences between the pups with male exposure from weaning to puberty and those without were that pups not exposed to males escalated to frank aggression and initiated sexual behavior much more quickly than pups with adult male exposure.[100] Most notably, pups with male exposure successfully integrated themselves into a new mixed-age and sex colony, at times achieving higher ranks than those held in their natal colony; whereas pups without male exposure completely failed at social integration in a new colony.[93]

Social buffering studies

Similar to the behavior patterns observed in primates,[101,102] guinea pig pups are more likely to explore in an open field while in visual (and possibly olfactory and auditory) contact with their mothers and littermates as opposed to when their mothers and littermates are absent.[103] While guinea pigs perceive short-term isolation in a novel environment as quite stressful, the amount of stress experienced can be buffered by the presence of familiar, and in some cases, unfamiliar social companions. Pre-weaning[72,89,104] pups and to a lesser degree periadolescents (after weaning but prior to onset of puberty)[72,104] vocalized less, locomoted more, and exhibited fewer "stress-induced sickness behaviors" when accompanied by their mothers in a clear, uncovered novel cage than when placed in the novel cage alone. In periadolescents, cortisol rose significantly after 60 minutes of isolation in an uncovered, novel environment, regardless of postweaning social grouping. However, when placed in the same novel environment with a cagemate (either their mother or littermate) or, for male periadolescents in particular, with an unfamiliar female, they vocalized at a much slower rate[104,105] and exhibited a dampened cortisol response.[89,104] The unfamiliar female exerts this social buffering effect despite the fact that they subject the pups to significantly more aggression than the pups' mothers.[106] Presence of an unfamiliar adult male does not have a similar buffering effect.[107] Social buffering also occurs in pair-bonded adult males, but only when their female partner accompanies them.[85,100] Adult females are somewhat less selective. Although, accompaniment by their pair-bonded male partner results in the greatest buffering effect, a familiar male with whom they are not bonded can also reduce their cortisol responses.[108]

Pre-natal stress

Maternal effects can influence the development of social behavior in guinea pig pups. Social instability during pregnancy and through lactation masculinizes social behavior in daughters[109–111] and infantilizes social behavior in sons.[112,113] These alterations in behavior likely reflect changes in the endocrine systems of both daughters and sons. Daughters of mothers exposed to an unstable social environment (UE) during pregnancy and lactation had higher circulating levels of testosterone,[114] higher sympathoadrenal system reactivity,[110] and upregulation in androgen and estrogen receptor responsiveness in limbic system neurons.[111] In contrast, UE sons had lower circulating testosterone levels,[114] higher HPA-axis activity, lower sympathoadrenal system reactivity,[112] and downregulation in androgen receptor responsiveness in limbic system neurons.[113] Although the mechanisms for these changes in behavior have not yet been completely identified, Kaiser and colleagues observed that UE mothers exhibited more defensive aggression toward males and lower circulating androgen levels than mothers housed in a stable social environment (SE) during pregnancy.[115] In sons, these alterations in behavior and endocrine profiles do not appear to impose long-term detrimental effects. Adult UE sons demonstrated competence at establishing stable social dominance hierarchies with SE sons, despite lower HPA-axis reactivity.[114] They also did not express any deficit in their ability to cope with an UE.[116] Research has yet to be conducted on UE daughters in this regard.

Welfare implications

Ironically, although the social behavior of male guinea pigs is significantly affected by isolation rearing and isolation or pair housing, under standard laboratory protocol, males are most likely to be housed either alone or in male–female pairs. However, the preceding studies on adult male effects imply that group housing of males can be a viable, and more welfare-friendly, alternative as long as male pups are reared through puberty with adult, sexually, and socially mature males. Furthermore, because males provided with individual shelters established stable dominance hierarchies more quickly than males provided with a single group shelter,[117] environmental enrichment using individual shelters may greatly facilitate group formation (see Figure 8.5).

Reproductive behavior

In general, male guinea pigs tend to be more sexually motivated than females, as indicated by the males' willingness

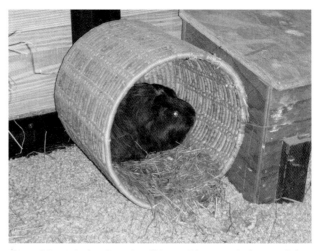

Figure 8.5   A single guinea pig utilizing a wicker waste basket as a shelter. (Photo courtesy of Lisa Nelson, VMD.)

to overcome obstacles and the speed with which they do so to gain access to a female. Males will scramble through an obstruction box more quickly when a female is placed in the goal box than if the goal box is empty.[118] While males denied sexual contact for at least 6 days will negotiate the obstruction box significantly more quickly.[119] Sex differences also emerge in hormone profiles. While sexual behavior is at its peak immediately after pairing males and females together, male and not female, plasma oxytocin levels rise. In contrast, female oxytocin levels appear to reflect the amount of social contact the pair engages in after sexual activity peaks. Both sexes do respond similarly, however, with a rise in oxytocin when an unfamiliar male is introduced.[119] The onset of puberty in males, and not females, is sensitive to photoperiod. Thus, male guinea pigs raised with a long photoperiod (L18:D6) reached puberty weight and plasma testosterone levels earlier than males reared with a short one (L6:D18).[120] Typically, breeding onset for females is between 2 and 3 months, while males begin breeding between 3 and 4 months of age.[18]

Females

Guinea pigs are capable of breeding throughout the year, with females entering estrus for approximately 8 hours[121] every 13–24 days and producing up to 4 litters per year. Considerable individual variation is seen in female guinea pig sexual behavior. However, three distinct stages in the cycle can be identified through behavior alone. When a female enters proestrus, as many as 2 days before estrus, she begins to perform many behaviors associated with male sexual behavior, including the "rumba", mounting and thrusting once mounted, and will direct these behaviors indiscriminately toward any guinea pig. In the meantime, she will continue to exhibit defensive aggression toward any courting male.[122] Commencement of estrus can be distinguished by a sudden spike in mounting behavior[123] followed by quiescence typified by the complete absence of defensive aggression. At this point, a guinea pig in estrus will readily assume the lordotic position in response to any tactile stimulation of her back or hindquarters. As estrus progresses, it becomes increasingly difficult to elicit lordosis.[122] While in estrus, a female is more likely to explore, investigate conspecifics, and scent-mark than she is either prior to or after estrus.[124,125] Estrus is immediately terminated by vaginal exposure to hormones in the male guinea pig ejaculate.[126] With the inception of diestrus, the female guinea pig will immediately resume defensive aggression toward courting males.[122]

Males

The male guinea pig sexual pattern typically begins with naso–anal investigation, where the male sniffs, licks, nuzzles, and occasionally nudges the perineal region of the female. Next, the male will follow the female with his nose touching her rump (chin-rump follow) and then perform a "rumba" slowly approaching the female with his head lowered, swaying his rump from side-to-side while emitting burble vocalizations, and everting his anal glands. Males may also perform rumping, where they attempt to raise one or both of their hind legs over the rump or back of the female. Often, the male will urinate while rumping. Finally, if the female assumes lordosis, the male will mount her, clasping her with his front legs and perform rapid pelvic thrusts to achieve intromission and ultimately ejaculation.[4] In most cases, males become satiated after a single ejaculation,[127] but this state can easily be reversed by introducing the male to a novel female.[128]

Although isolation rearing does not completely impair sexual performance in male guinea pigs, it can handicap it, with duration of isolation influencing the severity of the handicap. Males isolated through 17 days exhibited no deficit in sexual performance when tested with an unfamiliar female.[129] After isolation for 60 days, 30% of males failed to mount an unfamiliar female correctly.[129,130] Whereas, after 77 days of isolation, 70% of males failed to perform the mounting sequence correctly.[91,129,131] Incidentally, isolated male guinea pigs also express some inappropriate behaviors, such as headshaking and play-like leaps and hops, when exposed to an estrus female. The expression of these behaviors does not, however, interfere with sexual performance.[129,130] Some sort of contact, visual, olfactory, and/or auditory, appears to have a potentiating effect on male mounting behavior as males raised with a mesh partition preventing physical contact with their mother and littermates did not exhibit the same deficits.[129] Thus it appears as if isolation rearing exerts a negative influence on the normal organization of male sexual behavior.[131]

Male guinea pig sexual preferences appear to be relatively labile. Rearing male guinea pigs with a heterospecific surrogate (rat) caused those males to direct sexual behaviors toward adult female rats.[132] In addition, for periadolescent males, incest avoidance becomes overridden after only 1 day of separation from their mothers. In reunification tests performed 24 hours after separation, the male pups directed sexual behavior toward their mothers, with up to 63%[133] attempting incorrectly oriented mounts in contrast to 25% of males housed continuously with their mothers.[88]

Testosterone exerts significant effects on male sexual behavior, often by mediating arousal levels. In a study comparing plasma testosterone levels between resident and intruder males subsequent to an antagonistic encounter, higher plasma testosterone levels were found in the resident, regardless of the outcome of the encounter. The authors attribute this difference to the likelihood that the resident male, due to the intrusion in his home cage, remained vigilant for additional intrusions whereas the intruder male, by being returned to his undisturbed home cage did not.[134] In the periadolescent males described in the preceding paragraph, plasma testosterone levels rose in response to separation from their mothers.[133] Finally, Machatschke and colleagues described two male behavioral phenotypes: one that avoids male–male conflict (avoider) and one that does not (belligerent). In general, avoiders tended to be larger, have larger testis size, the same salivary corticosteroid levels, and lower baseline testosterone than belligerent males. Subsequent to social regrouping, the avoider males, when compared to belligerent ones, exhibited a higher initial testosterone response, with levels returning to their lower baseline levels by 6 days after group formation. In addition, avoider males secured greater reproductive success in the new groups than did the belligerent males.[135]

Maternal behavior

Gestation in the guinea pig lasts between 65 and 75 days and parturition is followed by postpartum estrus between 3.5 and 15 hours after parturition.[18,78] Litter sizes are typically between two and three pups, but may be as large as five.[18] Guinea pig pups are extremely precocious and emerge at birth fully furred with open eyes. Although capable of consuming solid food within hours following birth, weaning generally occurs when the pups are 14–21 days old.[18,78]

Generally speaking, mother guinea pigs nurse their pups more often[136] and nurse for longer periods per bout[137] during the day than night. As a consequence, they locomote more and maintain less physical contact with pups at night. Pups initiate most nursing bouts.[137] When nursing, mothers tend to assume a crouched position, while remaining immobile and are usually responsible for terminating nursing bouts. As female guinea pigs increase in parity, their mothering patterns change somewhat. Multiparous females allogroom, sniff, and perform nose–nose contact with their pups more through the first 10 days postpartum than do primiparous females. After sex differences in pup behavior emerge, around 14 days, multiparous females locomote less and maintain more ventrum contact with their pups than primiparous females. Multiparous females also perform more anogenital licking on their daughters than their sons after this point.[138] Rearing environment does not appear to affect maternal behavior. Neither hand rearing[138] nor isolation from birth[139] negatively impacted maternal behavior.

However, individual differences in mothering styles do exist. Although the mechanism responsible for mothering style differences has not been identified yet, Albers and colleagues have documented styles that differ based upon the level of affiliative, aggressive, and locomotor behavior.[140] Although no clear correlation has been established between mothering style and the willingness of pups to explore,[141] pups subjected to less frequent, but longer separations, from their mothers exhibited a greater propensity to explore.[142]

Using olfactory cues, females learn to discriminate their pups from other females' and pups seem to recognize their mothers based upon similar cues.[143] This ability contributes to the formation of loose reciprocal bonds between mother and pups. Thus, when presented with a choice between their own litter and another female's within the first 48 hours postpartum, mothers will spend more time near their own.[144] In addition, during the first few days postpartum, mothers will overcome obstacles in an obstruction test to gain access to their pups, but this motivation declines precipitously after 4 days.[145] Following 1½–2½ hours separation, mothers will approach their own litters first upon reintroduction. However, after this initial approach, both mother and pups do not restrict their interactions to one another. Instead, both will approach, investigate, and tolerate suckling by unrelated pups or attempt to nurse from unrelated females, respectively.[143]

Interestingly, guinea pig mothers appear to alter the amount of their maternal investment through nursing based predominantly upon their own and less so on pup condition.[146] In response to pups denied access to solid foods, and thus artificially increased pup nursing demand, mothers responded only by nursing for a longer proportion of time per day around weaning than mothers of control pups,[147] but food-restricted mothers actually postponed weaning by an average of 8 days when compared to control mothers, apparently in order to achieve a threshold pup weaning mass.[148]

Ingestive behavior

Although guinea pig pups have the ability to ingest solids immediately after birth, pups in semi-naturalistic outdoor enclosures do not begin consuming solids until 4 days postpartum, while in laboratory-reared guinea pigs complete

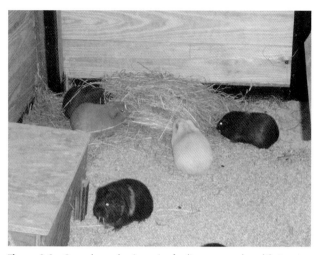

Figure 8.6 Group-housed guinea pigs feeding on grass hay. (Photo courtesy of Lisa Nelson, VMD.)

weaning occurs as late as 28 days. Guinea pigs housed in outdoor colonies will retain the same foraging patterns as wild cavies, foraging in loose social groups with daily peaks of feeding activity occurring at dawn and dusk.[82] Guinea pigs neither hoard nor cache food and will share large items (e.g., carrot) with other individuals in their foraging group.[80] As hindgut digesters, guinea pigs consume their own cecotropes from which they extract protein, B vitamins, and fiber.[18]

Guinea pigs can develop strong food preferences and aversions. They are more likely to consume food with which they have had previous experience and early experience with food types contributes to the formation of preferences for those food types.[149] At the opposite end of the spectrum, guinea pigs possess a natural aversion to tannin-producing plants and can learn to avoid other flavors paired with tannins.[150] This type of aversion learning occurs in guinea pigs as young as 1–2 days old.[151]

In captivity, guinea pigs require a fresh, clean source of water that should be provided *ad libitum*. Guinea pig diets ought to consist of 18–20% protein, 10–18% fiber, and 4% fat, plus high levels of folic acid. In addition, because guinea pigs lack L-gulonolactone oxidase, an enzyme that converts glucose to ascorbic acid, they require dietary supplementation of vitamin C.[18,19,78] All of these nutritional requirements are met in widely available commercial fortified guinea pig diets. Timothy hay can be used as a fiber supplement while fresh greens, fruit, and root crops can be utilized as foraging enrichments[19] (see Figure 8.6).

Common behavior problems: Diagnosis and treatment

Few behavioral problems are associated with guinea pigs. Occasionally, socially housed guinea pigs will exhibit low levels of barbering, that tends to be regarded as an expression of dominance.[78] Recently, Garner and colleagues have begun to challenge this hypothesis. Based upon their studies in mice, they could not establish a connection between relative dominance rank and performance of barbering. However, they did observe that barbering individuals exhibited symptoms akin to those seen in human subjects who perform trichotillomania, an abnormal repetitive behavior.[151] In light of these findings and the fact that isolation-reared male guinea pigs demonstrate aberrant headshaking, further examination of the mechanisms that trigger these abnormal behaviors may be warranted.

Handling and restraint

When handling guinea pigs, minimize stress by providing them with the maximum amount of support possible. Thus, if the purpose of handling is to transfer a guinea pig from cage-to-cage, encourage the guinea pig to enter a tunnel or tube and then transfer the guinea pig contained in the tunnel/tube. For purposes of health examinations, restrain the guinea pig by wrapping both hands around the guinea pig's chest. With the guinea pig restrained, place one hand under its hindquarters and reposition the fingers of the remaining hand so that one or two fingers support its collarbone, the remaining fingers support its chest, and the thumb wraps over its shoulder, and lift the guinea pig. To minimize struggling, bring the guinea pig against your chest. Allow the guinea pig a few moments to acclimatize before manipulating it further (*pers. obs.*).

References

1. Sachser N. Of domestic and wild guinea pigs: Studies in sociophysiology, domestication, and social evolution. *Naturwissenschaften* 1998;85:307–317.
2. Kunzl C, Kaiser S, Meier E et al. Is a wild mammal kept and reared in captivity still a wild animal? *Horm Behav* 2003;43:187–196.
3. Kunzl C, Sachser N. The behavioral endocrinology of domestication: A comparison between the domestic guinea pig (*Cavia aperea f. porcellus*) and its wild ancestor, the cavy (*Cavia aperea*). *Horm Behav* 1999;35:28–37.
4. Rood JP. Ecological and behavioural comparisons of three genera of Argentine cavies. *Anim Behav Monogr* 1972;5:3–83.
5. Baillie J. *Cavia aperea*. IUCN 2007 2007 IUCN Red List of threatened species. http://wwwiucnorg Downloaded on 09 September 2008, 1996.
6. Rood JP. Ecology and social behavior of the desert cavy (*Microcavia australis*). *Am Midl Nat* 1970;83:415–454.
7. Asher M, de Oliveira ES, Sachser N. Social system and spatial organization of wild guinea pigs (*Cavia aperea*) in a natural population. *J Mammal* 2004;85:788–796.
8. Asher M, Lippmann T, Epplen JT et al. Large males dominate: Ecology, social organization, and mating system of wild cavies, the ancestors of the guinea pig. *Behav Ecol Sociobiol* 2008;62:1509–1521.
9. Gade DW. Guinea pig in Andean folk culture. *Geogr Rev* 1967;57:213–224.
10. Granit R. Stimulus intensity in relation to excitation and pre- and post-excitatory inhibition in isolated elements of mammalian retinae. *J Physiol London* 1944;103:103–118.
11. Miles RC, Ratoosh P, Meyer DR. Absence of color vision in guinea pig. *J Neurophysiol* 1956;19:254–258.
12. O'Day K. Visual cells of the guinea pig. *Nature* 1947;160:648–648.
13. Szel A, Takacs L, Monostori E et al. Monoclonal antibody-recognizing cone visual pigment. *Exp Eye Res* 1986;43:871–883.
14. Szel A, Rohlich P. 2 cone types of rat retina detected by antivisual pigment antibodies. *Exp Eye Res* 1992;55:47–52.
15. Jacobs GH, Deegan JF. Spectral sensitivity, photopigments, and color-vision in the guinea-pig (*Cavia-porcellus*). *Behav Neurosci* 1994;108:993–1004.
16. Bridges CDB. Visual pigments of some common laboratory mammals. *Nature* 1959;184:1727–1728.
17. Parry JWL, Bowmaker JK. Visual pigment coexpression in guinea pig cones: A microspectrophotometric study. *Invest Ophthalmol Vis Sci* 2002;43:1662–1665.
18. Terril LA, Clemons DJ. *The Laboratory Guinea Pig.* Boca Raton: CRC Press, Ltd., 1997.
19. Townsend GH. Guinea-pig—General husbandry and nutrition. *Vet Rec* 1975;96:451–454.
20. Beauchamp GK, Magnus JG, Shmunes NT et al. Effects of olfactory bulbectomy on social-behavior of male guinea-pigs (*Cavia-porcellus*). *J Comp Physiol Psychol* 1977;91:336–346.
21. Ruddy LL. Discrimination among colony mates anogenital odors by guinea-pigs (*Cavia-porcellus*). *J Comp Physiol Psychol* 1980;94: 767–774.
22. Beauchamp GK, Martin IG, Wysocki CJ et al. Chemoinvestigatory and sexual-behavior of male guinea-pigs following vomeronasal organ removal. *Physiol Behav* 1982;29:329–336.
23. Beauchamp GK, Wysocki CJ, Wellington JL. Extinction of response to urine odor as a consequence of vomeronasal organ removal in male guinea-pigs. *Behav Neurosci* 1985;99:950–955.
24. Eisthen HL, Wysocki CJ, Beauchamp GK. Behavioral-responses of male guinea-pigs to conspecific chemical signals following neonatal vomeronasal organ removal. *Physiol Behav* 1987;41:445–449.
25. Beaucham GK. Attraction of male guinea-pigs to conspecific urine. *Physiol Behav* 1973;10:589–594.
26. Wellington JL, Beauchamp GK, Wojciechowskimetzler C. Stability of chemical communicants in urine—Individual identity and age of sample. *J Chem Ecol* 1983;9:235–245.
27. Carter CS, Marr JN. Olfactory imprinting and age variables in guinea-pig, *Cavia-porcellus*. *Anim Behav* 1970;18:238–244.
28. Jackel M, Trillmich F. Olfactory individual recognition of mothers by young guinea-pigs (*Cavia porcellus*). *Ethology* 2003;109:197–208.
29. Zechman JM, Martin IG, Wellington JL et al. Perineal scent gland of wild and domestic cavies—Bacterial-activity and urine as sources of biologically significant odors. *Physiol Behav* 1984;32: 269–274.
30. Beruter J, Beaucham GK, Muettert EL. Mammalian chemical communication—Perineal gland secretion of guinea-pig. *Physiol Zool* 1974;47:130–136.
31. Beaucham GK. Perineal scent gland and social dominance in male guinea-pig. *Physiol Behav* 1974;13:669–673.
32. Drickamer LC, Martan J. Odor discrimination and dominance in male domestic guinea-pigs. *Behav Process* 1992;27:187–194.
33. Upton M. The auditory sensitivity of guinea pigs. *Am J Psychol* 1929;41:412–421.
34. Horton GP. A quantitative study of hearing in the guinea pig (*Cavia cobaya*). *J Comp Psychol* 1933;15:59–73.
35. Heffner R, Heffner H, Masterton B. Behavioral measurements of absolute and frequency-difference thresholds in guinea pig. *J Acoust Soc Am* 1971;49:1888–1895.
36. Evans EF. Frequency-response and other properties of single fibers in guinea-pig cochlear nerve. *J Physiol London* 1972;226:263–287.
37. Petersen MR, Prosen CA, Moody DB et al. Behavioral-assessment of kanamycin-induced hearing-loss in guinea-pig. *J Acoust Soc Am* 1976;60:S80–S80.

38. Prosen CA, Petersen MR, Moody DB et al. Auditory-thresholds in guinea-pig determined by positive reinforcement methods. *J Acoust Soc Am* 1976;60:S87–S88.

39. Clough G. Environmental effects on animals used in biomedical research. *Biol Rev Camb Philos Soc* 1982;57:487–523.

40. Fay RR. Comparative psychoacoustics. *Hear Res* 1988;34:295–306.

41. Redies H, Sieben U, Creutzfeldt OD. Functional subdivisions in the auditory-cortex of the guinea-pig. *J Comp Neurol* 1989;282:473–488.

42. Anthony A, Ackerman E, Lloyd JA. Noise stress in laboratory rodents 1. Behavioral and endocrine response of mice, rats, and guinea pigs. *J Acoust Soc Am* 1959;31:1430–1437.

43. Anthony A, Harclerode JE. Noise stress in laboratory rodents 2. Effects of chronic noise exposures on sexual performance and reproductive function of guinea pigs. *J Acoust Soc Am* 1959;31:1437–1440.

44. Balcombe JP. Laboratory environments and rodents' behavioural needs: A review. *Lab Anim* 2006;40:217–235.

45. Bartussek H. A review of the animal needs index (ANI) for the assessment of animals' well-being in the housing systems for Austrian proprietary products and legislation. *Livest Prod Sci* 1999;61:179–192.

46. Baumans V. Environmental enrichment for laboratory rodents and rabbits: Requirements of rodents, rabbits, and research. *ILAR J* 2005;46:162–170.

47. Huntingford FA, Adams C, Braithwaite VA et al. Current issues in fish welfare. *J Fish Biol* 2006;68:332–372.

48. Krohn TC, Sorensen DB, Ottesen JL et al. The effects of individual housing on mice and rats: A review. *Anim Welf* 2006;15:343–352.

49. Millet S, Moons CPH, Van Oeckel MJ et al. Welfare, performance and meat quality of fattening pigs in alternative housing and management systems: A review. *J Sci Food Agric* 2005;85:709–719.

50. Prunier A, Bonneau M, von Borell EH et al. A review of the welfare consequences of surgical castration in piglets and the evaluation of non-surgical methods. *Anim Welf* 2006;15:277–289.

51. Rennie AE, Buchanan-Smith HM. Refinement of the use of non-human primates in scientific research. Part I: The influence of humans. *Anim Welf* 2006;15:203–213.

52. Rennie AE, Buchanan-Smith HM. Refinement of the use of non-human primates in scientific research. Part II: Housing, husbandry and acquisition. *Anim Welf* 2006;15:215–238.

53. Rennie AE, Buchanan-Smith HM. Refinement of the use of non-human primates in scientific research. Part III: Refinement of procedures. *Anim Welf* 2006;15:239–261.

54. Ritz CW, Fairchild BD, Lacy MP. Implications of ammonia production and emissions from commercial poultry facilities: A review. *J Appl Poult Res* 2004;13:684–692.

55. Stafford KJ, Mellor DJ. The welfare significance of the castration of cattle: A review. *N Z Vet J* 2005;53:271–278.

56. Tuyttens FAM. The importance of straw for pig and cattle welfare: A review. *Appl Anim Behav Sci* 2005;92:261–282.

57. Berryman JC. Guinea-pig vocalizations—Their structure, causation and function. *Z Tierpsychol—J Comparat Ethol* 1976;41:80–106.

58. Berryman JC. Social-behavior in a colony of domestic guinea-pigs—Aggression and dominance. *Z Tierpsychol—J Comparat Ethol* 1978;46:200–214.

59. Herman BH, Panksepp J. Ascending endorphin inhibition of distress vocalization. *Science* 1981;211:1060–1062.

60. Kyuhou S-i, Gemba H. Two vocalization-related subregions in the midbrain periaqueductal gray of the guinea pig. *Neuroreport: Int J Rapid Commun Res Neurosci* 1998;9:1607–1610.

61. Berryman JC. Guinea-pig responses to conspecific vocalizations—Playback experiments. *Behav Neural Biol* 1981;31:476–482.

62. Kober M, Trillmich F, Naguib M. Vocal mother–pup communication in guinea pigs: Effects of call familiarity and female reproductive state. *Anim Behav* 2007;73:917–925.

63. Pettijohn TF. Reaction of parents to recorded infant guinea pig distress vocalization. *Behav Neural Biol* 1977;21:438–442.

64. Tokumaru RS, Ades C, Monticelli PF. Individual differences in infant guinea pig pups isolation whistles. *Bioacoustics—Int J Animal Sound Record* 2004;14:197–208.

65. Harper LV. Role of contact and sound in eliciting filial responses and development of social attachments in domestic guinea pigs. *J Comp Physiol Psychol* 1970;73:427–435.

66. Pettijohn TF. Attachment and separation distress in the infant guinea-pig. *Dev Psychobiol* 1979;12:73–81.

67. Hennessy MB, Ritchey RL. Hormonal and behavioral attachment responses in infant guinea pigs. *Dev Psychobiol* 1987;20:613–625.

68. Ritchey RL, Hennessy MB. Cortisol and behavioral-responses to separation in mother and infant guinea-pigs. *Behav Neural Biol* 1987;48:1–12.

69. Hennessy MB. Both prevention of physical contact and removal of distal cues mediate cortisol and vocalization responses of guinea pig pups to maternal separation in a novel environment. *Physiol Behav* 1988;43:729–733.

70. Monticelli PE, Tokumaru RS, Ades C. Isolation induced changes in guinea pig *Cavia porcellus* pup distress whistles. *An Acad Bras Cienc* 2004;76:368–372.

71. Hennessy MB, Morris A. Passive responses of young guinea pigs during exposure to a novel environment: Influences of social partners and age. *Dev Psychobiol* 2005;46:86–96.

72. Hennessy MB, Moorman L. Factors influencing cortisol and behavioral responses to maternal separation in guinea pigs. *Behav Neurosci* 1989;103:378–385.

73. Hennessy MB, Deak T, Schiml-Webb PA. Stress-induced sickness behaviors: An alternative hypothesis for responses during maternal separation. *Dev Psychobiol* 2001;39:76–83.

74. Hennessy MB, Deak T, Schiml-Webb PA et al. Responses of guinea pig pups during isolation in a novel environment may represent stress-induced sickness behaviors. *Physiol Behav* 2004;81:5–13.

75. Hennessy MB, Becker LA, Oneil DR. Peripherally administered CRH suppresses the vocalizations of isolated guinea-pig pups. *Physiol Behav* 1991;50:17–22.

76. Wewers D, Kaiser S, Sachser N. Maternal separation in guinea-pigs: A study in behavioural endocrinology. *Ethology* 2003;109:443–453.

77. Anderson LC. Guinea-pig husbandry and medicine. *Vet Clin North Am Sm Anim Pract* 1987;17:1045–1060.

78. Lott DF. Intraspecific variation in the social-systems of wild vertebrates. *Behaviour* 1984;88:266–325.

79. King JA. Social-relations of the domestic guinea-pig living under semi-natural conditions. *Ecology* 1956;37:221–228.

80. Sachser N. Different forms of social organization at high and low population densities in guinea pigs. *Behaviour* 1986;97:253–272.

81. Fuchs S. Spacing patterns in a colony of guinea pigs: Predictability from environmental and social factors. *Behav Ecol Sociobiol* 1980;6:265–276.

82. Sachser N, Hendrichs, H. A longitudinal study on the social structure and its dynamics in a group of guinea pigs (*Cavia aperea f. porcellus*). *Saugetierkunde Mitteilungen* 1982;30:227–240.

83. Jacobs WW. Male–female associations in the domestic guinea pig. *Anim Learn Behav* 1976;4:77–83.

84. Sachser N, Durschlag M, Hirzel D. Social relationships and the management of stress. *Psychoneuroendocrinology* 1998;23:891–904.

85. Berryman JC, Fullerton C. A developmental study of interactions between young and adult guinea pigs (*Cavia porcellus*). *Behaviour* 1976;59:22–39.

86. Pettijohn TF. Social attachment of the infant guinea pig to its parents in a two-choice situation. *Anim Learn Behav* 1979;7:263–266.

87. Hennessy MB, Young TL, O'Leary SK et al. Social preferences of developing guinea pigs (*Cavia porcellus*) from the preweaning to the periadolescent periods. *J Comp Psychol* 2003;117:406–413.

88. Hennessy MB, Hornschuh G, Kaiser S et al. Cortisol responses and social buffering: A study throughout the life span. *Horm Behav* 2006;49:383–390.

89. Gaston MG, Stout R, Tom R. Imprinting in guinea pigs. *Psychon Sci* 1969;16:53–54.

90. Harper LV. The effects of isolation from birth on the social behaviour of guinea pigs in adulthood. *Anim Behav* 1968;16:58–64.

91. Kaiser S, Kirtzeck M, Hornschuh G et al. Sex-specific difference in social support—A study in female guinea pigs. *Physiol Behav* 2003;79:297–303.

92. Sachser N, Renninger SV. Coping with new social situations: The role of social rearing in guinea pigs. *Ethol Ecol Evol* 1993;5:65–74.

93. Stefanski V, Hendrichs H. Social confrontation in male guinea pigs: Behavior, experience, and complement activity. *Physiol Behav* 1996;60:235–241.

94. Levinson DM, Buchanan DR, Willis FN. Development of social behavior in the guinea pig in the absence of adult males. *Psychol Rec* 1979;29:361–370.

95. Willis FN, Levinson DM, Buchanan DR. Development of social behavior in the guinea pig. *Psychol Rec* 1977;27:527–536.

96. Sachser N. The ability to arrange with conspecifics depends on social experiences around puberty. *Physiol Behav* 1993;53:539–544.

97. Sachser N, Lick C. Social stress in guinea pigs. *Physiol Behav* 1989;46:137–144.

98. Sachser N, Lick C. Social experience, behavior, and stress in guinea pigs. *Physiol Behav* 1991;50:83–90.

99. Kaiser S, Harderthauer S, Sachser N et al. Social housing conditions around puberty determine later changes in plasma cortisol levels and behavior. *Physiol Behav* 2007;90:405–411.

100. Harlow HF. The nature of love. *Am Psychol* 1958;13:673–685.

101. Harlow HF, Suomi SJ. Nature of love-simplified. *Am Psychol* 1970;25:161–168.

102. Porter RH, Berryman JC, Fullerto C. Exploration and attachment behavior in infant guinea-pigs. *Behaviour* 1973;45:312–322.

103. Graves FC, Hennessy MB. Comparison of the effects of the mother and an unfamiliar adult female on cortisol and behavioral responses of pre- and postweaning guinea pigs. *Dev Psychobiol* 2000;36:91–100.

104. Hennessy MB, Mazzei SJ, McInturf SM. The fate of filial attachment in juvenile guinea pigs housed apart from the mother. *Dev Psychobiol* 1996;29:641–651.

105. Hennessy MB, Maken DS, Graves FC. Consequences of the presence of the mother or unfamiliar adult female on cortisol, ACTH, testosterone and behavioral responses of periadolescent guinea pigs during exposure to novelty. *Psychoneuroendocrinology* 2000;25:619–632.

106. Hennessy MB, O'Leary SK, Hawke JL et al. Social influences on cortisol and behavioral responses of preweaning, periadolescent, and adult guinea pigs. *Physiol Behav* 2002;76:305–314.

107. Sachser N, Kaiser S. Prenatal social stress masculinizes the females' behaviour in guinea pigs. *Physiol Behav* 1996;60:589–594.

108. Nagy ZM, Misanin JR. Social preference in the guinea pig as a function of social rearing conditions and age at separation from the mother. *Psychonom Sci* 1970;19:309–311.

109. Kaiser S, Sachser N. The social environment during pregnancy and lactation affects the female offsprings' endocrine status and behaviour in guinea pigs. *Physiol Behav* 1998;63:361–366.

110. Kaiser S, Kruijver FPM, Swaab DF et al. Early social stress in female guinea pigs induces a masculinization of adult behavior and corresponding changes in brain and neuroendocrine function. *Behav Brain Res* 2003;144:199–210.

111. Kaiser S, Sachser N. Social stress during pregnancy and lactation affects in guinea pigs the male offsprings' endocrine status and infantilizes their behaviour. *Psychoneuroendocrinology* 2001;26:503–519.

112. Kaiser S, Kruijver FPM, Straub RH et al. Early social stress in male guinea-pigs changes social behaviour, and autonomic and neuroendocrine functions. *J Neuroendocrinol* 2003;15:761–769.

113. Kemme K, Kaiser S, Sachser N. Prenatal maternal programming determines testosterone response during social challenge. *Horm Behav* 2007;51:387–394.

114. Kaiser S, Heemann K, Straub RH et al. The social environment affects behaviour and androgens, but not cortisol in pregnant female guinea pigs. *Psychoneuroendocrinology* 2003;28:67–83.

115. Kemme K, Kaiser S, Sachser N. Prenatal stress does not impair coping with challenge later in life. *Physiol Behav* 2008;93:68–75.

116. Nordlund A, Lidfors L, Lindh AS et al. Behavioural effects of the shelter design on male guinea pigs. *Scand J Lab Anim Sci* 2007;34:9–16.

117. Seward GH. Studies on the reproductive activities of the guinea pig: V. Specificity of sexual drive in the male. *Pedagog Semin J Genet Psychol* 1941;59:389–396.

118. Seward JP, Seward GH. Studies on the reproductive activities of the guinea pig: IV. A comparison of sex drive in males and females. *Pedagog Semin J Genet Psychol* 1940;57:429–440.

119. Wallner B, Dittami J, Machatschke I. Social stimuli cause changes of plasma oxytocin and behavior in guinea pigs. *Biol Res* 2006;39:251–258.

120. Bauer B, Womastek I, Dittami J et al. The effects of early environmental conditions on the reproductive and somatic development of juvenile guinea pigs (*Cavia aperea f. porcellus*). *Gen Comp Endocrinol* 2008;155:680–685.

121. Young WC, Dempsey EW, Myers HI. Cyclic reproductive behavior in the female guinea pig. *J Comp Psychol* 1935;19:313–335.

122. Young WC, Dempsey EW, Hagquist CW et al. Sexual behavior and sexual receptivity in the female guinea pig. *J Comp Psychol* 1939;27:49–68.

123. Birke LI. Object investigation by the oestrous rat and guinea-pig: The oestrous cycle and the effects of oestrogen and progesterone. *Anim Behav* 1979;27:350–358.

124. Birke LI. Some behavioural changes associated with the guinea-pig oestrous cycle. *Z Tierpsychol* 1981;55:79–89.

125. Roy MM, Goldstein KL, Williams C. Estrus termination following copulation in female guinea-pigs. *Horm Behav* 1993;27:397–402.

126. Young WC, Grunt JA. The pattern and measurement of sexual behavior in the male guinea pig. *J Comp Physiol Psychol* 1951;44:492–500.

127. Cohn DWH, Tokumaru RS, Ades C. Female novelty and the courtship behavior of male guinea pigs (*Cavia porcellus*). *Braz J Med Biol Res* 2004;37:847–851.

128. Gerall AA. An exploratory study of the effect of social isolation variables on the sexual behaviour of male guinea pigs. *Anim Behav* 1963;11:274–282.

129. Gerall HD. Effect of social isolation and physical confinement on motor and sexual behavior of guinea pigs. *J Pers Soc Psychol* 1965;2:460–464.

130. Valenstein ES, Riss W, Young WC. Experiential and genetic factors in the organization of sexual behavior in male guinea pigs. *J Comp Physiol Psychol* 1955;48:397–403.

131. Beaucham GK, Hess EH. Abnormal early rearing and sexual responsiveness in male guinea-pigs. *J Comp Physiol Psychol* 1973;85:383–396.

132. Maken DS, Hennessy MB. Rehousing periadolescent male guinea pigs (*Cavia porcellus*) apart from their mothers for 24 hours increases maternally directed sexual behavior and plasma testosterone. *J Comp Psychol* 1999;113:435–442.

133. Sachser N, Prove E. Short-term effects of residence on the testosterone responses to fighting in alpha male guinea pigs. *Agg Behav* 1984;10:285–292.

134. Machatschke IH, Bauer BE, Schrauf C et al. Conflict-involvement of male guinea pigs (*Cavia aperea f. porcellus*) as a criterion for partner preference. *Behav Ecol Sociobiol* 2008;62:1341–1350.

135. Schiml PA, Hennessy MB. Light dark variation and changes across the lactational period in the behaviors of undisturbed

mother and infant guinea-pigs (*Cavia-porcellus*). *J Comp Psychol* 1990;104:283–288.

136. Hennessy MB, Jenkins R. A descriptive analysis of nursing behavior in the guinea pig (*Cavia porcellus*). *J Comp Psychol* 1994;108:23–28.

137. Albers PCH, Timmermans PJA, Vossen JMH. Maternal behaviour in the guinea pig (*Cavia aperea f. porcellus*:): A comparison of multiparous, and primiparous, and hand reared primiparous mothers. *Netherlands J Zool* 1999;49:275–287.

138. Stern JJ, Hoffman BM. Effects of social isolation until adulthood on maternal behavior in guinea pigs. *Psychon Sci* 1970;21:15–16.

139. Albers PCH, Timmermans PJA, Vossen JMH. Evidence for the existence of mothering styles in guinea pigs (*Cavia aperea f. porcellus*). *Behaviour* 1999;136:469–479.

140. Albers PCH, Timmermans PJA, Vossen JMH. Is maternal behavior correlated with later explorative behavior of young guinea pigs (*Cavia aperea f. porcellus*)? *Acta ethol* 2000;2:91–96.

141. Albers PCH, Timmermans PJA, Vossen JMH. Effects of frequency and length of separation bouts between mother and offspring on later explorative behaviour of young guinea-pigs (*Cavia aperea f. porcellus*). *Behaviour* 2000;137:1487–1502.

142. Fullerton C, Berryman JC, Porter RH. On the nature of mother–infant interactions in the guinea-pig (*Cavia porcellus*). *Behaviour* 1974;48:145–156.

143. Porter RH, Fullerton C, Berryman JC. Guinea-pig maternal–young attachment behaviour. *Z Tierpsychol* 1973;32:489–495.

144. Seward JP, Seward GH. Studies on the reproductive activities of the guinea pig I. Factors in maternal behavior. *J Comparat Psychol* 1940;29:1–24.

145. Rehling A, Trillmich F. Weaning in the guinea pig (*Cavia aperea f. porcellus*): Who decides and by what measure? *Behav Ecol Sociobiol* 2007;62:149–157.

146. Laurien-Kehnen C, Trillmich F. Lactation performance of guinea pigs (*Cavia porcellus*) does not respond to experimental manipulation of pup demands. *Behav Ecol Sociobiol* 2003;53:145–152.

147. Laurien-Kehnen C, Trillmich F. Maternal food restriction delays weaning in the guinea pig, *Cavia porcellus*. *Anim Behav* 2004;68:303–312.

148. Reisbick SH. Development of food preferences in newborn guinea-pigs. *J Comparat Physiol Psychol* 1973;85:427–442.

149. Lichtenstein G, Cassini MH. Behavioural mechanisms underlaying food aversion in guinea pigs. *Etologia* 2001;9:29–34.

150. Kalat JW. Taste-aversion learning in infant guinea pigs. *Dev Psychobiol* 1975;8:383–387.

151. Garner JP, Dufour B, Gregg LE et al. Social and husbandry factors affecting the prevalence and severity of barbering ("whisker trimming") by laboratory mice. *Appl Anim Behav Sci* 2004;89:263–282.

9

The mouse

Naomi Latham

Introduction

The house mouse has had a long and turbulent relationship with humans. Considered a serious agricultural and urban pest by many, it has become an enormously useful "tool" in scientific research, and has also found a warmer place in our affections as a companion animal. In order to ensure that we provide captive mice with suitable environments, we need to understand their natural biology and behavior. Therefore, this chapter will include: a brief review of the history of the mouse's relationship with humans, the sensory biology and natural life history of the free-living house mouse, and some of the common behavior problems exhibited by captive mice. Together, this information should enable those who keep and care for mice to offer them the best possible housing and management in keeping with their basic behavioral needs.

History of the mouse

The house mouse

The house mouse (*Mus musculus*) originated in the steppes of Central Asia (the word *mouse* is thought to be derived from a Sanskrit word meaning *to steal*), and has been associated with hominid dwellings since the Middle Pleistocene, 230,000 years ago.[1] The relationship between house mice and humans was sealed with the development of agriculture around 9000 BC.[1] Since then the house mouse has spread around the world with human migration, and is now found in every temperate and tropical region except tropical Africa.[2,3]

Free-living house mice continue to have a close relationship with humans. They are often found in man-made environments such as barns, farm-buildings, and houses, and such populations are termed *commensal* (literally *sharing one's table*).[3–5] The remarkable adaptability of mice means that they are able to inhabit almost any man-made environment. House mice have been found living in meat storage freezers at $-10°C$ (10°F),[6] and even temperatures of $-30°C$ ($-20°F$);[7] in coal mines at depths of over 548 m (1800 ft);[7,8] in tombs;[9] and one mouse was even found in a sealed biscuit barrel after 14 months.[10] However, some house mice have lessened their links with humans and live in more natural environments such as woods, forests, and fields, and these populations are here termed *feral*.[4]

Fancy (and other pet) mice

Fancy mice (the word "fancy" being used in terms of its old English meaning—"hobby") have been kept and bred for hundreds of years. The earliest records relating to breeding different colors of mice appear to date back to Japan in the 1700s, when a booklet was produced by Chobei Zenya (a Kyoto money exchanger) titled "The Breeding of Curious Varieties of the Mouse."[11,12] However, mice did not become popular as pets in Europe until the 1800s.

Colored mice were brought from the Far East to Europe during the 1800s, and in 1892 the first class for fancy mice was held at a small livestock show in Oxford.[13] Three years later (in 1895) the National Mouse Club was formed in the United Kingdom, and in 1897 the club organized its first "mouse only" show in East London.[13] Less is known about how fancy mouse breeding spread to North America. As in Europe, it is thought that captured house mice were being kept and bred as pets, but that early American fancy mice breeds may have been derived from individuals acquired from mouse colonies at scientific research institutions.[12] An American fancy mouse breeders' club first appeared in the 1950s and the American Fancy Mouse and Rat

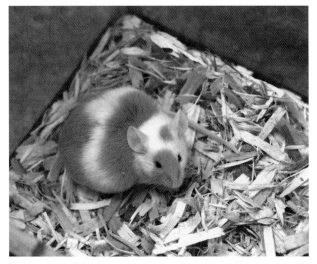

Figure 9.1   A piebald mouse commonly referred to as a fancy mouse in the pet trade. (Photo courtesy of Heather Mohan-Gibbons.)

Table 9.1   Website details for fancy mouse clubs in the United Kingdom, Sweden, Poland, Australia, and United States

UK	The National Mouse Club (www.nationalmouseclub.co.uk)
Sweden	Swedish Mouse Club (www.svemus.org)
Poland	Polish Mouse Club (pzhmmr.w.interia.pl)
Australia	New South Wales Fancy Rat and Mouse Club (nswfrmc.org/index.htm)
USA	American Fancy Rat and Mouse Association (www.afrma.org)

Association was born in 1983 (Figure 9.1). Fancy mouse clubs can now be found all over the world, and web site details for a few of these are listed in Table 9.1.

Sensory biology

The world of the mouse is dominated by smell. Mice have 3 times as many olfactory receptors as humans[14] and 1% of their genome is devoted to odor discrimination.[15] Olfactory cues are detected by receptors in the nasal olfactory epithelium, and by the vomeronasal organ in the roof of the mouth.[16] Odor cues are crucially important in social communication and are also heavily used in detecting and assessing food and predators. There is even evidence that odor gradients may be used to anticipate edges and drops.[17]

Mice have a well-developed sense of hearing. They have large, mobile ears and a wide auditory range, extending from approximately 80 Hz to over 100 kHz, although they are most sensitive to sounds between 15 and 20 kHz and around 50 kHz.[18] Thus mice are sensitive to sounds above the audible range of humans (ultrasounds). Mice are also more sensitive to sudden bursts of noise, and are thought

to find sound pressure levels aversive at lower levels (about 20 dB lower) than humans.[18] Mice use both audible and ultrasounds in intra-specific communication, the former particularly during aggressive interactions, and the latter particularly during courtship behavior and by pups.

Mice are very sensitive to touch. Their whiskers (*tactile vibrissae*) act as a "poor man's radar" in dark conditions, allowing mice to avoid obstacles and run freely in places where light levels are extremely low.[19,20] The input from each individual whisker is mapped in a whisker barrel, a specialized region of the brain's somatosensory cortex.[16] The guard hairs on the body are also used to sense overhead cover, and when moving along walls.[7,21] Tactile contact is important to mice who attempt to maintain body contact with solid objects as much as possible (*thigmotaxic behavior*), especially when anxious.[22]

Mouse vision is fairly well-developed, but visual acuity is poor compared with that of humans—although mice are very sensitive to movement and changes in light intensity. Mice also have a very wide field of vision as a result of their eyes being positioned on the sides of the head.[25] Their retinas are composed of about 97% rods,[23] giving them sensitive monochrome vision in dim light but making color perception poor.[16,20] Unlike humans, mice are able to see ultraviolet (UV) wavelengths due to the density of UV sensitive cones, particularly in the ventral area of their retina.[23] It is not clear to what extent mice use their UV sensitivity under natural conditions, especially since mice are primarily nocturnal, but it is an intriguing possibility that they may use it in assessing the age of conspecific urine marks. Pest control companies often state that fresh urine appears blue–white under UV light while older urine appears yellow–white.

Taste in mice appears to be broadly similar to that of humans, although they do not respond to some compounds which taste sweet to us[21] and will also ingest substances which humans find disgustingly bitter, for example Bitrex.[24] Taste is used to identify food type and quality, and is crucial as mice are unable to vomit if food proves dangerous.[24]

Activity and locomotor behavior

Mice are primarily crepuscular or nocturnal,[10] but their activity patterns may be altered by factors such as the timing of food availability,[25] lighting patterns and human activity in man-made environments,[26] and reproductive state—for example, the timing of activity bouts may become much more flexible during lactation.[27] Little is known about how much time free-living mice actually spend active or the duration of discreet activity bouts. In the laboratory, mice are active for less than 50% of the 24-hour day.[28] Here, activity bouts often last no more than 2–3 hours, with the longest of these usually occurring following lights-out, while shorter activity bouts then occur during the remainder of the dark period and intermittently during the light period (N. Latham, unpublished data). However, while free-living mice also exhibit discreet activity bouts,[26] this estimate of the total amount of time spent active is likely to be somewhat conservative for free-living mice since non-captive environments are far more demanding.

House mice are creatures of habit, especially *commensal* mice living in man-made environments, where territories or home ranges tend to be smaller than those of their *feral* counterparts.[29] When out and about mice use visual landmarks to navigate around their environment[30] and repeatedly follow familiar routes, leading to well-worn runways.[7] Wherever possible, mice display thigmotaxic behavior ("wall-hugging"), following barriers and walls. However, mice are extremely agile and their movements are certainly not limited to the ground. Mice are excellent climbers, able to scale vertical brickwork or bark; they are proficient jumpers, able to leap over 30 cm (12 in.) vertically and 2.5 m (8.2 ft) downward without harm; and they are capable swimmers, but are susceptible to hypothermia in cold water.[7] Indeed a number of authors have noted that mice use raised vantage points in order to monitor conspecific activity, and potentially also to detect approach by predators.[22,28] However, mice generally avoid areas that have been cleared of vegetation, exposed areas, or areas that are regularly disturbed by human activity.[21,31] Routine movements around their (three-dimensional) environment allow mice to build up a detailed, continually updated map of their domain. This not only ensures that mice exhibit good homing abilities over large distances up to several hundred meters from their nest site,[21] but commensal mice often acquire such habitual locomotor patterns that, if disturbed, they can return to the safety of their nest with minimal sensory input.[12,32] However, the degree to which mice develop and rely upon such routine formation varies. For example, feral mice with large home ranges may only traverse a small portion of their range each night.[33] Interestingly, in the laboratory, mice selected for low aggression (and thus more closely resembling this characteristic in feral than commensal mice) also show less use of routines.[34,35]

Regular, predictable movement around the environment also serves a number of other functions, for example, it allows the investigation of olfactory cues used in communication. Mice use olfactory cues to communicate information about age, sexual status, relatedness, and individual identity.[20,36] Many of these cues are contained in the urine (although important cues are also present in feces and plantar gland secretions), and because the volatile signaling pheromones are bound to non-volatile major urinary proteins (MUPs—which act as a slow-release mechanism), these urinary odor cues may last for up to 2 days.[37–39] These cues are particularly important in territorial, sexual, and parental behavior.

Mice may also use regular movements around their environment to investigate olfactory cues associated with

predators. Feral mice may be predated by owls, weasels, feral cats, snakes, and even toads,[40–42] while one of the main predators of commensal mice is the domestic cat.[43,44] The presence of predators can have marked effects on the behavior of mice. For example, exposure to predator odors can increase anxiety-related behaviors in laboratory mice and avoidance of tainted areas.[45,46] However, other studies have found that the presence of predator odors have no significant effect on foraging behavior (indeed removing vegetation was more effective at reducing foraging behavior),[47] and synthetic predator odors are not particularly effective as agricultural repellents for wild mice.

Periods of inactivity are spent in sheltered nests which provide protection against predators and adverse weather conditions. In feral environments, nests are usually constructed in underground burrows and are lined with grass, hair, or feathers.[3] Mice are efficient tunnelers, but they also take advantage of burrows dug by other animals,[4,48] and if the ground is too hard or poorly drained for burrowing, feral mice will construct their nests above ground.[40,49] In commensal environments, mice build spherical or bowl-shaped surface nests consisting of a loose outer paper or rag-based structure and lined with finer shredded material.[12,50] The amount of material used in nest construction often increases as ambient temperatures decrease,[51,52] and nests can have extremely effective thermoregulatory effects—even at outside temperatures of −3°C (27°F), the temperature within a nest can be more than 17°C (63°F).[53] Mice typically nest either alone or with the breeding partner and family group (termed a *deme*): although under adverse conditions (e.g., extreme cold) even highly territorial individuals will nest with other mice, including subordinates that they normally attack.[26,54]

Body care

Grooming behavior has been well-documented in rodents and normally follows a cephalocaudal progression such that the self-grooming sequence[55] progresses as follows:

- paw licking,
- nose/face grooming (stokes along the snout),
- head washing (semi-circular movements over the top of the head and behind ears),
- body grooming/scratching (body fur licking and scratching the body with the hind paws),
- leg licking and tail/genitals grooming (licking of the genital area and tail).

Grooming occurs commonly in the transition between inactivity and active periods. It then also occurs sporadically during activity bouts and, in captivity, mice can spend a large proportion of their time budget (17%) performing these behaviors.[28] Self-grooming is important for hygiene and insulation,[16] while allo-grooming helps to maintain social relationships.[38,56] Grooming can occur particularly intensively after eating and may then, during allo-grooming, assist the transfer of information about food stuffs.[16,57] Grooming behavior is also elicited by stressors, and in contrast to the complete "low stress comfort" grooming sequences associated with the preceding examples, stress-induced grooming is characterized by frequent bursts of rapid, short, interrupted grooming sequences.[55,58]

Ingestive behavior

Foraging behavior is incorporated into regular movements around the mouse's environment. Mice eat up to 20% of their body weight daily, consuming about 200 small meals per night from up to 30 food sites.[3,21,59,60] Mice are omnivores, but show a preference for foods high in fat and protein.[6,7] Mice also acquire food preferences early in life from their mothers and exhibit preferences for foods eaten by recently encountered conspecifics.[61] The diet of commensal mice is often determined by the nature of their environment, for example grain in grain stores,[9] while the diet of feral mice includes cereals, grasses, roots, and seeds.[3] House mice also exhibit predatory behavior, eating live insects and their larvae.[62,63] Mice are also known to predate upon seabird chicks, and may pose a threat to the survival of some bird species on islands where the house mouse has inadvertently been introduced.[64] Although house mice can be very aggressive and territorial males will fight to the death,[26] mice do not generally appear to be prone to cannibalizing the bodies of other adult mice. Thus, laboratory studies have shown that group-housed but not isolated mice show an aversion to eating the dead bodies of adult conspecifics,[65] and indeed that females are less likely to eat the flesh of dead conspecifics than males.[66]

Mice generally acquire their water requirements from their food, if feeding on a diet with a moisture content of at least 15%, but they will drink free water if it is available, and require additional water if living in hot, arid environments or feeding on a dry or protein-rich diet.[21,67]

Social behavior (and territoriality)

The social structure and territorial behavior of house mouse populations varies according to the animals' environment. In feral conditions both male and female mice may hold loosely defended territories (or ranges). While ranges of individuals within either of the sexes tend not to overlap, male and female ranges may overlap, sometimes completely, even if the respective male and female are not a breeding pair.[35,68,69] Home range sizes vary with the density of available food, with maximum reported densities ranging from one mouse per three square meters[70] or 33 m^2 (108 ft^2) in fields of grain,[71] to an average of 6000 m^2 (19,685 ft^2) in forests,[35] to an incredible 80,000 m^2 (262,467 ft^2) in the wheat lands of Australia.[72] Due to the varying nature of

feral habitats, the home ranges of feral mice often fluctuate greatly in size, shape, and even location with seasonal changes in habitat quality.[69,73] In commensal environments, territories are typically only held by males and territory sizes are much smaller. Thus, some authors report that commensal mice may not venture more than a meter or two from their nest site.[7,31] A study by Southern[10] found that territories ranged between 2 and 6 m^2 (6.5−19.6 ft^2), and the pest control literature reports that commensal mice rarely travel more than 10 m (32 ft) from their nest site.[7,74] In contrast to the loosely defended, somewhat flexible home ranges of feral mice, commensal males tend to divide the available space into strictly defended territories with minimal overlap.[22,75] Breeding females establish nest sites within a male territory, and the breeding pair and their offspring all participate in defending territorial boundaries against neighboring demes. However, some young mice, typically smaller animals, never establish their own territory. Life for these individuals is particularly tough as they must continually avoid aggressive encounters with territory-holding mice, and they are restricted to poor nest sites and food sources—although some are able to adapt their behavior patterns so that they minimize contact with the territorial deme members.[26]

Territorial boundaries often occur at physically and/ or visually striking features of the environment.[26,76,77] Territory ownership is signaled, particularly by dominant males, via regularly refreshed urine marks along the borders of their territory.[8,40] These marks are also laid down throughout the rest of the territory, especially on conspicuous objects and favored nesting and feeding sites.[78,79] Dominant males may even venture into neighboring territories to over-mark the urine marks of their competitors, as fresh urine marks signal competitive ability.[17,80] However, this generally occurs less in feral than commensal populations due to the larger size of feral ranges and the fact that only selected regions, such as the best nesting and feeding sites, are strictly defended.[16,69] Urine marks are laid down so regularly that mice become surrounded by the familiar scent of the territorial male. Indeed, in commensal populations urine marks may be deposited so frequently that, mixed with grease and dust, they form "pillars" many millimeters high.[7,17,75] Dominant males will often tolerate marks from juveniles and females, since juvenile urine lacks the aggression-eliciting properties of adult male urine, and female urine contains an aggression-inhibiting factor.[81] However, dominant males generally do not tolerate the urine marks of other adult males. This may explain why, in contrast to the extensive urine marking by dominant animals, subordinate males typically produce less urine[82] and, in captivity at least, tend to pool their urine away from the dominant animal.[83]

If two males encounter each other within the territory the dominant male will initiate an aggressive interaction, chasing the intruder and biting at his rump and tail.[84]

The lengths to which the dominant male pursues this chase and the severity of the attack can vary according to factors including the identity of the intruder, population density, the complexity of the physical environment, and the distribution of resources (i.e., whether they are clumped or scattered). Thus, for example, if the intruder is a neighboring territory holder in a high-density (typically a commensal) population the pursuit may last to the territorial boundary, at which point the roles of the animals reverse, and the intruder (now the territory holder) becomes the aggressor. If the intruder is a subordinate or nomadic non-territory holder, he may be chased beyond the boundaries of the original territory and then across successive territories held by respective territorial males, and possibly also other members of the demes.[26] In such situations, if the intruder is unable to escape or hide from the territorial male he is likely to suffer serious, and potentially fatal, injuries in the attack.[26,57,85] Thus, subordinate males in high-density populations may change their activity patterns in order to avoid dominant males, for example, by becoming active during the day[22,26] or by exhibiting more cautious behavior when entering a dominant male's territory.[86] In contrast, males in lower-density (typically feral) populations tend to be more tolerant of familiar intruders. Here, territorial males initially establish their dominance over rivals through a series of brief chases. If the rival male indicates his subordinate status by rearing on his hind paws, raising his forepaws and exposing his belly,[16] the rival is then likely to be tolerated on subsequent occasions—although favored nesting and feeding sites may still be strictly defended.[4,87] Population density, resource distribution, and environmental complexity also affect the nature and duration of aggressive encounters by influencing how easily males can defend resources within their territories or how successfully subordinate animals are able to escape or hide from aggressive attacks.[88,86] In addition to these environmental factors, genetic factors may also play a role. Thus, laboratory studies have shown that two extremes can be bred from feral mice: aggressive mice exhibiting short attack latencies and less aggressive mice exhibiting long attack latencies.[36,37,87] However, it is not yet clear whether commensal and feral animals differ systematically in these traits, nor whether this reflects differences in adaptive strategies in different types of environment.

Reproductive behavior

Once mice are established within a territory they can begin the process of starting a family. Mice are rapid and prolific breeders in good quality environments—that is, where there is ample food, nest sites, and nesting material. Thus, in man-made environments breeding can occur year-round, while breeding may be more seasonal in feral populations.[5,89] If resources are abundant the pest control literature estimates that a reproductive female may produce up to 10 litters (totaling roughly 50 pups) a year.[7,90] Indeed, a reproductive female may spend most of her life bearing and rearing pups.

House mice can form pair bonds or they may be polygamous, whereby the dominant males and females may both mate with numerous partners.[3,91,92] Females may be brought into reproductive state, if they are in good physical condition, by exposure to volatile components of male urine—the so-called Whitten effect.[93] Females' estrous cycles last between 4 and 6 days (although this can be extended in groups of females—the so-called Lee-Boot effect[93]). During estrus, receptive females mate with their partner or even a number of males, showing an attraction for unfamiliar males (those less likely to be directly related to themselves).[91,92] Indeed polyandry has been found to increase post-birth survival of pups.[94] However, while mice of both sexes may mate with a number of individuals, they are selective about potential partners, and will reject some animals altogether.[91] Females select mates based on a number of attributes, including: their social status, which may already be known from odor cues around their environment, and his rate of ultrasonic calling[95] their "maleness," which they assess by his preputial odor;[36,96] aspects of health and fitness, such as the absence of parasitic infections, high parasite resistance, and the absence of potentially lethal genetic traits.[97–99] Another important feature is whether he has the same major histocompatibility complex, which is assessed via urinary cues[100]—although prolonged inbreeding may reduce (and even eliminate) natural variability in the major histocompatibility complex.[101] Males also appear to display some mate choice, preferring unfamiliar females to close female relatives;[102] and "feminized" females with shorter anogenital distances,[103,104] which can be assessed through urinary cues.[105] By exhibiting such preferences, animals can reduce the chances of breeding with closely related individuals (and the adverse effects of inbreeding) and potentially increase the success of their offspring. Laboratory studies have shown that females allowed to mate with a preferred mate produce more litters (than those mated with non-preferred males), and their offspring perform better in dominance contests and nest-building.[106] Similar results are obtained when males are mated with preferred and non-preferred females.[107]

Courtship is initiated by the female indicating sexual motivation through ear-wiggling, hopping, and darting movements and ultrasonic vocalizations.[16] The male responds by investigating the female, in particular her genital odors, and producing his own ultrasonic "songs."[108] The male then mounts the female from the rear, grasping her flanks with his front paws. Copulation consists of a series of discrete mounts by the male which lead to intromission and finally ejaculation. However, copulatory behavior can be variable in its duration and the number of intromissions prior to ejaculation, and this has an impact upon the number of pups born, with an increasing number of intromissions being found to correlate positively with subsequent litter size.[109] Following ejaculation the male remains fully intromitted for a further 13–25 seconds during which he clutches the female with all four limbs and may fall to his side.[110] Following this, the male grooms his genitals and shows little attention to the female,[16] while the female often retreats away from the male in order to control the pace of copulation.[111] Successful copulation can be identified by a waxy vaginal plug, which remains in place for approximately 24 hours. Implantation occurs 5 days after fertilization, but can be delayed for up to 12 days in lactating females.[3] If females are exposed to an unfamiliar male's urine following fertilization fetal resorption may occur—the so-called Bruce effect.[93]

Gestation usually lasts between 19 and 21 days[3] during which the female constructs a nest in preparation for the birth of her pups. These nests, sometimes referred to as brood or maternal nests, are roughly 2–3 times larger and more complex than normal "sleeping" nests (being enclosed with one or two entrances).[112] Females in cold climates build the most complex nests, particularly those with prior breeding experience.[113] Good nests can be extremely effective, as noted earlier, and well-built nests can significantly improve the survival of offspring.[114] However, nest building behavior by one pregnant female can elicit the behavior in others, leading to damage to the nest (if nesting material is not abundant) as each female attempts to use the material for her own nest.[57] In addition to nest-building, pre-parturient females can also exhibit other behavioral changes. For example, some females may become more aggressive (a behavioral change that persists following the birth of the pups), particularly toward non-reproductive individuals, vigorously defending their nests and biting intruders' heads and bellies.[84,115] Maternal aggression has been linked to suckling stimulation from the pups following parturition.[116] This increase in aggression may be necessary if females are to defend their nests, and subsequently their pups[117,118]—although females may find it impossible to defend their nest if they must repel large numbers of conspecifics.[26]

Mouse pups are usually born at night, and if the female is undisturbed she will remain in the nest cleaning the pups after each birth.[3,5] The pups each weigh about 1 g (0.03 oz), and are blind, deaf, and completely hairless, except for small whiskers on the muzzle.[3,119] Females will give birth to four to eight pups per litter, typically with equal numbers of males and females.[3,42] However, a number of reproductive females may nest together and even nurse their young communally if the pups are very similar in age. This may be an adaptive strategy, increasing the reproductive output of females, perhaps by improving thermoregulation and nest defense.[112,120]

Maternal behavior and mouse development

During the first few weeks, the pups are reliant on their mother (and communal carers) for temperature regulation, food, and to stimulate defecation.[40,121] The pups stimulate parental behaviors, such as nursing, retrieval, and grooming, through specific vocal cues including audible squeals and clicks and ultrasounds:[122] with ultrasounds being further split into pure ultrasounds (which elicit pup approach and retrieval), broadband ultrasonic calls indicating injury, and low-frequency "wriggling" calls eliciting licking and other maternal behaviors.[123,124] These calls are crucial in maintaining maternal behaviors as the performance of these behaviors decreases rapidly during the first week after birth, partly as a result of the mother spending more and more time away from the litter performing other behaviors such as feeding, grooming herself, and dozing.[123] As reviewed by Latham,[29] several studies have found that the quality of maternal care pups receive has numerous other effects on their success later in life. For example, the amount of milk pups receive influences their weight at weaning, aggressiveness, and territorial success; and the amount of licking and grooming they receive influences their stress responsiveness during adulthood and the amount of maternal behavior female pups perform for their pups when they themselves become mothers.

The pups grow and develop rapidly during the weeks following their birth. They develop pigmentation within a few days, and start growing fur within a week. They begin to show auditory responses between about 4 and 11 days, and can identify their mother's odor by 12 days.[81] The pups first open their eyes between days 12 and 15, although they continue to keep them tightly shut while in the nest until day 15, but their vision is not fully developed for a further 2 weeks.[81] Pups start trying solid food at roughly 17 days,[119] but they have already learned about the food eaten by their mother from olfactory and gustatory cues they have been exposed to through grooming and their mother's milk.[125] Around this time mice also start exploring their wider environment. Their first exploratory trips are brief, and usually accompanied by one of their parents,[26] but as they grow in confidence the young mice make longer, unchaperoned, and more playful trips away from the nest, continuing to learn from the behavior of older, more experienced mice.[26,62] By the time the mice are 3–4 weeks old they have increased their weight to 9 g, they are able to regulate their own body temperature, and are nutritionally independent of their mothers.[42,119]

The young mice remain in their natal territory for several more weeks, but around 5–6 weeks the family relationships begin to change, and this is triggered by the onset of sexual maturity.[21,88] Females generally mature earlier than males, but the timing of puberty can be influenced by a variety of environmental and social factors. Thus, females may delay puberty if they are living in crowded or cold conditions, while exposure to odor cues or the presence of the opposite sex may advance puberty in both males and females (the so-called Vandenbergh effect [in females]).[93] Young males, once mature, become more aggressive,[3] and in turn are the subject of more aggressive behavior from their fathers.[8] As a result, many young males leave the familial nest to search for their own territory,[3] but some may remain as subordinate animals awaiting an opportunity to overthrow their father and take over the territory.[59,88] Young females also face this choice, but are at less risk of aggression. Many will always remain subordinate to the breeding female(s), and will never have young of their own. However, they may help the breeding female(s) rear subsequent litters, and some may eventually succeed in becoming breeders themselves.[42,126]

Lifespan and death under natural conditions

House mice have a potential lifespan of approximately 2 years.[8] However, in addition to the risks of injury and death due to aggressive actions of conspecifics, mice face numerous other hazards. Cold conditions and lack of food during winter are the most serious threats to mouse survival, and predation will claim many more lives. As a result, the average lifespan of house mice is often only about 3–12 months.[3,50,69]

Using house mouse biology and behavior to inform housing and husbandry for pet mice

The importance of understanding species' natural biology and behavior in informing practices for caring for captive animals has been acknowledged for many years.[127] There are numerous books and Internet sites (e.g., www.miceandrats. com and www.fancymice.info/index.htm) that provide the basic instructions for housing and caring for mice. The following section will go into more detail about how the sensory biology and behavior of mice may inform our decisions about housing and husbandry.

Sensory biology

Sensory differences between mice and humans must be taken into account when deciding where and how to house mice. While mice use the same five basic senses as humans, there are dramatic differences in prioritization and acuity of those senses between the two species—most notably the predominance of olfaction in murine communication and their investigation of their environment. Like laboratory mice,[18,29] this has a number of implications for mice kept as pets. Thus, for example, routine cage-cleaning removes all of the territorial and group membership odors from cages, which may be one of the reasons why an increase in aggression is often observed following cage-cleaning (in laboratory studies of male mice, at least):[128] and may help to explain why returning some nesting material (which is likely to contain group odors) following cleaning can help to reduce aggression, while returning substrate material (which is likely to contain territorial scents) may increase

agonistic behavior.[128] This enhanced olfactory sensitivity may also mean that mice find household smells, such as cleaning products or even strong perfumes, unpleasant. Even scented pet bedding may have anxiogenic effects on rodents[129] and as a prey species, pet mice may also find scents from other pets (particularly carnivorous pets such as cats and dogs) aversive.

Similarly, the differences in auditory sensitivity must be considered. Mice hear ultrasounds well above frequencies audible to humans, and ultrasounds are produced by numerous household appliances, from running taps to televisions and computer screens, some at very high sound pressures.[130] Thus, if mice are housed near sources of ultrasound they may find ambient noise levels unpleasant, noises of which humans may be completely unaware— perhaps similar to humans living in a room in which a vacuum cleaner is regularly (or even permanently) switched on.

Mice generally avoid brightly lit areas, and bright lighting may even cause retinal damage in certain types of mice, particularly albino lines.[121] Thus, mice should not be housed in brightly lit environments. In addition, their sensitivity to ultraviolet wavelengths means that mice may see the world very differently from humans. While it is not currently clear to what extent ultraviolet wavelengths are used by this predominantly nocturnal species, it has been suggested that being housed in environments without UV wavelengths may distort or shift all color perception (like humans looking at a psychedelic picture).[18] No studies to date have investigated whether mice show a preference for lighting conditions that include UV wavelengths, but studies in poultry (which are also UV sensitive) have found such a preference.[131]

The thigmotaxic (wall-hugging) behavior of mice should also be taken into account when designing the cage environment. Thus, laboratory studies have shown that mice prefer subdivided cages to cages that are not divided,[132] and a preference for nest boxes that are small and angular to ones that are larger and circular.[133]

Other aspects of the sensory environment must also be considered. For example, mice do not like draughts, and although they can withstand cool environments they must be provided with appropriate nesting materials in order to ensure that they can build effective thermoregulatory nests (as is shown in Figure 9.2).

Environment and natural behaviors

Given that the smallest natural mouse territory is roughly 2 m² (6.5 ft²), practical mouse cages will only ever be a tiny fraction of the size of a free-living mouse's environment. Fancy mouse handbooks recommend that a single or pair of mice require a cage measuring at least 30 × 20 × 15 cm length × width × height (11.8 × 7.8 × 5.9 in.).[9,134] Cages should have a solid base since mice prefer solid to grid floors[135] and can be constructed from glass or plastic. Where cages have sections enclosed by wire bars, the bars must

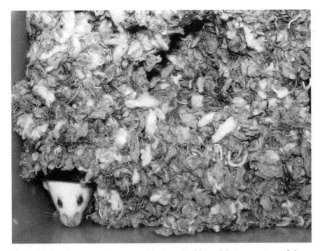

Figure 9.2 A mouse in a cage with deep bedding. (Photo courtesy of the author.)

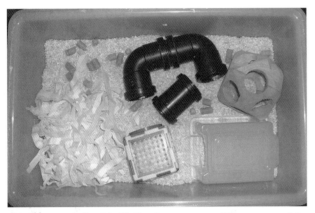

Figure 9.3 A well-enriched habitat for a pet mouse. (Photo courtesy of the author.)

not be set more than 8 mm apart (considerably less in breeding cages) since mice can squeeze through these small gaps. Some pet books also indicate that cages may be made from wood[9] but these may absorb smells and so are generally not recommended. Cages should be large enough to ensure that mice have adequate space for locomotor behavior—including opportunities for climbing and vertical movement. Pet shops sell a wide variety of cages suitable for mice, and these come in an increasingly unusual variety of shapes and colors. While these cages may at first sight appear somewhat gimmicky (and impractical for a large mouse colony), interestingly they may meet a number of needs of mice that could be less well-served by "standard" plastic base/mesh top cages. For example, the cage is compartmentalized, allowing the mice to use different areas for different purposes (e.g., distinct latrine and sleeping areas), and the tunnel systems allow vertical locomotion and are particularly suitable for a highly thigmotaxic species (Figure 9.3).

All mouse cages should contain a manipulable substrate, such as sawdust or wood-shavings (although the former should be avoided in hairless varieties of mouse, since the small particles can enter the eyes and cause health

problems). If possible the substrate should be suitable for and deep enough to allow burrowing behavior, since captive mice retain the ability to burrow and are motivated to do so if provided with suitable opportunities.[136] All cages should also contain nesting material. This has already been mentioned with regards to the need to provide mice with adequate opportunities for thermoregulation. However, nesting is also a highly motivated natural behavior, and mice are motivated to gain access to environments containing nesting material.[135,137] The provision of adequate nesting material is particularly important for breeding females prior to parturition, when these animals are highly motivated to build complex nests.

Further natural (or naturalistic) and motivated behaviors can also be encouraged by providing other enrichments. Thus, gnawing blocks can satisfy the motivation to gnaw, and can help to prevent overgrowth of the incisor teeth (which grow throughout life in mice). If left unchecked, these overgrown teeth can result in mice becoming unable to eat. Gnawing may also be encouraged through the provision of chewable shelters—which range from simple cardboard structures to more elaborate, edible homes.

Extended locomotor behavior can also be encouraged (albeit in an artificial manner) through the provision of running wheels within cages and exercise balls. Wheel running behavior has stimulated much debate in laboratory animal studies. Mice are highly motivated to perform this behavior and will run enormous distances (several kilometers per night) if provided with a wheel.[138] However, the behavior shares similarities with the physical characteristics of stereotypic behaviors, highly repetitive behaviors that often stem from frustration, and hence are commonly used as indicators of poor welfare.[138–140] Moreover, recent research has shown that running wheels may increase aggression and disrupt social hierarchy in group-housed mice,[141] and hence should be monitored carefully in grouped animals (although they may be rewarding enrichments where animals must be housed singly).

Numerous items are available for increasing complexity within cages. The addition of structures within cages can be beneficial for thigmotaxic species (see earlier), but may also have additional benefits. For example, structural complexity may enable males to hide from aggressive cage-mates; they may allow mice to use different areas of the cage for different purposes (e.g., using a partitioned area as a latrine); and they may allow breeding females to retreat from males in order to control the pace of copulation. However, the behavior of mice must be monitored in complex cages, because adding structural complexity may also increase the visual boundaries within the cage and the ease with which specific areas can be defended, and so potentially increases territorial (and escape-related) behavior in group-housed males.[142,143]

Pet mice require approximately 8–10 g (0.28–0.35 oz) of food per day, and foraging behavior and "gustatory enrichment" can be encouraged through the provision of a wide range of food types. There are a variety of commercially available diets for pet mice which usually include a mix of seeds, nuts, and dried vegetables (e.g., sweetcorn and flaked peas), and scattering the mix in clean substrate can be a simple foraging enrichment. Seed mixes can also be topped up once or twice a week with fresh fruits and vegetables (but avoid watery salad leaves such as lettuce as these can induce diarrhea), and even occasionally with small amounts of cooked meat or even small mealworms.[9,134,144]

With regards to their social environment, although free-living mice tend to live in extended family groups, their ability to breed rapidly and prolifically means that this natural social grouping is usually impractical for captive mice. However, like many captive animals, mice benefit from social housing and so guidelines often state that they should be kept in same-sex pairs or groups.[19] Mice can be sexed relatively easily by examining the groin area, with the distance between the urethra and the anus being greater in males than females, and females having two rows of distinct nipples down their abdomen. Due to the rapid maturation of mice, sexing should be carried out following weaning (and/or confirmed at the time of purchase).

Females are less aggressive, and so group housing for non-reproductive individuals generally produces few problems. Males, on the other hand, while far more docile than their free-living counterparts can be intensely aggressive, particularly following disruptive events such as cage-cleaning or if they have been mated with a female.[128] Thus, mated males almost certainly need to be housed singly if they are not housed with a breeding partner in between matings. The inability to escape or hide from aggression by the dominant male can lead to serious, and potentially fatal, injuries in subordinate animals. It may also have less dramatic, but nonetheless serious, effects such as increasing escape-related behavior (such as bar-biting) and urine retention (which may lead to kidney problems) in subordinate animals. Breeding males may also exhibit infanticidal behavior toward pups, and so their behavior must be monitored closely if they are allowed to remain with their breeding partner following the birth of the litter (although as discussed earlier, males are less prone to infanticide if they have been housed with their partner since mating and if the litter is born in their "territory").

Handling

Mice can be tamed to accept human handling, but as a small prey species they are naturally nervous initially. Mice should be picked up by gently grasping the base of the tail (NOT the tip, as this may be painful for the mouse and can result in damage to the tail) and sliding the other hand under the body to support their weight. If particularly nervous individuals must be picked up, it may be easier to entice these mice into a tube first and lift the tube.

Mice can also be socialized so that, in time, they readily interact with their owner (although mice will only interact to a limited extent compared to other larger rodent species, such as rats). Full instructions for the socialization process can be found on mouse web sites (such as www.fancymice.info/handling.htm). Briefly, the socialization process begins by habituating the mouse to the owner's presence and smell (e.g., sitting quietly with one hand in the cage). The mouse may then be "bribed" to start venturing onto the owner's hand by removing the food for several hours and then placing the hand in the cage with some favorite tit-bits on it. As the socialization process continues, the mouse will become increasingly bold, exploring further and further up the arm. With regular handling, the mouse should become accustomed to interacting with its owner.

Common behavioral problems

In addition to the behavioral problems associated with inappropriate housing and management, there are three specific behavioral problems that should be mentioned, and the first of these is aggression. Aggression can be a serious welfare concern in male mice, and there are two possible solutions to aggressive behavior. Either the subordinate animal that is the object of the dominant animal's aggression can be removed and re-housed, or the aggressor may be removed. Here, it is likely that the removed animal will subsequently need to be housed singly. Although single-housing is not generally recommended, studies investigating whether single-housing impairs welfare produce inconsistent results,[145] and mice that are singly-housed show an aversion to artificial social stimuli (e.g., via the provision of a mirror),[146] even though mirrors appear to be beneficial in other social species.[147,148]

Abnormally repetitive stereotypic behaviors are prevalent in captive mice as well as many other captive animals.[149] Stereotypic behaviors are commonly used as behavioral welfare indicators since they often stem from frustrated attempts to perform natural, motivated behaviors (although other causal factors can blur the relationship between stereotypic behavior and welfare[150]). For example, bar-biting in mice stems from attempts to escape from the cage perhaps due to the desire to escape from an aggressive cage-mate[150] and stereotypic digging in another common rodent pet species, the gerbil, stems from the motivation for a naturalistic burrow.[151] These behaviors therefore reflect that the environment is generally aversive, or that there is a specific environmental deficit. Observing the form of the stereotypic behavior may give an indication as to the nature of the underlying problem, and observing changes in stereotypic behavior following environmental changes (e.g., following the addition of environmental enrichments) may indicate whether welfare has improved, although the following *caveats* apply. Firstly, stereotypic behaviors may be harder to disrupt if they become a habit, or if they act as a substitute for a naturally rewarding behavior[149] and secondly, changes in other behaviors (e.g., aggression) should also be monitored to ensure that these are not adversely affected by environmental changes.[139]

A common behavioral problem in laboratory mice, and also reported in fancy mice, is barbering, also known as "whisker trimming" and the "Dalila effect"[152,153]—this latter name referring to the behavior of Delilah toward Samson in the Biblical story (I. Whishaw, *pers. comm.*).

Barbering behavior involves the removal of the whiskers and/or other areas of body fur (usually of cage-mates, but self-barbering can occur). Interestingly, although the plucking of fur appears to be painful,[152] mice continue to allow themselves to be barbered even if they are allowed to retreat from the barber.[154] Laboratory studies suggest that the behavior may have a number of causes, including dominance behavior, sexual over-grooming, and as a response to stress.[153] The behavior can also be influenced by aspects of the physical and social environment, such as cage material and whether animals are housed with siblings or non-siblings.[155] However, more recently, barbering has also been suggested as a potential model of trichotillomania (an obsessive compulsive behavior) in humans[156] (Figure 9.4). Unfortunately, the only method of preventing the behavior appears to be the removal of the barber.

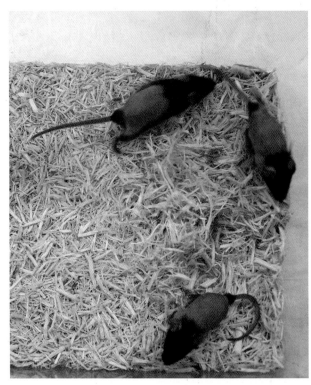

Figure 9.4   Young mice that have been barbered by their mother. (Photo courtesy of Joseph Garner and Aaron Kiess.)

References

1. Brothwell D. The pleistocene and holocene archaeology of the house mouse and related species In: Berry R, ed. *Biology of the House Mouse.* London: Academic Press, 1981;1–14.
2. Schwartz E, Schwartz H. The wild and commensal stocks of the house mouse *Mus musculus* Linnaeus. *J. Mammal* 1943;24:59–72.
3. Berry R. The natural history of the house mouse. *Field Stud* 1970;3:219–262.
4. Gray S, Hurst J. Competitive behaviour in an island population of house mice, *Mus domesticus.* *Anim Behav* 1998;56:1291–1299.
5. Pelikán J. Patterns of reproduction in the house mouse In: Berry R, ed. *Biology of the House Mouse.* London: Academic Press, 1981; 205–230.
6. Laurie E. The reproduction of the house mouse (*Mus musculus*) living in different environments. *Proc Roy Soc B* 1946;133:248–282.
7. Iivonen H, Nurminen L, Harri M, Tanila H, Puoliväli J. Hypothermia in mice tested in Morris water maze. *Behav Brain Res* 2003;141:207–213.
8. Bronson F. The reproductive ecology of the house mouse. *Quart Rev Biol* 1979;54:265–299.
9. Henwood C. *Fancy Mice.* New Jersey: TFH Publications, Inc., 1995.
10. Southern H. *Control of Rats and Mice. Vol. 3: House Mice.* Oxford: Clarendon Press, 1954.
11. La Madeleine B. Not so generic mice: Japanese companies venture into the transgenic mouse trade. *Japan, Inc* 2006;Summer 2006 Available at: http://findarticles.com/p/articles/mi_m0NTN/is_/ai_n26946947?tag=artBody;col1. Accessed Nov 30, 2008.
12. AFRMA. The history of fancy mice. Available at: http://wwwafrmaorg/rminfo4bhtm. Accessed Nov 30, 2008.
13. National Mouse Club. A brief history of the National Mouse Club. Available at: http://wwwnationalmouseclubcouk/historyhtml. Accessed Nov 30, 2008.
14. Buck L. Deconstructing smell. Available at: http://wwwhhmiorg/research/investigators/buckhtml. Accessed Nov 30, 2008.
15. Chess A. Scientists use smell to decipher the secrets of brain function. Available at: http://wwwwimitedu/nap/pdfs/Directors_Report/DirReport2000/dir_chesspdf. Accessed Nov 30, 2008.
16. Crawley J. *What's Wrong with my Mouse? Behavioural Phenotyping of Transgenic and Knockout Mice.* Chichester: Wiley-Liss and Sons, Inc., 2000.
17. Hurst J. The network of olfactory communication operating in populations of wild house mice In: MacDonald D, Müller-Scharze D, Natynczuk S, eds. *Chemical Signal in Vertebrates 5.* Oxford: Oxford University Press, 1990;401–414.
18. Olsson A, Nevison C, Patterson-Kane E et al. Understanding behaviour: The relevance of ethological approaches in laboratory animal science. *AABS* 2003;81:245–264.
19. Jennings M, Batchelor G, Brain P et al. Refining rodent husbandry: The mouse. *Lab Anim* 1998;32:233–259.
20. Lawlor M. A home for a mouse. *Hum Inn Alt Anim Exp* 1994;8:569–573.
21. Meehan A. *Rats and Mice: Their Biology and Control.* Tonbridge, Kent: Brown Knight and Truscott Ltd., 1984.
22. Mackintosh J. Behaviour of the house mouse In: Berry R, ed. *Biology of the House Mouse.* London: Academic Press, 1981;337–366.
23. Calderone J, Jacobs G. Regional variations in the relative sensitivity to UV-light in the mouse retina. *Vis Neurosci* 1995;12:463–468.
24. Rentokil. Research and development information. Available at: http://www.jm.rentokil.com/en/residential-customers/rodents/mice/index.html. Accessed Nov 30, 2008.
25. Dell'Omo G, Ricceri L, Wolfer D et al. Temporal and spatial adaptation to food restriction in mice under naturalistic conditions. *Behav Brain Res* 2000;115:1–8.
26. Crowcroft P. *Mice All Over.* London: Foulis, 1966.
27. Perrigo G. Food, sex, time and effort in a small mammal: Energy allocation strategies for survival and reproduction. *Behaviour* 1990;114:1–4.

28. Baumgardner D, Ward S, Dewsbury D. Diurnal patterning of eight activities in 14 species of muroid rodent. *Anim Learn Behav* 1980;8:322–330.

29. Latham N, Mason G. From house mouse to mouse house: The behavioural biology of free-living *Mus musculus* and its implications in the laboratory. *AABS* 2004;86:261–289.

30. Alyan S. Conditions for landmark-based navigation in the house mouse, *Mus musculus*. *Anim Behav* 2004;67:171–175.

31. Proctor D. *Grain Storage Techniques—Evolution and Trends in Developing Countries*. Rome: FAO Agricultural Services, 1994.

32. Fentress J. Dynamic boundaries of patterned behaviour: Interaction and self organisation In: Bateson P, Hinde R, eds. *Pers Ethol*. New York: Plenum Press, 1976;135–169.

33. Fitzgerald B, Karl B, Moller H. Spatial organisation and ecology of a sparse population of house mice (*Mus musculus*) in a New Zealand forest. *J Anim Ecol* 1981;50:489–518.

34. Benus R, Bohus R, Koolhaas J et al. Behavioural differences between artificially selected aggressive and non-aggressive mice: Response to apomorphine. *Behav Brain Res* 1991;43:201–208.

35. Koolhaas J, Korte S, De Boer S et al. Coping styles in animals: Current status in behavior and stress-physiology. *Neurosci Biobehav Rev* 1999;23:925–935.

36. Brown R. The rodents II: Suborder Myomorpha In: Brown R, MacDonald D, eds. *Social Odours in Mammals*. Oxford: Clarendon Press, 1985;345–417.

37. Beynon R, Hurst J. Making sense (and diagnostic use) of scents. *Business: The Quarterly Magazine of the Biotechnology and Biological Sciences Research Council* 2000;July:22–23.

38. Hurst J, Payne C, Nevison C et al. Individual recognition in mice mediated by major urinary proteins. *Nature* 2001;414:631–634.

39. Mucignat-Caretta C, Caretta A. Chemical signals in male house mice urine: Protein bound molecules modulate interactions between sexes. *Behaviour* 1999;136:331–343.

40. Berry R, Bronson F. Life history and bioeconomy of the house mouse. *Biol Rev* 1992;67:519–550.

41. Elton C. *Voles, Mice and Lemmings: Problems in Population Dynamics*. Oxford: Clarendon Press, 1942.

42. Medina F, Lopez-Darias M, Nogales M et al. Food habits of feral cats (*Felis silvestris catus* L.) in insular semiarid environments (Fuerteventura, Canary Islands). *Wildlife Res* 2008;35:162–169.

43. Gomez M, Priotto J, Provensal M et al. A population study of house mice (*Mus musculus*) inhabiting different habitats in an Argentine urban area. *Int Biodet Biodeg* 2008;62:270–273.

44. Woods M, McDonald R, Harris S. Predation of wildlife by domestic cats *Felis catus* in Great Britain. *Mamm Rev* 2003;33:174–188.

45. Kemble E, Bolwahnn B. Immediate and long-term effects of novel odors on risk assessment in mice. *Physiol Behav* 1997;61:543–549.

46. Dell'Omo G, Alleva E. Snake odor alters behavior, but not pain sensitivity in mice. *Physiol Behav* 1994;55:125–128.

47. Powell F, Banks P. Do house mice modify their foraging behaviour in response to predator odours and habitat? *Anim Behav* 2004;67:753–759.

48. Triggs G. The population ecology of house mice (*Mus domesticus*) on the Isle of May, Scotland. *J Zool* 1991;225:455–459.

49. Baker R. A study of rodent populations on Guam, Mariana Islands. *Ecol Mon* 1946;16:393–408.

50. Nowak R. *Walker's Mammals of the World*. London: John Hopkins University Press, 1999.

51. Lynch C, Possidente B. Relationships of maternal nesting to thermoregulatory nesting in house mice (*Mus musculus*) at warm and cold temperatures. *Anim Behav* 1978;26:1136–1143.

52. Barnett S, Hocking W. Are nests built for fun? Effects of alternative activities on nest-building by wild house mice. *Behav Neural Biol* 1981;31:73–81.

53. Barnett S, Munro K, Smart J, Stoddart R. House mice bred for many generations in two environments. *J Zool Lond* 1975;177:153–169.

54. Batchelder P, Kinney R, Demlow L et al. Effects of temperature and social interactions on huddling behavior in *Mus musculus*. *Physiol Behav* 1983;31:97–102.

55. Kalueff A, Tuohimaa P. Contrasting grooming phenotypes in C57BL/6 and 129S1/SvImJ mice. *Brain Res* 2004;1028:75–82.

56. Brain P, Benton D. Conditions of housing, hormones and aggressive behavior. In: Svare B, ed. *Hormones and Aggressive Behavior*. New York: Plenum Press, 1983;349–372.

57. Brown R. Social behavior, reproduction and population changes in the house mouse (*Mus musculus* L.). *Ecol Mon* 1953;23:217–240.

58. Kalueff A, Tuohimaa P. Grooming analysis algorithm for neurobehavioural stress research. *Brain Res Prot* 2004;13:151–158.

59 Potter M. *Control of Mice: Cooperative Extension Service*, University of Kentucky, 1994.

60. Rowe F. Wild house mouse biology and control In: Berry R, ed. *Biology of the House Mouse*. London: Academic Press, 1981; 575–590.

61. Choleris E, Guo C, Liu H et al. The effect of demonstrator age and number on duration of socially induced food preferences in house mouse (*Mus domesticus*). *Behav Proc* 1997;41:69–77.

62. Landry S. The rodentia as omnivores. *Qu Rev Biol* 1970;45:351–372.

63. Whitaker J. Food of *Mus musculus, Peromyscus maniculatus* and *Peromyscus leucopus* in Vigo County, Indiana. *J Mamm* 1966;47:473–486.

64. Wanless R, Angel A, Cuthbert R et al. Can predation by invasive mice drive seabird extinctions? *Biol Let* 2007;3:241–244.

65. Carr W, Schwartz D, Chism E et al. A natural food aversion in Norway rats and in house mice. *Behav Neural Biol* 1981;31:314–323.

66. Wuensch K. Sex differences in the flesh-eating preferences of wild house mice. *Physiol Behav* 1990;47:389–391.

67. Fertig D, Edmonds V. The physiology of the house mouse. *Sci Am* 1969;221:103–110.

68. Berry R, Jakobson M. Vagility in an island population of the house mouse. *J Zool* 1974;173:341–354.

69. Krebs C, Kenney A, Singleton G. Movements of feral house mice in agricultural landscapes (Abstract only). *Aus J Zool* 1995;43:293–302.

70. Brown P, Singleton G, Tann C et al. Increasing sowing depth to reduce mouse damage to winter crops. *Crop Prot* 2003;22:653–660.

71. Dickman C. Rodent ecosystem relationships: A review. In: Zhang Z, Hinds L, Singleton G, Wang Z, eds. *Rodent Biology and Management*. Canberra: Australian Centre for International Agricultural Research, 1999;127–128.

72. Chambers I, Singleton G, Krebs C. Movements and social organisation of wild house mice (*Mus domesticus*) in the wheatlands of northwestern Australia. *J Mamm* 2000;81:59–69.

73. Torre I, Bosch M. Effects of sex and breeding status on habitat selection by feral house mice (*Mus musculus*) on a small Mediterranean island. *Zeit Sauget* 1999;64:176–186.

74. Surgeoner G. *Rodent Control in Livestock Facilities*. Guelph: Queen's Printer for Ontario, 1986.

75. MAFF. *Code of Practice for the Prevention of Rodent Infestations in Poultry Flocks*. London: MAFF Publications, 1996.

76. Mackintosh J. Factors affecting the recognition of territory boundaries by mice (*Mus musculus*). *Anim Behav* 1973;21:464–470.

77. Mackintosh J. The experimental analysis of overcrowding In: Ebling F, Stoddart D, eds. *Population Control by Social Behaviour*. London: Institute of Biology, 1978;157–180.

78. Hurst J. The functions of urine marking in a free-living population of house mice *Mus domesticus*. *Anim Behav* 1987;35:1433–1442.

79. Hurst J. The priming effects of urine substrate marks on interactions between male house mice *Mus musculus domesticus* Schwarz & Schwarz. *Anim Behav* 1993;45:55–81.

80. Eklund A. The effects of inbreeding on aggression in wild male house mice (*Mus domesticus*). *Behaviour* 1996;133:883–901.

81. Smith J. Senses and communication In: Berry R, ed. *Biology of the House Mouse*. London: Academic Press, 1981;367–393.

82. Drickamer L. Rates of urine excretion by house mouse (*Mus domesticus*)—Differences by age, sex, social status and reproductive condition. *J Chem Ecol* 1995;21:1481–1493.

83. Desjardins C, Maruniak J, Bronson F. Social rank in house mice: Differential revealed by ultraviolet visualization of urinary marking patterns. *Science* 1973;182:939–941.

84. Brain P, Parmagiani S. Variation in aggressiveness in house mouse populations. *Biol J Linn Soc* 1990;41:257–269.

85. Calaresu G. Effects of early experience and status on social interactions of male wild house mice *Mus musculus* L. *Mouse News* 1979;4:25–26.

86. Jensen S, Gray S, Hurst J. Excluding neighbours from territories: Effects of habitat structure and resource distribution. *Anim Behav* 2005;69:785–795.

87. Van Zeegeren K. Variation in aggressiveness and the regulation of numbers in house mouse populations. *Neth J Zool* 1980;30:635–770.

88. Jensen S, Gray S, Hurst J. How does habitat structure affect activity and use of space among house mice? *Anim Behav* 2003;66:239–250.

89. Pech R, Hood G, Singleton G et al. Models for predicting plagues of house mice (*Mus domesticus*). In: Zhang Z, Hinds L, Singleton G, Wang Z, eds. *Rodent Biology and Management*. Canberra: Australian Centre for International Agricultural Research, 1999;81–112.

90. Timm R. *Pest Notes: House Mouse*. Oakland: University of California Agriculture and Natural Resources Publications, 2000;7483.

91. Patris B, Baudoin C. Female sexual preferences differ in *Mus spicilegus* and *Mus musculus domesticus*: The role of familiarisation and sexual experience. *Anim Behav* 1998;56:1465–1470.

92. Wright S, Brown R. Maternal behavior, paternal behavior, and pup survival in CD-1 albino mice (*Mus musculus*) in three different housing conditions. *J Comp Psychol* 2000;114:183–192.

93. Koyama S. Primer effects by conspecific odors in house mice: A new perspective in the study of primer effects on reproductive activities. *Horm Behav* 2004;46:303–310.

94. Firman R, Simmons L. Polyandry, sperm competition and reproductive success in mice. *Behav Ecol* 2008;19:695–702.

95. Nyby J, Dizinno G, Whitney G. Social status and ultrasonic vocalizations of male mice. *Behav Biol* 1976;18:285–289.

96. Scott J, Pfaff D. Behavioral and electrophysiological responses of female mice to male urine odors. *Physiol Behav* 1970;5:407–411.

97. Ehman K, Scott M. Urinary odour preferences of MHC congenic female mice: *Mus domesticus*: Implications for kin recognition and detection of parasitised males. *Anim Behav* 2001;62:781–789.

98. Lenington S, Coopersmith C, Williams J. Genetic basis of mating preferences in wild house mice. *Am Zool* 1992;32:40–47.

99. Kavaliers M, Colwell D, Braun W et al. Brief exposure to the odour of a parasitized male alters the subsequent mate odour responses of female mice. *Anim Behav* 2003;65:59–68.

100. Jordan W, Bruford M. New perspectives on mate choice and the MHC. *Heredity* 1998;81:127–133.

101. Cheetham S, Smith A, Armstrong S et al. Limited variation in the major urinary proteins of laboratory mice. *Physiol Behav* 2008;96:253–261.

102. Hayashi S, Kimura T. Degree of kinship as a factor regulating preferences among conspecifics in mice. *Anim Behav* 1983;31:81–85.

103. Drickamer L. Intra-uterine position and anogenital distance in house mice: Consequences under field conditions. *Anim Behav* 1996;51:925–934.

104. Palanza P, Parmagiani S, Vom Saal F. Urine marking and maternal aggression of wild female mice in relation to anogenital distance at birth. *Physiol Behav* 1995;58:827–835.

105. Drickamer L, Robinson A, Mossman C. Differential responses to same and opposite sex odors by adult house mice are associated with anogenital distance. *Ethology* 2001;107:509–519.

106. Drickamer L, Gowarty P, Homes C. Free female mate choice in house mice affects reproductive success and offspring viability and performance. *Anim Behav* 2000;59:371–378.

107. Gowarty P, Drickamer L, Schmid-Holmes S. Male house mice produce fewer offspring with lower viability and poorer performance when mated with females they do not prefer. *Anim Behav* 2003;65:95–103.

108. Holy T, Guo Z. Ultrasonic songs of male mice. *PLoS Biol* 2005;3:e386.

109. DeCatanzaro D. Duration of mating relates to fertility in mice. *Physiol Behav* 1991;50:393–395.

110. Hull E, Dominguez J. Sexual behavior in male rodents. *Horm Behav* 2007;52:45–55.

111. Johansen J, Clemens L, Nunez A. Characterization of copulatory behavior in female mice: Evidence for paced mating. *Physiol Behav* 2008;95:425–429.

112. Weber E, Olsson I. Maternal behaviour in *Mus musculus* sp.: An ethological overview. *AABS* 2008;114:1–22.

113. Wolfe J, Barnett S. Effects of cold on nest-building by wild and domestic mice, *Mus musculus* L. *Biol J Linn Soc* 1977; 9:73–85.

114. Bult A, Lynch C. Nesting and fitness: Lifetime reproductive success in house mice bidirectionally selected for thermoregulatory nest-building behavior. *Behav Genet* 1997;27:231–240.

115. Vom Saal F, Franks P, Boechler M et al. Nest defense and survival of offspring in highly aggressive wild Canadian female house mice. *Physiol Behav* 1995;58:669–678.

116. Svare B, Gandelman R. Postpartum aggression in mice: The influence of suckling stimulation. *Horm Behav* 1976;7:407–416.

117. Maestripieri D, Alleva E. Maternal aggression and litter size in the female house mouse. *Ethology* 1990;84:27–34.

118. Elwood R, Nesbitt A, Kennedy H. Maternal aggression in response to the risk of infanticide by male mice, *Mus domesticus*. *Anim Behav* 1990;40:1080–1086.

119. König B, Markl H. Maternal care in house mice. I. The weaning strategy as a means for parental manipulation of offspring quality. *Behav Ecol Sociobiol* 1987;20:1–9.

120. Manning C, Dewsbury D, Wakeland E et al. Communal nesting and communal nursing in house mice, *Mus musculus domesticus*. *Anim Behav* 1995;50:741–751.

121. Clough G. Environmental effects of animals used in biomedical research. *Biol Rev* 1982;57:487–523.

122. Elwood R, McCauley P. Communication in rodents: Infants to adults In: Elwood R, ed. *Parental Behaviour of Rodents*. New York: John Wiley & Sons Ltd., 1983;127–149.

123. Ehret G, Bernecker C. Low-frequency sound communication by mouse pups (*Mus musculus*): Wriggling calls release maternal behaviour. *Anim Behav* 1986;34:821–830.

124. Ehret G. Infant rodent ultrasounds—A gateway to the understanding of sound communication. *Behav Genet* 2005;35:19–29.

125. Valsecchi P, Moles A, Mainardi M. Transfer of food preferences in mice (*Mus domesticus*) at weaning—The role of maternal diet. *Boll Zool* 1993;60:297–300.

126. Gerlach G. Dispersal mechanisms in a captive wild house mouse population (*Mus domesticus* Rutty). *Biol J Linn Soc* 1990;41:271–277.

127. Dawkins M. *Animal Suffering: The Science of Anim Welf*. London: Chapman and Hall, 1980.

128. Van Loo P, Kruitwaggen C, Van Zutphen L et al. Modulation of aggression in male mice: Influence of cage cleaning regime and scent marks. *Anim Welf* 2000;9:281–295.

129. Fleming P. Scented products for domestic animals: A cause for concern? *UFAW Annual Report 2004–2005*, 2005.

130. Sales G, Milligan S, Khirnykh K. Sources of sound in the laboratory animal environment: A survey of the sounds produced by procedures and equipment. *Anim Welf* 1999;8:97–115.

131. Moinard C, Sherwin C. Turkeys prefer fluorescent light with supplementary ultraviolet radiation. *AABS* 1999;64:261–267.

132. Chamove A. Cage design reduces emotionality in mice. *Lab Anim* 1989;23:215–219.

133. Buhot-Averseng M. Nest box choice in the laboratory mouse: Preference for nest boxes differing in design (size and/or shape) and composition. *Behav Proc* 1981;6:337–384.

134. Mays N. *Your First Mouse*. Portsmouth: Kingdom Books, 1999.

135. Van de Weerd H, Van Loo P, Van Zutphen L et al. Strength of preference for nesting material as environmental enrichment for laboratory mice. *AABS* 1998;55:369–382.

136. Sherwin C, Haug E, Terkelsen N et al. Studies on the motivation for burrowing by laboratory mice. *AABS* 2004;88:343–358.

137. Roper T. Self-sustaining activities and reinforcement in the nest-building behaviour of mice. *Behaviour* 1975;50:40–58.

138. Sherwin C. Voluntary wheel running: A review and novel interpretation. *Anim Behav* 1998;56:11–27.

139. Mason G. Stereotypic behaviour in captive animals: Fundamentals, and implications for welfare and beyond. In: Mason G, Rushen J, eds. *Stereotypic Animal Behaviour: Fundamentals and Applications to Welfare*. Wallingford: CAB International, 2006;325–351.

140. Latham N, Würbel H. Wheel running: A common rodent stereotypy? In: Mason G, Rushen J, eds. *Stereotypic Animal Behaviour: Fundamentals and Applications to Welfare*. Wallingford: CAB International, 2006; 91–92.

141. Howerton C, Garner J, Mench J. Effects of a running wheel-igloo enrichment on aggression, hierarchy linearity, and stereotypy in group-housed male CD-1 (ICR) mice. *AABS* 2008;115:90–103.

142. Haemisch A, Voss T, Gartner K. Effects of environmental enrichment on aggressive behavior, dominance hierarchies, and endocrine states in male DBA/2J mice. *Physiol Behav* 1994;56:1041–1048.

143. Nevison C, Hurst J, Barnard C. Strain-specific effects of cage enrichment in male laboratory mice (*Mus musculus*). *Anim Welf* 1999;8:361–379.

144. McKeown C. Feeding your mice. Available at: http://wwwfancymiceinfo/ feeding1htm. Accessed Nov 30, 2008.

145. Krohn T, Sorenson D, Ottesen J et al. The effects of individual housing on mice and rats: A review. *Anim Welf* 2006;15:343–352.

146. Sherwin C. Mirrors as potential environmental enrichment for individually housed laboratory mice. *AABS* 2004;87:95–103.

147. Mills D, Davenport K. The effect of a neighbouring conspecific versus the use of a mirror for the control of stereotypic weaving behaviour in the stable horse. *Anim Sci* 2002;74:95–101.

148. Zotte A, Princz A, Matics Z et al. Rabbit preference for cages and pens with or without mirrors. *AABS* 2009;116:273–278.

149. Mason G, Latham N. Can't stop, won't stop: Is stereotypy a reliable animal welfare indicator? *Anim Welf* 2004;13:S57–S69.

150. Nevison C, Hurst J, Barnard C. Why do male ICR(CD-1) mice perform bar-related (stereotypic) behaviour? *Behav Proc* 1999;47:95–111.

151. Wiedenmayer C. Causation of the ontogenic development of stereotypic digging in gerbils. *Anim Behav* 1997;53:461–470.

152. Sarna J, Dyck R, Whishaw I. The Dalila effect: C57BL6 mice barber whiskers by plucking. *Behav Brain Res* 2000;108:39–45.

153. Kalueff A, Minasyan A, Keisala T et al. Hair barbering in mice: Implications for neurobehavioural research. *Behav Proc* 2006;71:8–15.

154. Van den Broek F, Omzight C, Beynen A. Whisker trimming behaviour in A2G mice is not prevented by offering means of withdrawal from it. *Lab Anim* 1993;27:270–272.

155. Garner J, Dufour B, Gregg L et al. Social and husbandry factors affecting the prevalence and severity of barbering ("whisker trimming") by laboratory mice. *AABS* 2004;89:263–282.

156. Garner J, Weisker S, Dufour B et al. Barbering (fur and whisker trimming) by laboratory mice as a model of human trichotillomania and obsessive-compulsive spectrum disorders. *Comp Med* 2004;54:216–224.

10

Rats

Anne Fullerton Hanson and Manuel Berdoy

History

The Norway rat (*Rattus norvegicus*) does not come from Norway, but owes its name to its formal Linnaean nomenclatural description by Berkenhourt (1769) who mistakenly believed that the species came from Norway. Fossil records indicate that the Norway rat originated in the plains of Asia, probably in what is now Northern China.[1–3] The rat's behavioral, social, and feeding adaptability allowed it to colonize new environments, including buildings and ships in a human-dependent association called commensalism. This association has contributed directly to its spread to other parts of the world by following routes of human migration and the rat has now colonized all continents except Antarctica.

The Norway rat was the first mammalian species to be domesticated for scientific research, with work dating to before 1828. The first recorded captive breeding colony for rats was established in 1856.[3] White (i.e., albino) rats of European origin were brought to America at the end of the 19th century and became the foundation stock of American laboratory rats.[4] In 2004 the rat joined the very select group of mammals (with mice, in 2002, and men in 2001) to have its genome sequenced.[5]

Behavior of wild rats

The rat can arguably be described as the jack of all trades and, contrary to the idiom, the master of several, as a key to its ecological success resides in its behavioral, social, and feeding adaptability.[6]

The social and mating systems of rats depend on their population density, which in turn is determined by the richness of the environment. In poor environments with sparsely distributed food, such as the rural environment, feral rat populations exist at low densities and rats are territorial and polygynous.[6–8] One male rat monopolizes the burrows of females. He defends a territory, keeping other males away from the burrows and the surrounding area, and he mates only with the females of his group.

In rich environments, where food is abundant and clumped (such as urban areas), commensal rats can live at high densities. Rat colonies can act as "information centers" where rats can learn from the feeding experience of other individuals in the colony[9] (see "Ingestive behavior"). In stable environments, dominance hierarchies (which can be remarkably stable) develop, particularly amongst males.[7,9,10] The male social system becomes despotic instead of territorial and the mating system becomes polygynandrous. Males no longer defend female burrows, as there are too many male intruders for a single territorial male to fend off. When a female comes into heat, a group of males rushes her and mates with her sequentially, with little or no overt competition.[10,11] Males may mate with multiple estrous females, and females with multiple males in a type of scramble competition.

Socially dominant males do, however, gain a subtle reproductive advantage over subordinate males. Dominant males achieve more ejaculations and continue mating with females longer than subordinate males.[6,11,12] This increases the chance that the dominant male's sperm will fertilize more of the female's eggs, and thus more of the resulting litter will be his.[13]

For the females' part, mating with multiple males may increase the chance of fertilization. It may also provide paternity uncertainty, which may reduce the chance of infanticide by males once the litter is born (Table 10.1(m)). Copulation reduces male infanticidal behavior starting several weeks later, at a time that roughly coincides with the birth of the male's young.[14,15]

Table 10.1 Relevant online resources

Two websites maintained by the authors (www.ratbehavior.org and www.ratlife.org) contain a wide range of factual and visual data on rat biology and behavior. The following lists some of the web sections that provide additional information relevant to sections presented in the text.

Wild rat behavior:
(a) Wild rat behavior: www.ratbehavior.org/WildRats.htm
(b) For an example of cat avoidance: see section "Cat Alert" in www.ratlife.org

Sensory systems:
(c) Olfactory system: www.ratbehavior.org/RatOlfaction.htm
(d) The rat's whiskers: www.ratbehavior.org/RatWhiskers.htm and www.ratbehavior.org/HearingWhiskers.htm
(e) Auditory system: www.ratbehavior.org/rathearing.htm
(f) Visual system: www.ratbehavior.org/RatVision.htm

Communication:
(g) Urine marking: www.ratbehavior.org/UrineMarking.htm
(h) To hear rat vocalizations: www.ratbehavior.org/norway_rat_vocalizations.htm and section "Ultrasounds" in www.ratlife.org

Locomotion:
(i) To see galloping: see section "Release" in www.ratlife.org

Social behavior:
(j) Play: www.ratbehavior.org/RatPlay.htm
(k) Aggression: www.ratbehavior.org/Aggression.htm
To view aggressive interactions between rats: see section "Social Hierarchy" in www.ratlife.org
(l) To see a video of a rat's eyes boggling: www.ratbehavior.org/Eyeboggle.mov

Reproduction and development:
(m) To view reproductive behavior in a dense wild rat colony, see sections "Smells and Sex" and "Multiple Partners" in www.ratlife.org.
(n) To see rat reproductive behavior with ear vibration: see section "Smells & Sex" in www.ratlife.org
(o) To see a mother rat with her new pups: see sections "Birth & Death" and "Stepping Out" in www.ratlife.org
(p) To see footage of an infanticidal male and learn more about infanticide: see section "Birth & Death" in www.ratlife.org and the article at www.ratbehavior.org/infanticide.htm
(q) Developmental data can be found in: www.ratbehavior.org/Stats.htm

Feeding:
(r) How young and adult rats make choices about what to eat: see sections "Stepping Out" and "More Balanced Diet" in www.ratlife.org and www.ratbehavior.org/FoodChoices.htm
(s) The rat's inability to vomit: www.ratbehavior.org/vomit.htm

Female rats may raise their young alone[16,17] or up to six reproductive females may share a burrow, usually each with a separate nest chamber, although sometimes they will raise their young together in a single nest.[18] When the offspring are weaned, the young males disperse.

Wild rat aggressive behavior involves fighting, chasing, biting, boxing, and flight. Wild rats do not display some of the agonistic behaviors seen in domestic rats, such as the sidling posture and the supine (lying on the back) posture. Most agonistic encounters between wild rats are brief and end in the flight of the defeated rat.[19] The difference between wild and domestic rat aggressive behavior is probably due to the confined environment of the cage, which leads to escalated conflicts and the necessity of protracted self-defense in close quarters.

Senses

Rats evolved in and continue to live in environments that are rich in non-visual stimuli. They live in burrows and are active at night and during twilight hours. They rely on their senses of smell, touch, and hearing far more than vision.

Olfaction

Rats have a highly developed olfactory system and a keen sense of smell. Almost every aspect of a rat's life is guided by its sense of smell (Table 10.1(c)). The sequencing of the rat genome which estimated a staggering 2070 genes and pseudogenes involved with olfaction[5] suggests that we are a long way from unraveling the complexity of the rat's olfactory world.

Rats possess two olfactory systems: the olfactory epithelium in the nose, and the vomeronasal organ. Air enters the rat's nostrils and flows past a patch of skin, the *olfactory epithelium*, rich with smell receptors. It has been estimated that rats have between 500 and 1000 olfactory receptors.[20] Odor particles in the air bind to receptors on olfactory neurons that project into the olfactory epithelium.

The accessory olfactory system, called the vomeronasal organ, is situated in a pouch off the nasal cavity. Unlike the olfactory epithelium of the nose, this dead-end position means that air can't flow into it.[21] When a rat sniffs and licks, molecules from the environment stick to its moist nose and dissolve. The molecules are then transported to the vomeronasal organ suspended in mucus. The vomeronasal organ detects non-volatile chemicals and pheromones found in the urine and other secretions;[22] it is critical in mate attraction, courtship, copulation, aggression, and parental care.[23]

Finally, rats use smells to avoid predators in the wild and it is noteworthy that even after many generations of never having contact with a cat, domesticated rats still have an innate aversion to cat odors (Table 10.1(b)).[24]

Touch

The rat perceives its immediate environment with its whiskers, or vibrissae (Figure 10.1). The rat moves its whiskers back and forth several times per second (Hz) brushing them against the substrate and nearby objects.[25] Whisker movements range from small twitches at a rate of 7–12 Hz[26] to large, rhythmic sweeps at a rate of 5–9 Hz during active exploration.[27,28] The rat uses its whiskers to determine the position, distance, size, texture, and shape of objects it encounters in its immediate environment.[29] The rat's whiskers are as sensitive as human fingertips[27] and the rat gains a highly detailed picture from its tactile exploration. Whiskers can detect wind and slight breezes, which may

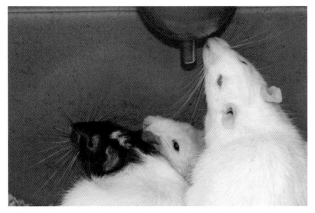

Figure 10.1   A close up of rats' long vibrissae. (Photo courtesy of M. C. Tynes, copyright 2010.)

help rats orient underground. Whiskers also apparently aid swimming by detecting the surface of the water: rats without whiskers easily drown.[30,31] Whiskers are used socially as well. During agonistic encounters, when two rats stand face to face, the defending rat attempts to keep whisker-to-whisker contact with the aggressive rat and this helps avoid an attack on the head.[32] Whiskers are continuously replaced throughout life. They regenerate after they are plucked or trimmed.[33]

Hearing

Rats can detect and emit sounds in the ultrasonic range. The human ear can detect frequencies up to 20 kHz, but rats can hear up to 90 kHz, with peak sensitivity in the range of 10–50 kHz.[34] The bulk of rat vocal communication occurs at frequencies beyond the human's range of hearing (Table 10.1(h)).

Mammals pinpoint the source of sound using several types of cues (Table 10.1(e)). The first two types of localization cues use the fact that mammals have two ears separated by the width of the skull: a sound coming from the left will reach the left ear slightly before the right ear, and the sound will be louder in the left ear than the right. The brain uses the time delay and difference in loudness to pinpoint the source of sound in space in the left–right plane. The third type of cue involves the outer ear (pinna). Sounds coming from the front of the ear will be louder than those coming from the back. Also, the sound is modified as it passes over the ear's many bumps and convolutions, and will therefore sound different depending on whether it comes from above or below. Therefore, the outer ear helps localize sound in space in the front–back and up–down planes.[35] Small animals, such as rats, have only a short distance between their ears, so they have less time delay to work with than large animals. Rats are therefore not as good at pinpointing sources of sound as large animals.[36]

Albinism does not appear to affect hearing in rats. Albino rats can localize sounds,[37] discriminate between sounds of different frequency and intensity,[38] and have the same hearing range as pigmented rats.[39]

Vision

The rat's vision is much poorer than a human's, but is adequate for the rat's needs as a nocturnal and crepuscular burrow-dwelling rodent (Table 10.1(f)).

The rat eye has relatively poor optics. It also has no fovea or area centralis. The photoreceptors in the retina consist of 99% rods and 1% cones.[40] In the human eye 5% of the photoreceptors are cones,[41] and the human fovea contains only cones.

Rats have typical mammalian dichromatic vision, with a twist; one of their two cone types is sensitive to ultraviolet light, thus they perceive ultraviolet wavelengths in addition to blues and greens in the visible spectrum. The second cone type detects medium wavelengths. Without the third cone type (that humans have) for detecting long wavelength light, they cannot see reds. Rats can be trained to distinguish between ultraviolet wavelengths, blues, and greens, but under normal circumstances they do not appear to attend to color differences, focusing instead on brightness cues.[42]

The function of ultraviolet vision in rodents is not well-understood and is currently an active area of research.[43] Ultraviolet vision may enable rats to see urine marks in addition to being able to smell them.[44] Ultraviolet vision may also be useful during the twilight hours, when rats are active but visible light is dim.[45]

Normally pigmented rats have poor visual acuity— about 1.5 cycles/degree (equivalent to 20/600 vision) meaning they cannot see well at long distances. However, at close range, rats are able to see objects in considerable detail.[46–48]

Albino rats have unpigmented irises that do not block light well, so they cannot control levels of incoming light. Albinos lack the pigmented epithelium that lines the back of the retina and absorbs light that has passed through the photoreceptor layer. Without it, light inside the eye is reflected back, which degrades the retinal image and leads to retinal degeneration over time. Albino rats also have abnormal neural connections to the visual cortex from the retina, which may affect visual processing. The visual acuity of albinos is much worse than normally pigmented rats, around 0.5 cycles/degree[46,48] roughly equivalent to 20/1200 vision.

Like many prey species, rats have laterally placed eyes giving them a large field of vision but only a small binocular field; thus their binocular depth perception (more often associated with predators) is poor. Rats use motion parallax to estimate depth by bobbing their heads up and down.[49] The poor visual acuity of albino rats further contributes to their poor visual depth perception.[50] Pet owners often note that albino rats bob their heads and sway frequently; these movements may represent the albino rat's attempt to increase its depth perception using motion parallax.

As rats age beyond 2 years, the retina loses many of its cells. Parts of the retina and capillaries that feed it become enlarged and thickened.[51] Therefore, rats over 2 years of age probably do not see as well as younger rats.

Communication

Olfactory communication

As social nocturnal animals, it is not surprising that olfaction plays a crucial role in almost every aspect of a rat's life, sometimes even before birth. As is the case with many rodents,[52] olfactory signals that emanate from the animals' body (sebaceous glands), breath, urine, and feces convey a great range of information whose subtlety we may never fully comprehend.

Perhaps the most readily visible form of olfactory signaling is urine marking (Table 10.1(g)). Rats deposit small drops of urine (scent marks) in their environment and on conspecifics. Urine marking is an important form of chemical communication that contains information about the species, sex, age, reproductive status, sexual availability, social status, individual identity, current stress level of the animal that produced it, and the time elapsed since the urine mark was deposited.[21,53]

All rats urine-mark, but males mark more than females or neutered males. Adult rats mark more than juveniles and dominant males mark the most. Adult males mark at all times, but adult female marking is cyclical; females mark most the night before they ovulate.[54–56]

Urine marking has multiple functions. Environmental marking is a sexual advertisement and attractant to rats of the opposite sex. Female rats prefer the urine of males with high testosterone levels[55,57] and may use male urine to help them select a mate from multiple males. Female rats mark their environment the night before they ovulate in order to advertise their availability and receptivity to males at a time when they are most likely to conceive.[57]

Rats may also use urine marks as a habitat labeling system. Urine marks may help the rat to create and maintain optimum levels of the rat's own odor,[58] to navigate through its environment,[59] to create an index of spatial knowledge,[60] and to increase the confidence of the resident rat.[61]

Rats also mark over preferred foods. These urine marks attract other rats to that food source and function as one of the methods of social transmission of food preferences[62] (see "Ingestive behavior").

Rats mark each other by crawling over each other and depositing a drop or two of urine on the other rat's fur. Females appear to mark males with different amounts of urine to identify and select the male they prefer.[63] Male rats readily mark other males. Dominant males mark subordinates more than vice versa.[64]

Rats also mark their human owners. The function of human marking is unknown but may be a form of environmental marking.

Vocal communication

Rats emit a variety of squeaks and chirps within the range of human hearing, but the bulk of their vocal communication occurs in the ultrasonic range, from 20 to 70 kHz.[34]

Rats have two types of ultrasonic calls. The first type is a 35–70 kHz short, chirp-like call that is associated with vigorous activity, high levels of arousal, and during social contact such as play, aggression (e.g., during the introduction of two males), and copulation. In some cases it seems to make the females more likely to be sexually receptive. The second type of call is a 22 kHz long call associated with sexual behavior and aggression, such as after ejaculation, after defeat in an aggressive encounter, at the end of a painful stimulus, and when exposed to a predator.[34] Rats may also use ultrasound for short range echolocation.[65,66]

Rats also emit vocalizations in the audible range. Infants produce broadband vocalizations in response to pain or when being groomed.[34] Adults emit a variety of chirps and squeaks, usually during agonistic encounters. Adults also emit a scream or shriek in contexts of fear or pain, such as in response to a predator, during a fight, during pain, or when the nest is approached by a strange rat.[67]

Rats chatter or brux their teeth, a non-vocalized sound produced by grinding the front incisors together. Rats chatter their teeth during times of stress, such as during pain[68] or agonistic encounters. Anecdotally, rats brux their teeth softly at times of relaxation and pleasure such as when being gently stroked.

Body care

Rats spend up to half their waking hours engaged in grooming[69] and a ruffled coat can be the sign of stress and/or disease. Self-grooming is a complex, organized behavior whose function is to clean and maintain the fur and skin. Grooming movements include wiping, licking, and scratching.

A grooming sequence proceeds from nose to tail. It begins with paw-licking or face-washing and proceeds to rubbing and licking the fur around the head, neck, body, and tail.[70] Single grooming actions such as scratching or direct grooming of the trunk may also occur. Beyond a hygienic environment, rats do not need any special accessories to engage in grooming.

Rats can sometimes exhibit alarming looking dark-red tears and nasal secretions that look like dried blood. This is known as chromodacryorrhoea (red or "bloody" tears). The coloration, however, is not blood nor is it sign of disease per se. The staining is caused by the Harderian gland, a modified tear gland located behind the eyeball that produces a porphyrin-rich secretion which normally lubricates the eye (and may possibly also play a role in protection from light levels).[71,72] When the rat is stressed, however, this secretion can overflow, producing crusty dots or a ring around the eye. It may sometimes appear at the nose as the secretion flows down the nasolacrimal duct. Thus the staining is a non-specific indication of stress, either caused by social and/or environmental conditions or by internal factors.[72,73]

Locomotion

The rat uses the same basic gaits as all quadrupeds: the walk, the trot, and the gallop.

Rats use a lateral walk with the following stride order: left hindlimb, left forelimb, right hindlimb, right forelimb.[74] Two or three limbs are in contact with the ground at all times. The limbs act as struts, with the body rising and falling during each step.[75] The walk is the rat's slowest gait, ranging between 0 and 55 cm/sec.[74]

To increase speed beyond the walk, quadrupeds incorporate an aerial phase into the gait. This switch results in the trotting gait, in which the legs act as springs instead of struts. Only two limbs at a time contact the ground. The legs move together in diagonal pairs: right forelimb and left hindlimb, left forelimb and right hindlimb. During a very fast trot the rat may jump from one diagonal pair to the other, becoming briefly airborne. Rats trot at speeds of 55–90 cm/sec.[74,75]

Galloping, or bounding, is the quadruped's fastest gait (Table 10.1(i)). To increase speed beyond the trot, the rat must extend the trunk. The rat jumps from the hindlimbs to the forelimbs, then brings the hindlimbs under the body and stretches forward on the forelimbs.[75] One, two, or no limbs are on the ground at any given time. The faster the gallop, the more synchronized the limbs. Rats gallop at speeds over 80 cm/sec.[74,76]

The rat's cage should be as large as the owner can afford and maintain. When given a choice between a large and a small cage, rats prefer the larger cage.[77] Standard laboratory rat cages (47.6 × 26 × 21 cm [18.75 × 10.25 × 8.25 in.] for a small size, 50 × 40.6 × 21 cm [20 × 16 × 8.25 in.] for a large one) are considered small for pet rats and are best used temporarily (e.g., for a mother and a litter, for a sick or elderly rat, or as a transport cage). An adult rat stands on its hind legs frequently, so its permanent cage should be tall enough to allow for this behavior. Lawlor[78] suggests a minimum height of 30 cm (11.8 in.) to accommodate this behavior. Rats also prefer more complex environments, with interior walls and platforms, to simple ones of the same size.[79] Inside the cage, rats should have suitable bedding for nest-building and nest boxes or refuges for hiding.[80]

Aquariums and wire cages offer two larger options for housing pet rats. Aquariums are inexpensive, warm, and easily cleaned. They also offer good visibility and prevent bedding from being scattered outside the cage. However, aquariums are heavy and offer poor air circulation that may result in condensation and heat in warm weather. A 10-gallon aquarium is the minimum for a pair of females or a single male.[81]

Wire cages are a common choice. Wire cages are lightweight, well-ventilated, and provide many opportunities for enrichment. However, they can be difficult to clean and rats may scatter shavings outside the cage. They come in a large number of shapes and sizes. Horizontal surfaces should be solid for greater comfort[82] or should have wire of no more than 0.5 × 0.5 in. to prevent foot entrapment.[81]

Aging rats may lose mobility and balance and may no longer be able to climb ramps or stand on their hind legs to reach food or water. Older rats may therefore need to have their cages modified so they can continue to move about, eat, and sleep in comfort. Food bowls for aging rats should be heavy and have a low lip. Water bottles should be lowered. Smooth, slippery ramps may need to be replaced with textured ramps that provide more traction. Eventually, food, water, and shelter may need to be moved to the bottom floor of the cage.

Social behavior

Rats engage in a number of affiliative social behaviors. They groom each other, play together, and sleep huddled next to each other (Figure 10.2). They also crawl under and walk over each other, sometimes depositing small drops of urine.[67]

Play

Young rats play-fight together from age 5 weeks to around age 5–6 months (Table 10.1(j)). Play-fighting involves attempts to touch another rat's nape, which, if successfully contacted, is rubbed gently with the snout.[83]

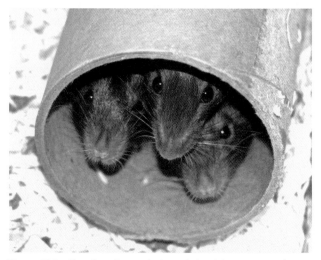

Figure 10.2   Three juvenile rats sharing a shelter. (Photo courtesy of Heather Mohan-Gibbons, copyright 2010.)

As young male rats approach social maturity at around 5–6 months of age their fighting becomes serious, with chasing, sidling, and biting. One rat emerges as a consistent winner. In this way a stable, long-term dominance hierarchy emerges between males.[10,84]

Aggression

Aggression between rats is a normal part of colony life (Table 10.1(k)). It is seen most frequently during the establishment of a new colony, when young rats approach social maturity (around 5–6 months of age) and begin to establish long-term dominance hierarchies, during the introduction of a strange rat to an existing colony, and during pregnancy and lactation. Once the colony is stable, aggression between colony members is rare.[10,85]

In an aggressive encounter, the goal of the aggressor is to inflict a bite on its opponent's lower back or flank. The opponent retaliates with defensive bites directed at the aggressor's face.[86]

During a typical aggressive encounter, the aggressor sidles toward his opponent in a lateral orientation. In response, the opponent stands on his hind feet, fans out his whiskers, and faces the aggressor. The rats may appear to stand motionless for some time in this configuration, though each rat is in fact making multiple small movements that are countered by small movements of the other.[87] The aggressor may also rear on his hind feet and the two rats may stand facing each other (Figure 10.3), nearly nose to nose, making vertical movements of their forepaws.[88] In this position, the defending rat's whiskers and face get in the way of the attacking rat. As long as the defender can maintain whisker-to-whisker contact he is never bitten.[89]

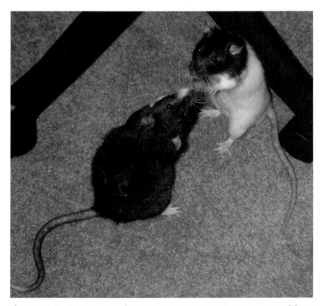

Figure 10.3 Two rats stand nose to nose in an agonistic encounter. (Photo courtesy of Anne F. Hanson.)

Either rat can break the stalemate. The aggressor may press forward laterally and lunge at the opponent's flank, destabilizing the opponent. The opponent may flee or roll supine. Flight may be followed by a chase. Flight is a problematic option for a caged rat because it opens the rump to further attack. The opponent may also break the stalemate by rolling supine. The supine position protects the rump but leaves the opponent poorly positioned to fend off further attack.[90] The supine position may be more frequent in small enclosures where flight is less of an option.[91] The aggressor may lie on top of the opponent and may attempt to gain access to the back to inflict a bite. Piloerection and tooth chattering are frequently observed during aggressive encounters.[92]

Aggressive encounters end when the opponent escapes, or when the aggressor stops displaying aggression and moves away. The opponent may continue to lie in a supine position for minutes after the aggressor has left.[88]

Rats in established colonies tend to attack intruders, and can do so with great violence. However, aggression toward intruders is not automatic and the intensity of the attack is variable.

Resident rat aggression toward intruders depends on the familiarity of the surroundings, the presence of an escape chamber, the age of the residents, the age of the intruders, and the age and sex of the rats in the colony. In mixed-sex colonies, the socially dominant male attacks intruders far more than females and subordinate males do.[32,85,92] In all-female colonies females do attack intruders, and as with males, one female tends to account for most of the attacks.[93] Rats tend to be more aggressive toward intruders in their home cage than two strange rats are toward each other in a neutral area.[94] The presence of an escape chamber in the home cage also reduces fighting: the intruder tends to run to the chamber and defend itself from the inside.[89]

Aggression levels also depend on the age of the resident males. Young males, of less than 6 or 7 months of age, show less aggression toward intruders. Aggression toward intruders increases up to age 20 months.[85] Aggression of resident males toward intruders is enhanced in the presence of intact female rats[95] and nursing young,[96] and reduced in the presence of young juvenile rats.[97]

Thor and Flannelly[98] introduced juveniles of different ages to resident adult males, and found that the resident adult males rarely attacked 21- to 40-day old juveniles. The resident males attacked almost all 41- to 60-day old juveniles after considerable posturing and sniffing, and attacked 61- to 80-day old juveniles almost immediately.

Maternal aggression is a normal behavior associated with parenting and protection of vulnerable young. A pregnant or lactating mother rat may attack intruders (other rats, humans, or other animals). Maternal aggression may include a lunging attack, typically directed at the neck or back of an intruding rat. The mother rat may also bite, sidle, or kick. Intruders usually respond by assuming an upright posture or rolling supine.[99] Maternal aggression is present but occurs infrequently at the end of pregnancy, increases after the birth of the litter, and peaks during the 9th day of lactation, after which it declines.[99] Maternal aggression wanes as the young grow older, and the mother rat eventually returns to normal levels of aggression.

Reproductive behavior

Female rats have a 4 to 5 day estrous cycle. It consists of 2 days of diestrus, followed by a 12–18 hour proestrus phase, then a 24–36 hour estrus period.[100]

The onset of sexual receptivity occurs shortly after nightfall at the end of proestrus (approximately the third day), and precedes ovulation by 4–6 hours. Sexual receptivity persists for 12–20 hours, depending on whether the female mates. If the female rat does not mate, her sexual receptivity lasts up to 20 hours, after which the cycle begins anew.[101]

Sexual behavior in the female rat occurs during her period of sexual receptivity. The female rat wanders beyond her customary home range and actively seeks males. She disperses her scent by rubbing her sides and anal region on objects in her environment, and dragging her genital–anal region along the ground.[54]

If the female rat engages in sexual behavior, her sexual receptivity is abbreviated,[102] and her ovulation is followed by an additional luteal phase during which implantation can occur if her eggs are fertilized. The luteal phase lasts for 12 days, after which the placenta takes over responsibility for maintaining hormonal support of the pregnancy. If the mating was infertile, the female may experience a 12-day period of anestrus, called pseudopregnancy.[101]

When the female encounters a male, they may approach each other, touch noses, and exchange genital inspections. The female may solicit sexual behavior from the male by approaching, presenting, hopping, darting, running away, and ear wiggling accompanied by ultrasonic vocalizations (Table 10.1(m and n)).[6]

The male mounts the female from the rear and clasps her flanks (Figure 10.4). If the female is sexually receptive, this stimulation results in her assuming a reflexive posture called *lordosis*. When in lordosis, the female presses her chest to the ground, arches her back, raises her coccyx, and deflects her tail to allow the male to gain intromission. Without lordosis, intromission is impossible. The whole contact takes only a few seconds. The male may intromit multiple times before ejaculation occurs.[101]

After ejaculation, the male enters a post-ejaculatory refractory period that lasts 2–5 minutes. During this time, he may groom or nap. Once he recovers he usually mates again.[101]

The male rat will mate any time that he comes into contact with a receptive female.[101] Male rats that attempt to mount a female who is not sexually receptive are unsuccessful: the female walks away or kicks the male off.[54]

A copulatory plug of gelatinous material from the seminal fluid is left in the vagina for 12–24 hours. It then falls out and can be used to determine that mating has occurred.

Postpartum and postweaning estrus

Female rats experience a postpartum estrus on the first evening that occurs at least 10 hours after giving birth.[103] However, eggs fertilized during the postpartum estrus may not implant right away due to a lactation-induced delay.[104] Female rats that conceive during postpartum estrus may therefore go through an extended gestation of 32 days rather than the normal 21–22 days.[14]

After the postpartum estrus, the female rat does not come into heat again until after the weaning of the litter. This estrus is called *postweaning estrus* and it occurs about 29 days after giving birth.[14]

Male rat fertility after neutering

It takes at least 8 days for male rats to become sterile after neutering.[105] In a natural experiment, a rat rescue organization, Rattenvermittlung (part of Club der Rattenfreunde Schweiz), placed neutered males in cages with females 10 days after surgery. Over 100 males have been neutered and placed in this way and no pregnancies have occurred (C. Schenk, *pers. comm.*).

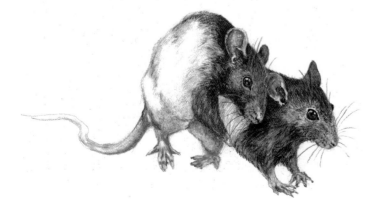

Figure 10.4 Rats copulating. (Original artwork by Jennifer L. Sobie)

Maternal behavior

Norway rat pups are born in litters of 8–16 hairless pups (Table 10.1(o)). Their eyes open a couple of weeks after birth, and they start exploring the nest. Pups remain with their mothers until weaning, 22–30 days after birth.[106] Young rats become able to breed at about 5 weeks of age (Table 10.1(q)),[107] so litters should be separated into same-sex age groups before then, in order to avoid accidental pregnancies.

Three to five days before birth, the female rat builds a substantial nest by carrying nesting material to the nest site in her mouth and patting and shaping it with her forefeet. The maternal nest is typically open at the top until the pups are born, whereupon she adds more material, first covering the pups then shaping the structure to create a domed cavity within the nest. After about 10 days post-parturition, the cavity is enlarged and left open to the outside, with progressively lower walls.[67]

At the onset of parturition, the female rat lies stretched out during waves of muscular contractions. During delivery, the mother sits with her head between her hind legs and licks each infant as it emerges. She pulls off the amniotic sac, bites through the umbilical cord, eats the placenta, and cleans the pup. Once birth is complete, the mother rat engages in the three major components of maternal rat behavior: she retrieves the pups to the nest, mouths and licks them, and adopts a nursing posture over them. She also engages in nest-building and nest defense.[67,108]

Pup licking is an important component of maternal behavior. It has significant effects on the emotionality,[109] cognition,[110,111] and physiology[112] of developing pups. There are two types of pup licking: body licking and anogenital licking, which both play an important role in pup development.[106] Body licking is observed before and between retrievals and during nursing, while anogenital licking occurs when pups are nursing on their backs. Anogenital licking ensures pup urination and defecation and plays a role in the sexual development of the male pup.[113]

Ingestive behavior

Rats, as omnivores, can exploit many different kinds of food resources. This breadth of diet has enabled rats to live in a wide variety of environments. However, being an omnivore poses special risks: each individual has many choices about what to eat, and the wrong choice could be fatal.

Rats must learn what is safe to eat. They are generally neophobic (fearful of novel situations or objects) when it comes to trying novel foods. Presenting the same food over multiple days may induce the rat to try a new food.[6,114]

It is now well-known that rats' feeding *preferences* can be socially transmitted. The ability to gather information from the experience of other conspecifics is of course an important advantage for omnivores (including humans) who are faced with a wide variety of potential foods in their environment. Social learning about food preferences occurs at many different times during a rat's life. Before birth and early in life, fetal and infant rats detect odor-bearing particles from the mother's diet through the placental barrier or in the mother's milk, and subsequently prefer those foods. Weanling rats that are in the process of eating solid foods for the first time use adult rats as guides. They forage where adults are foraging or where adults have previously scent marked. Older rats that forage on their own are influenced by interactions with other rats as well. They smell foods on the fur and breath of other rats and strongly prefer the foods those (healthy) rats had previously eaten: this is called the "Demonstrator Effect" (Table 10.1(r)).[115]

When a rat encounters a food item, the rat picks it up with a characteristic set of movements (Figure 10.5). The rat first sniffs the food and touches it with its whiskers, then takes the food in its mouth and sits back on its haunches and transfers the food to its forepaws. The rat grasps and manipulates the food with its fingertips.[116]

Like all rodents, rats are coprophagic, that is eat their own feces. Rats do not possess the enzyme systems to digest fiber. Thus they rely on recycling feces to harness the caloric value of bacterial fermentation in the cecum and colon, as well as important vitamins that have been synthesized by microorganisms in their lower intestinal tracts.

Rats also learn what not to eat. They have extremely sensitive learned food aversions. If a food makes the rat feel ill, it scrupulously avoids that food in the future.[117] Unlike food *preferences*, however, food aversions do not seem to be able to be socially transmitted.

If the rat does eat something that makes it feel nauseous, it cannot vomit (Table 10.1(s))[118] but it does have an alternative to vomiting, called pica. Pica is the consumption of non-foods like clay. When a rat feels ill it may eat clay, dirt, or even hardwood bedding.[119] These substances may help dilute the toxin's effect on the body.[120]

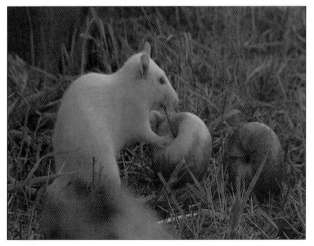

Figure 10.5 A rat investigating a food item. (Photo courtesy of the authors.)

Gnawing

The rat's incisors grow constantly. Incisors are worn down and kept sharp by gnawing and bruxing, also called *thegosis*. Rat incisors have hard enamel on the front surface of the tooth and soft dentin at the back, so the incisors wear at an angle.[121]

Rats do not require special objects to gnaw on for their dental health. Rats will wear their teeth down through contact with hard foods and through bruxing. Overgrowth of the incisors is probably a consequence of malocclusion.[122] However, rats are attracted to chewable objects, so these can be provided as a source of behavioral enrichment. Chmiel and Noonan[123] found that rats enjoyed chewing on $9 \times 9 \times 2$ cm blocks of spruce wood and 4.5 cm diameter balls of birch wood for their study.

Rats enjoy exploring the environment outside the cage and such activity can be an important form of environmental enrichment. However, beware that rats allowed to range freely outside the cage can be very destructive. If it is not possible to keep an eye on them at all times, ensure that such an environment is "rat proofed" for the protection of the rat and the owner's personal property.

Common behavior problems: Diagnosis and treatment

Male aggression

Aggression is a normal part of rat behavior, particularly amongst males, but in colonies with highly aggressive males this may escalate to fighting that leads to injury. The confined environment of the cage prevents the losers from fleeing from a fight, which may lead to an escalation of conflict. The cage also prevents continuously harassed subordinate rats from leaving the colony altogether.

Appropriate cage design may reduce levels of aggression. The cage should be large enough to allow the rats enough space to flee from conflict and avoid each other. All shelves and cage furniture (e.g., nestboxes, platforms) should have at least two exits to prevent any rat from being cornered, which could lead to an escalation of conflict. Providing multiple desirable resources such as food bowls and soft places to sleep may also reduce conflict.

In colonies with persistent or violent aggression problems, neutering is an effective and permanent solution that still enables the rats to live together. Castration reduces inter-male aggression. Castration of the dominant male decreases his aggression and status. An intact subordinate male may become dominant in his place.[124] If all rats in a group are neutered, they behave less aggressively toward each other.[125] Castration of resident male rats may not completely eliminate aggression, however, particularly toward new rats. Castrated rats rarely initiate an aggressive encounter with an intruder, but will display aggression if provoked[126] and will fight effectively.[127]

If neutering is not an option, the aggressor can be separated into a permanent, separate cage from the rest of the colony.[128]

Introducing new rats to an existing colony

Introducing a new rat to an existing colony may provoke aggression from resident rats, especially introducing new male rats to an existing male colony. In fact, aggression is so likely in these circumstances that the introduction of a new rat was the standard way to study rat aggression in the laboratory at one time.

The smoothest introductions occur when both the residents and new rats are very young, before any of them have entered puberty.[128] Puberty occurs at 39–47 days for male rats and 34–38 days for female rats.[104] The aggression of male resident rats toward newcomers increases steadily with resident age.[85,129]

To reduce the chance of aggression during introductions involving older rats, introduce the rats gradually to each other in a neutral area (such as an empty bathtub) under close supervision. Rats tend to be less aggressive toward each other when they meet in a neutral area.[127]

Aggression toward humans

Rats may bite their human owners. Most bites are defensive bites, in which the rat lunges forward, delivers a bite on an outstretched finger, and retreats. A rat that is being picked up may also turn and bite the owner.

Defensive bites may be motivated by fear. To accustom a fearful rat to human handling, the owner should handle the rat regularly and gently stroke it, give it treats, and carry it around (e.g., for 15 minutes per day).

Defensive bites may also be motivated by cage defense. A rat may be quite gentle outside the cage, but defensive and prone to bite when approached inside. To remove a defensive rat from its cage, the owner can try leaving the cage door open and allow the rat to walk outside on its own. The owner can also pick up the rat's nestbox with the rat inside, place the nestbox on a safe surface outside the cage (such as a table) and allow the rat to emerge.

Some pregnant or lactating female rats may also bite defensively. This behavior usually disappears when the babies are weaned.

Not all bites are defensive, however. Some bites are offensively aggressive. Some aggressive males may engage the human owner in an agonistic encounter and may sidle, piloerected and chattering, toward the human's hand. The rat may deliver a bite during this interaction. Neutering the rat, which reduces intraspecific aggression,[124,127] may decrease the incidence of this type of aggression being directed toward humans as well.

Lastly, some bites may be accidental. A rat may bite when startled from a sound sleep or when grabbed unexpectedly. The owner should give the rat some warning in the form of a soft noise before picking the rat up, and should move slowly and calmly.

A rat may also accidentally bite a finger inserted between the bars of the cage, especially if treats are regularly fed through the bars. To avoid having a finger mistaken for food, it is best never to feed rats through the bars of the cage.

Infanticide

Most maternal cannibalism occurs in the first 24 hours after birth and tapers off steeply during the first week.[130] Infanticide occurs for a variety of reasons:

1. Mothers may kill deformed or wounded offspring or their littermates.[130–132]
2. Mothers that are stressed (e.g., by excessive noise, rough handling, or too frequent cage cleaning) may consume their litters.[133]
3. Malnourished mothers may cannibalize their young. For example, obesity,[134] protein deficiency,[135] and vitamin deficiency (B12)[136] have all been found to increase the incidence of infanticide.
4. Mothers that have an abnormal birth experience, such as premature birth[137] or Caesarian section,[138] are more likely to kill their offspring than females who give birth vaginally to full-term litters.

Rats other than the mother rat may kill offspring. Male rats, like the males of many mammal species, tend to kill litters that are not their own,[14] possibly to hasten the mother's return to estrus. Unrelated nulliparous females may also kill newborn rats.[139]

To avoid infanticide and another pregnancy immediately after giving birth, it is best to remove other rats from the cage before the mother gives birth.

Urine marking

Neutering reduces urine marking in male rats, but may not eliminate it entirely. Price[140] and Taylor et al.[141] found that neutering reduces urine marking to about 20–22% of pre-castration levels.

Unusual behavior

Swaying and head bobbing—Albino rats (and occasionally pigmented rats) may sway from side to side or may bob their heads up and down repeatedly. This is a normal behavior and is probably an attempt to determine depth via motion parallax.

Eye boggling—A rats' eyes may vibrate rapidly in and out of the eye socket in time to a rapid bruxing action of the teeth. This is a normal behavior and is associated with both stress and, anecdotally, with pleasure (Table 10.1(c)).

Ear vibration—A female rat rapidly vibrates her ears when she is in behavioral estrus. It seems that females engage in ear wiggling to solicit sexual behavior from male rats (Table 10.1(n)).

Tail writhing or wagging—The rat's tail moves sinuously on the ground and may bang on the floor. The movement may involve the entire tail, or as little as the tail tip. Tail writhing may indicate a high degree of tension or excitement. For example, lactating females have been observed writhing their tails during aggressive encounters with each other.[142]

Handling

A tame rat should be lifted with one or two hands around the rat's chest. The rat's hindquarters should be supported with the second hand or with an arm. Unless absolutely necessary, avoid picking a rat up by its tail. This is more stressful for the rat, and in extreme cases (although very rare) the skin may de-glove (never hold the tail at its distal end).

A skittish rat can be picked up by placing the palm of the hand on the rat's back swiftly and firmly, with the middle and index fingers on either side of the rat's neck. Wrap the thumb, ring finger, and pinkie around the middle of the rat. Control the hind legs with the other hand or a towel. This hold will control the head and will prevent the rat from turning to deliver a bite. It will also prevent the rat from backing out of a grip.

To deliver oral medication, the best method is to mix the medication in a small amount of palatable food. The owner may need to try a variety of foods and ratios of medication to food before finding a combination that the rat will eat.

If mixing the medicine with a palatable food does not work, the rat may be wrapped in a towel with the head protruding from one side, allowing the delivery of liquid medication by syringe. The owner should hold the rat close to his chest and insert the tip of the syringe in the side of the mouth, behind the incisors. The tip of the syringe should be angled toward the back of the throat, and the plunger depressed slightly to administer a small quantity of medication. It may take several attempts to deliver the entire dose.

References

1. Meng J, Wyss AR, Dawson MR et al. Primitive fossil rodent from inner Mongolia and its implications for mammalian phylogeny. *Nature* 1994;370:134–136.
2. Musser GG, Carleton MD. Family Muridae. In: Wilson DE, Reader DM, eds. *Mammal Species of the World: A Taxonomic and Geographic Reference.* 2nd ed. Washington, DC: Smithsonian Institution Press, 1993;501–756.
3. Hedrich HJ. History, strains, and models. In: Krinke GJ, Bullock GR, eds. *The Laboratory Rat (Handbook of Experimental Animals),* 2000;3–16.
4. Castle WE. The domestication of the rat. *Genetics.* 1947;33:109–117.

5. Rat Genome Sequencing Project Consortium. Genome sequence of the brown Norway rat yields insights into mammalian evolution. *Nature* 2004;428:493–516.

6. Berdoy M, Drickammer LC. Comparative social organization and life history of *Rattus* and *Mus*. In: Wolff J, Sherman PW, eds. *Rodent Societies: An Ecological & Evolutionary Perspective*. Chicago: University of Chicago Press, 2007;380–392.

7. Barnett SA. An analysis of social behaviour in wild rats. *Proc. Zool. Soc. Lond* 1958;130:107–152.

8. Lott D. Intraspecific variation in the social systems of wild vertebrates. *Behav* 1984;88:266–325.

9. Berdoy M. Making decisions in the wild: Constraints, conflicts and communication in foraging rats. In: Galef BG, Jr., Valsechhi P, eds. *Behavioural Aspects of Feeding*. Ettore Majorana International Life Science Series, Vol. 12. Switzerland: Harwood Academic Publishers, 1994;289–313.

10. Berdoy M, Smith P, Macdonald DW. Stability of social status in wild rats: Age and the role of settled dominance. *Behav* 1995;132:193–212.

11. Moore J. Population density, social pathology, and behavioral ecology. *Primates* 1999;40:5–26.

12. Thor DH, Carr WJ. Sex and aggression: Competitive mating strategy in the male rat. *Behav Neur Biol* 1979;26:261–265.

13. Lanier D, Estep DQ, Dewsbury DA. Role of prolonged copulatory behavior in facilitating reproductive success in a competitive mating situation in laboratory rats. *J Comp Physiol Psychol* 1979;93:781–792.

14. Mennella JA, Moltz H. Infanticide in rats: Male strategy and female counter-strategy. *Physiol Behav* 1988;42(1):19–28.

15. Huck UW, Soltis RL, Coopersmith CB. Infanticide in male laboratory mice: Effects of social status, prior sexual experience, and bias for discrimination between related and unrelated young. *Anim Behav* 1982;30:1158–1165.

16. Telle HJ. Bietrag zur Kenntnis der Verhaltensweise von Ratten vergleichend dargestellt bei, *Rattus norvegicus* und *Rattus rattus*. *Zeit Zool* 1966;53:129–196. (Available in English translation as Technical Translation 1608, Translation Section National Science Library, National Research Council of Canada, Ottawa, Ontario, Canada.)

17. Schultz LA, Lore RK. Communal reproductive success in rats (*Rattus norvegicus*): Effects of group composition and prior social experience. *J Comp Psychol* 1993;107(2):216–222.

18. Steiniger, F. Bietrag zur Soziologie und Sonstigen Biologie der Wanderrate. *Zeit Tierpsychol* 1950;7:356–379.

19. Robitaille JA, Bovet J. Field observations on the social behavior of the Norway rat, *Rattus norvegicus* (Berkenhout). *Biol Behav* 1976;1:289–308.

20. Buck L, Axel R. A novel multigene family may encode odorant receptors: A molecular basis for odor recognition. *Cell* 1991;65(1):175–187.

21. Agosta WG. *Chemical Communication: The Language of Pheromones*. New York: *Scientific American Library*, 1992;4–9.

22. Brennan PA. The vomeronasal system. *Cell Moll Life Sci* 2001;58(4):546–555.

23. Bradbury JW, Vehrencamp SL. Principles of animal communication. Sunderland, MA: Sinauer Associates, Inc.1998;311–312.

24. Berdoy M, Webster JP, Macdonald DW. Fatal attractions in rats infected with *Toxoplasma gondii*. *Proc Royal Soc Lond Series B* 2000;267:1591–1594.

25. Welker WI. Analysis of sniffing of the albino rat. *Behav* 1964;12:223–244.

26. Semba K, Komisaruk BR. Neural substrates of two different rhythmical vibrissal movements in the rat. *Neurosci* 1984;12:761–774.

27. Carvell GE, Simons DJ. Biometric analysis of vibrissal tactile discrimination in the rat. *J Neurosci* 1990;10:2638–2648.

28. Berg RW, Kleinfeld D. Rhythmic whisking by rat: Retraction as well as protraction of the vibrissae is under active muscular control. *J Neurophysiol* 2003;89:104–117.

29. Dyck RH. Vibrissae. In: Whishaw IQ, Kolb B, eds. *The Behavior of the Laboratory Rat: A Handbook with Tests*. New York: Oxford University Press, 2004;81–89.

30. Ahl AS. The role of vibrissae in behavior: A status review. *Vet Res Commun* 1986;10:245–268.

31. Meyer ME, Meyer ME. The effects of bilateral and unilateral vibrissotomy on behavior within aquatic and terrestrial environments. *Physiol Behav* 1992;51(4):877–880.

32. Blanchard RJ, Blanchard DC, Takahashi T et al. Attack and defense behavior in the albino rat. *Anim Behav* 1977;25:622–634.

33. Oliver RF. Histological studies of whisker regeneration in the hooded rat. *J Embryol and Exp Morphol* 1966;16:231–244.

34. Sokoloff G, Blumberg MS. Vocalization. In: Whishaw IQ, Kolb B, eds. *The Behavior of the Laboratory Rat: A Handbook with Tests*. New York: Oxford University Press, 2004;371–382.

35. Hofman PM, Van Riswick JGA, Van Opstal AJ. Relearning sound localization with new ears. *Nature* 1998;1(5):417–421.

36. Kelly JB, Phillips DP. Coding of interaural time differences of transients in auditory cortex of *Rattus norvegicus*: Implications for the evolution of mammalian sound localization. *Hear Res* 1991;55(1):39–44.

37. Heffner RS, Heffner HE. Sound localization in wild Norway rats (*Rattus norvegicus*) *Hear Res* 1985;19(2):151–155.

38. Syka J, Rybalko N, Brozek G et al. Auditory frequency and intensity discrimination in pigmented rats. *Hear Res* 1996;23(4):3207–3213.

39. Kelly JB, Masterson B. Auditory sensitivity of the albino rat. *J Comp Physiol Psychol* 1977;91(4):930–936.

40. LaVail MA. Survival of some photoreceptors in albino rats following long-term exposure to continuous light. *Invest Ophthalmol Vis Sci* 1976;15:64–70.

41. Hecht E. *Optics*. 2nd ed. Reading, MA: Addison Wesley, 1987.

42. Jacobs GH, Fenwick JA, Williams GA. Cone-based vision of rats for ultraviolet and visible lights. *J Exp Biol* 2001;204(14):2439–2446.

43. Gouras P, Ekesten B. Why do mice have ultra-violet vision? *Exp Eye Res* 2004;79(6):887–892.

44. Desjardins C, Maruniak JA, Bronson FH. Social rank in house mice: Differentiation revealed by ultraviolet visualization of urinary marking patterns. *Science* 1973;182:939–941.

45. Hut RA, Scheper A, Daan S. Can the circadian system of a diurnal and a nocturnal rodent entrain to ultraviolet light? *J Comp Physiol* 2000;186:707–715.

46. Prusky GT, Harker KT, Douglas RM et al. Variation in visual acuity within pigmented, and between pigmented and albino rat strains. *Behav Brain Res* 2002;136(2):339–348.

47. Prusky GT, West PW, Douglas RM. Behavioral assessment of visual acuity in mice and rats. *Vision Res* 2000;40(16):2201–2209.

48. Prusky GT, Douglas RM. Vision. In: Whishaw IQ, Kolb B, eds. *The Behavior of the Laboratory Rat: A Handbook with Tests*. Oxford University Press, 2004;49–59.

49. Legg CR, Lambert S. Distance estimation in the hooded rat: Experimental evidence for the role of motion cues. *Behav Brain Res* 1990;41(1):11–20.

50. Schiffman HR, Lore R, Passafiume J et al. Role of vibrissae for depth perception in the rat (*Rattus norvegicus*). *Anim Behav* 1970;18:290–292.

51. Weisse I. Changes in the aging rat retina. *Ophthalmic Res* 1995;27 (Suppl 1):154–163.

52. Roberts SC. Scent marking. In: Wolff J, Sherman PW, eds. *Rodent Societies: An Ecological and Evolutionary Perspective*. Chicago: University of Chicago Press, 2007;254–266.

53. Brown RE. Mammalian social odors: A critical review. *Adv Study Behav* 1979;10:10–162.

54. Calhoun JB. *The Ecology and Sociology of the Norway Rat. US Public Health Service Publication No. 1008*. Washington, DC: US Government Printing Office, 1963.

55. Brown RE. Odor preference and urine marking scales in male and female rats: Effects of gonadectomy and sexual experience on responses to conspecific odors. *J Comp Physiol Psychol* 1977;91(5): 1190–1206.

56. Birke LI. Scent-marking and the oestrous cycle of the female rat. *Anim Behav* 1978;26:1165–1166.

57. Taylor GT, Haller J, Regan D. Female rats prefer an area vacated by a high testosterone male. *Physiol Behav* 1982;28(6):953–958.

58. Hopp SL, Timberlake W. Odor cue determinants of urine marking in male rats *Rattus norvegicus*. *Behav Neural Biol* 1983;37(1): 162–172.

59. Wallace DG, Gorny B, Whishaw IQ. Rats can track odors, other rats, and themselves: Implications for the study of spatial behavior. *Behav Brain Res* 2002;131(1–2):185–192.

60. Harley CW, Martin GM, Skinner DM et al. The moving fire hydrant experiment: Movement of objects to a new location re-elicits marking in rats. *Neurobiol Learn Mem* 2001;75(3):303–309.

61. Adams DB. The relation of scent-marking, olfactory investigation, and specific postures on the isolation-induced fighting of rats. *Behav* 1976;56(1–2):286–297.

62. Galef BG, Beck M. Aversive and attractive marking of toxic and safe foods by Norway rats. *Behav Neural Biol* 1985;43:298–310.

63. Taylor GT, Haller J, Bartko G, et al. Conspecific urine marking in male-female pairs of laboratory rats. *Physiol Behav* 1984; 32(4): 541–546.

64. Taylor GT, Griffin M, Rupich R. Conspecific urine marking in male rats (*Rattus norvegicus*) selected for relative aggressiveness. *J Comp Psychol* 1988;102(1):72–77.

65. Rosenzweig MR, Riley DA, Krech D. Evidence for echolocation in the rat. *Science* 1955;121:600.

66. Kaltwasser MT, Schnitzler HU. Echolocation signals confirmed in rats. *Z Saugetierkd* 1981;46:394–395.

67. Barnett SA. *The Rat: A Study in Behavior*. Chicago: University of Chicago Press, 1975.

68. Rosales VP, Ikeda K, Hizaki K et al. Emotional stress and brux-like activity of the masseter muscle in rats. *Eur J Orthod* 2002; 24(1):107–117.

69. Bolles RC. Grooming behavior in the rat. *J Comp Physiol Psychol* 1960;53:306–310.

70. Richmond G, Sachs BD. Grooming in Norway rats: The development and adult expression of a complex motor pattern. *Behav* 1978;75:82–96.

71. Hugo J, Krijit J, Vokurka M, Janousek V. Secretory response to light in rat Harderian gland: Possible photoprotective role of Harderian porphyrin. *Physiol Biophys* 1987;6:401–404.

72. Sakai T. The mammalian Harderian gland: Morphology, biochemistry, function and phylogeny. *Arch Histol Jap* 1981;44:299–333.

73. Harkness JE, Ridgeway MD. Chromodacryorrhea in laboratory rats (*Rattus norvegicus*): Etiologic considerations. *Lab Anim Sci* 1980;30:841–844.

74. Gillis GB, Biewener AA. Hindlimb muscle function in relation to speed and gait: *In vivo* patterns of strain and activation in a hip and knee extensor of the rat (*Rattus norvegicus*). *J Exp Biol* 2001;204:2712–2731.

75. Muir GD. Locomotion. In: Whishaw IQ, Kolb B, eds. *The Behavior of the Laboratory Rat: A Handbook with Tests*. New York: Oxford University Press, 2004;150–161.

76. Muir GD, Whishaw IQ. Red nucleus lesions impair overground locomotion in rats: A kinetic analysis. *Eur J Neurosci* 2000;12: 1113–1122.

77. Patterson-Kane EG. Cage size preference in rats in the laboratory. *J Appl Anim Welf Sci* 2002;5(1):63–72.

78. Lawlor M. The size of rodent cages. In: Guttman, HN, ed. *Guidelines for the Well-Being of Rodents in Research*. Bethesda, MD: Scientist Center for Animal Welfare, 1990;19–28.

79. Anzaldo AJ, Harrison PC, Riskowski GL, Maghirangi RG, Gonyou HW. Increasing welfare of laboratory rats with the help of spatially enhanced cages. *Anim Welf Inform Centre Newslett* 1994; 5(3):1–5.

80. Baumans V. Environmental enrichment for laboratory rodents and rabbits: Requirements of rodents, rabbits, and research. *ILAR J*. National Research Council, Institute of Laboratory Animal Resources 2005;46(2):162–170.

81. AFRMA. A house for your mouse (or rat). American fancy rat and mouse association, 2000; Last viewed June, 2009. http://www.afrma. org/house4mousep1.htm.

82. Manser CE, Morris TH, Broom DM. An investigation into the effects of solid or grid cage flooring on the welfare of laboratory rats. *Lab Anim* 1995;29(4):353–363.

83. Pellis SM, Pellis VC. Play-fighting differs from serious fighting in both target of attack and tactics of fighting in the laboratory rat *Rattus norvegicus*. *Aggress Behav* 1987;13:227–242.

84. Pellis SM, Pellis VC. Role reversal chances during the ontogeny of play-fighting in male rats: Attack vs. defense. *Aggress Behav* 1991; 17:179–189.

85. Blanchard RJ, Flannelly KJ, Blanchard DC. Life-span studies of dominance and aggression established colonies of laboratory rats. *Physiol Behav* 1988;43(1):1–7.

86. Blanchard DC, Blanchard RJ. The colony model of aggression and defense. In: Dewsbury DA, Ed. *Contemporary Issues in Comparative Psychology*. Sunderland, MA: Sinauer Associates, Inc. 1990; 410–430.

87. Blanchard DC, Blanchard RJ. Environmental targets and sensorimotor systems in aggression and defense. In: Cooper SJ, Hendrie CA, eds. *Ethology and Psychopharmacology*. New York: John Wiley and Sons, 1994;133–157.

88. Miczek KA, de Boer SF. Aggressive, defensive, and submissive behavior. In: Whishaw IQ, Kolb B, eds. *The Behavior of the Laboratory Rat: A Handbook with Tests*. New York: Oxford University Press, 2004;344–352.

89. Takahashi LK, Grossfield S, Lore RK. Attack and escape in the laboratory rat: A modification of the colony-intruder procedure. *Behav Neural Biol* 1980;29:512–517.

90. Pellis SM, Pellis VC. Play and fighting. In: Whishaw IQ, Kolb B, eds. *The Behavior of the Laboratory Rat: A Handbook with Tests*. New York: Oxford University Press, 2004;298–306.

91. Boice R, Adams N. Degrees of captivity and aggressive behavior in domestic Norway rats. *Bull Psychon Soc* 1983;21:149–152.

92. Takahashi LK, Blanchard RJ. Attack and defense in laboratory and wild Norway and black rats. *Behav Proc* 1982;7:49–62.

93. Blanchard DC, Fukunaga-Stinson C, Takahashi LK et al. Dominance and aggression in social groups of male and female rats. *Behav Proc* 1984;9:31–48.

94. Thor DH. Intraspecific aggression in rats and dimensions of the enclosure. *Psychol Rep* 1976;38:1253–1254.

95. Flannelly KJ, Lore RK. The influence of females upon aggression in domesticated male rats (*Rattus norvegicus*). *Anim Behav* 1977;25:38–51.

96. Lore R, Luciano D. Attack stress induces gastrointestinal pathology in domesticated rats. *Physiol Behav* 1977;18:743–745.

97. Taylor GT, Weiss J. Presence of intact and gonadectomized juveniles and the reduction of fighting between adult male rats. *Physiol Behav* 1982;29:1019–1023.

98. Thor DH, Flannelly KJ. Age of intruder and territorial-elicited aggression in male Long–Evans rats. *Behav Biol* 1976;17:237–241.

99. Erskine MS, Barfield RJ, Goldman BD. Intraspecific fighting during late pregnancy and lactation in rats and effects of litter removal. *Behav Biol* 1978;23:206–218.

100. Nelson RJ. *An Introduction to Behavioral Endocrinology*. Sunderland, MA: Sinauer Associates, 1995;611.

101. Jenkins WJ, Becker JB. Sex. In: Whishaw IQ, Kolb B, eds. *The Behavior of the Laboratory Rat: A Handbook with Tests.* Oxford University Press, 2004;307–320.

102. Bennett AL, Blasberg ME, Blaustein JD. Mating stimulation required for mating-induced estrous abbreviation in female rats: Effects of repeated testing. *Horm Behav* 2002;42(2):206–211.

103. Gilbert AN, Rosenwasser AM, Adler AM. Timing of parturition and postpartum mating in Norway rats: Interaction of an interval timer and a circadian gate. *Physiol Behav* 1985;34:61–63.

104. Mantalenakis SJ, Ketchel MM. Frequency and extent of delayed implantation in lactating rats and mice. *J Reprod Fertil* 1966;12:391–394.

105. Pholpramool C, Sornpaisarn L. Fertility and electrolyte composition of the rat cauda epididymal plasma and spermatozoa before and after castration. *Contraception* 1980;22(6):673–681.

106. Rees SL, Lovic V, Fleming AS. Maternal behavior. In: Whishaw IQ, Kolb B, eds. *The Behavior of the Laboratory Rat: A Handbook with Tests.* New York: Oxford University Press, 2004;287–297.

107. Engelbregt MJT, Houdijk MECAM, Popp-Snijders C et al. The effects of intra-uterine growth retardation and postnatal under-nutrition on onset of puberty in male and female rats. *Pediatr Res* 2000;48:803–807.

108. Hudson RY, Cruz A, Lucio J et al. Temporal and behavioral patterning of parturition in rabbits and rats. *Physiol Behav* 1999;66:599–604.

109. Francis DD, Meaney MJ. Maternal care and the development of stress responses. *Curr Opin Neurobiol* 1999;9:128–134.

110. Liu DJ, Diorio J, Day JC, Francis DD, Meaney MJ. Maternal care, hippocampal synaptogenesis and cognitive development in rats. *Nature Neurosci* 2000;3:799–806.

111. Lovic V, Fleming AS. Artificially reared female rats show reduced prepulse inhibition and deficits in the attentional set-shifting task—Reversal of effects with maternal-like licking stimulation. *Behav Brain Res* 2004;148(1–2):209–219.

112. Kuhn CM, Schanberg SM. Responses to maternal separation: Mechanisms and mediators. *Int J Dev Neurosci* 1998;16(3–4):261–270.

113. Moore CL. Maternal contributions to the development of masculine sexual behavior in laboratory rats. *Dev Psychobiol* 1984;17:347–356.

114. Clifton PE. Eating. In: Whishaw IQ, Kolb B, eds. *The Behavior of the Laboratory Rat: A Handbook with Tests.* New York: Oxford University Press, 2004;197–206.

115. Galef BG. Social enhancement of food preferences in Norway rats: A brief review. In: Hayes CM, Bennett G, eds. *Social Learning in Animals: The Roots of Culture.* San Diego: Academic Press, 1996;49–64.

116. Whishaw IQ. Prehension. In: Whishaw IQ, Kolb B, eds. *The Behavior of the Laboratory Rat: A Handbook with Tests.* New York:Oxford University Press, 2004;162–170.

117. Garcia JR, Koelling A. Relation of cue to consequence in avoidance learning. *Psychon Sci* 1966;4:123–124.

118. Hatcher RA. The mechanism of vomiting. *Physiol Rev* 1924;4:479–504.

119. Mitchell D, Wells C, Hoch N et al. Poison-induced pica in rats. *Physiol Behav* 1976;17(4):691–697.

120. Phillips TD. Dietary clay in the chemoprevention of aflatoxin-induced disease. *Toxicol Sci* 1999;52(2 Suppl):118–126.

121. Addison WHF, Appleton JL. The structure and growth of the incisor teeth of the albino rat. *J Morphol* 1915;26:42–96.

122. Miles AE, Grigson C. Overgrowth of teeth. In: Miles AE, Grigson C, eds. *Colyer's Variations and Diseases of the Teeth of Animals.* Revised edition. Cambridge, UK: Cambridge University Press, 2003;692.

123. Chmiel DJ, Noonan M. Preference of laboratory rats for potentially enriching stimulus objects. *Lab Anim* 1996;30(2):97–101.

124. Albert DJ, Walsh ML, Gorzalka BB et al. Testosterone removal in rats results in a decrease in social aggression and a loss of social dominance. *Physiol Behav* 1986;36:401–407.

125. Stewart J, Palfai T. Castration, androgens and dominance status in the rat. *Psychon Sci* 1967;7(1):1–2.

126. Christie MH, Barfield RJ. Effects of castration and home cage residency on aggressive behavior in rats. *Horm Behav* 1979;13:85–91.

127. Barfield RJ, Busch DE, Wallen K. Gonadal influence on agonistic behavior in the male domestic rat. *Horm Behav* 1972;3:247–259.

128. Committee on Rodents. Rodents. In: *Laboratory Animal Management: A Series.* Washington, DC: National Academies Press, 1996.

129. Takahashi LK, Lore R. Intermale and maternal aggression in adult rats tested at different ages. *Physiol Behav* 1983;29:1013–1018.

130. Schardein JL, Petrere JA, Hentz DL et al. Cannibalistic traits observed in rats treated with a teratogen. *Lab Anim* 1978;12(2):81–83.

131. Reynolds RD. Preventing maternal cannibalism in rats. *Science* 1981;213(4512):1146.

132. Helander HF, Bergh A. How to avoid maternal cannibalism after neonatal surgery in rats. *Experientia* 1980;36(11):1295–1296.

133. Lane-Petter W. Cannibalism in rats and mice. *Proc Roy Soc Med* 1968;61:1295–1296.

134. Wehmer F, Bertino M, Jen KL. The effects of high fat diet on reproduction in female rats. *Behav Neural Biol* 1979;27:120–124.

135. Babicky A, Novakova V. Protein malnutrition of the lactating female rat: Effect on maternal behaviour and spontaneous weaning of young rats. *Physiol Bohemoslov* 1986;35(5):456–463.

136. Hankin L. The control of filicidal cannibalism by vitamin B12. *J Nutrition* 1960;71:188–190.

137. Vickery BH. Studies on the effects of altered timing of parturition in the rat. *Prostaglandins Med* 1979;2(2):141–154.

138. Stern JM. Parturition influences initial pup preferences at later onset of maternal behavior in primiparous rats. *Physiol Behav* 1985;35(1):25–31.

139. Peters LC, Sist TC, Kristal MB. Maintenance and decline of the suppression of infanticide in mother rats. *Physiol Behav* 1991;50(2):451–456.

140. Price EO. Hormonal control of urine-marking in wild and domestic Norway rats. *Horm Behav* 1975;6(4):393–397.

141. Taylor GT, Bartko G, Farr S. Gonadal hormones and conspecific marking in male rats. *Horm Behav* 1987;21(2):234–244.

142. Adams N, Boice R. A longitudinal study of dominance in an outdoor colony of domestic rats. *J Comp Psychol* 1983;97(1):24–33.

11

Gerbils

A. Dawn Faircloth Parker and Valarie V. Tynes

Introduction

Among pet rodents, the gerbil is easily one of the most endearing. Although there are many species that are informally referred to as "gerbils," the one used most often in research and seen most frequently in the pet trade is *Meriones unguiculatus*, the Mongolian gerbil. They are fascinating creatures with traits, features, and behaviors that make them desirable pets and well suited for many research needs.

Taxonomy

The Mongolian gerbil is in the class Mammalia, order Rodentia, family Muridae, and subfamily Gerbillinae. Although there is some discrepancy in the literature it is generally agreed that this subfamily is further divided into 14–16 genera containing about 100–111 species, any of which can correctly be designated as "gerbils."[1-3] The genus *Meriones* includes the popular Mongolian gerbil, the Shaw's jird (*Meriones shawi*), and 14 other less commonly encountered species.

Among hobbyists, the term "jird" is typically used to refer to the Shaw's jird (*Meriones shawi*), whereas "gerbil" generally denotes the Mongolian gerbil (*Meriones unguiculatus*). Other names for the Mongolian gerbil are clawed jird, desert rat, clawed bird, or sand rat.[4] For the remainder of this chapter, *Meriones unguiculatus* will be the primary focus. Unless otherwise noted, the term "gerbil" will hence refer to the common Mongolian gerbil.

Appearance and physical characteristics

Larger than mice yet smaller than rats, fully grown Mongolian gerbils typically weigh between 70 and 130 g (0.15–0.03 oz), and measure between 22 and 30 cm (9–12 in.) in length including the tail. Females are slightly smaller than males, but are otherwise similar in appearance. Unlike rats, gerbils have fur completely covering their long tails, which are almost as long as their bodies.[5]

Gerbils can now be found in a multitude of coat colors and patterns, primarily due to their popularity and subsequent selective breeding by hobbyists. Still, the majority of gerbils one will encounter are of the wild "agouti" type (Figure 11.1), which appears as a golden brown to the naked eye.[5] The hair on the abdomen is off-white and underneath, the skin is darkly pigmented. This agouti pattern is thought to have been beneficial for camouflage in their native environments. One might also see gerbils in solid black, white, and over 20 other existing colors.

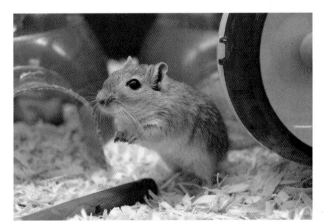

Figure 11.1 An agouti-colored gerbil.

Origin

Members of the subfamily Gerbillinae are found in many deserts, grasslands, and other arid habitats throughout Asia, Africa, and India. Mongolian gerbils are predominantly native to the inner Mongolian regions of China, which experience drastic temperature fluctuations and very low levels of precipitation. In these environments, temperature may fluctuate from 50° (120°F) to lows of 40° below 0°C (−40°F), and some years see less than 22 cm (9 in.) of rain.[6] Due to some very unique anatomical features and their adaptations to such challenging climates, the Mongolian gerbil is able to tolerate wide temperature ranges and water shortages.

Circadian activity rhythms and life span

There have been conflicting findings over the years regarding the true circadian activity rhythms of gerbils. Some recent literature suggests that they are strictly nocturnal.[7] Other investigators find them to be primarily diurnal[8,9] and still others find that they exhibit crepuscular behavior patterns.[6,10] This confusion may stem from the fact that in the wild, gerbils adjust their surface behavior patterns in accordance with the ambient temperature. During the hot months gerbils will be mostly nocturnal and during the cold months, diurnal. When temperatures are moderate they will be mostly crepuscular.[11] Studies have also shown that in the laboratory, gerbil activity patterns are readily influenced by human activities and they may be particularly sensitive to noise in their environment.[7] This ability to adapt quickly to changes in their environment is just one more feature that has allowed the Mongolian gerbil to thrive in their harsh native environment.

Unlike hamsters, gerbils do not hibernate, but instead store food on which to subsist during cold winters.[6,12] Life span is 2–4 years.[8] They breed readily, are hardy animals, and have a stable conservation status.[13]

Behavior of wild ancestors

When looking back at the wild ancestors of today's domesticated gerbil, there are several unique behaviors that stand out. Notable is the extended family social structure in which wild gerbils live, made up of a single, monogamous breeding pair and their offspring of varying ages. It has been observed that the adult female of the breeding pair is often promiscuous, entering neighboring territory and soliciting copulations from the resident male which may serve to improve reproductive success by increasing genetic variability.[6] Social suppression of sexual maturation appears to prevent sub-adults from breeding while they remain in their natal nest.[6,14] It is theorized that they assist in providing for and raising the nursing pups, and in doing so they may improve their parenting skills.[15] In order to become a breeding animal, the sub-adults must either wait for the dominant animal to disappear, or leave their natal group to join or form a new territory. Since this may be very difficult in a harsh environment with a high density population, it is more likely that they will increase their inclusive fitness by staying in their natal group, helping to raise their siblings, while they continue to mature.[15,16] Population density in one study area was noted to range from 42 to 90 animals/hectare (21–45/acre).[6]

Gerbils spend the largest portion of their time budget digging.[9] They construct narrow but elaborate underground tunnels with multiple entrances, as well as chambers where they breed, nest, and store food. The underground lifestyle of the gerbil is another adaptation to their harsh environment. They remain underground during extreme climactic conditions and can escape underground to avoid predation. Typically, the breeding burrow is constructed in the center of their territory.[6]

Gerbils are very territorial and will defend the borders of their territory, primarily against adult intruders. Territory defense is performed most often by the adult breeding male and consists primarily of attempts to chase intruders out of the territory. Territories are marked by adult gerbils using their ventral scent gland (see "Communication") along the borders and near the main burrow systems.[6] Larger males and larger family groups are able to maintain larger territories containing more resources.[6]

Senses and communication

Senses

Gerbils are unique amongst other small rodents in that they hear low frequency sounds better than high frequency sounds. They are more sensitive to speech sounds than pure tones and this human-like auditory sensitivity makes them excellent animal models for human auditory research.[17] In addition, the gerbil is able to localize sounds quite well, a very useful adaptation for a prey species.[18]

Little has been documented regarding the visual capabilities of gerbils, but it appears that they have relatively good vision and can be trained to perform several different visual discrimination tasks.[19] Their visual acuity is better than that of the hamster[19] but it is believed that they have poor long-distance vision.[12]

As is the case with most social species, olfaction and olfactory cues play an important role in the social behavior of the gerbil. It has been demonstrated that male Mongolian gerbils can distinguish between the urine and ventral gland secretions of different individuals.[20] However, they apparently cannot differentiate between feces, ear swabs, or saliva that originates from more than one animal.[20] Nevertheless, gerbils have demonstrated an ability to discriminate their partner's urine from that of other gerbils. They also emit more ultrasound vocalizations in the presence of their partner's odor.[21] Male gerbils spend more time investigating ventral gland secretions than urine, suggesting that urine is simply of lesser importance in conspecific identification. Gerbils live in a very arid habitat so urine would be a costly form of communication. They do not use urine to mark their territory and it is likely that urine plays a less important role in olfactory communication than ventral gland secretions.[20]

While the gerbil is likely to have a vomeronasal organ, little is documented about what role a vomeronasal organ or pheromones may play in their behavior.

Communication

Gerbils utilize several mechanisms to communicate, of which "marking behavior" is well known and studied. Gerbils press their abdominal, or ventral scent gland against objects along the borders of their territory, within their territory, and when exploring novel environments, leaving a visible, waxy, yellow sebaceous secretion.[9,22] One can locate this scent gland by looking for the hairless area along the ventral midline. The gland is normally more prominent in males than in females, and both sexes will experience gross and histological changes as they age.[23,24] Males typically mark more than females and the behavior is androgen-dependant. The behavior decreases dramatically in males after castration.[24,25] Studies show that marking by gerbils is an innate rather than a learned behavior.[26] As the animals age, the communicatory function of marking behavior appears to wane but the behavior continues.[24,26]

Marking behavior is differentiated in the literature from "marking-like" behavior, which has been shown to be non-communicatory, and non-androgen dependent.[23] Marking-like behavior is characterized by a slight spreading of the fore and hind legs combined with a lowering of the abdomen onto the substrate. This behavior has been observed as early as 19 days of age, before the ventral scent gland is fully developed and capable of producing secretions. Male and female gerbils perform this behavior at almost identical rates.[23] True marking behavior, characterized by the development of the scent gland and the actual deposition of secretions by rubbing the scent gland on objects, is exhibited by males as early as day 40 and females by day 50.[23]

Female gerbils have been noted to greatly increase their frequency of marking during estrus.[9] They also occasionally scent mark pups for retrieval.[9,27] Group members will also participate in mutual marking, where one animal crawls over or under the other, pressing its body closely to the other. Two individuals may do this to each other several times in a single bout, circling under and over each other repeatedly.[9] Thus scent marking behavior may serve to promote family cohesion and decrease aggression by spreading a "family scent" throughout the territory.[9]

Another important means of communication occurs via the exocrine secretions of the Harderian gland, as they are distributed from the nares to the body surface by means of grooming. These secretions appear to function as affiliative or attractant pheromones and conspecifics are stimulated to investigate and lick the areas of the face where the secretions are spread. There is no evidence that gerbils vocalize when grooming or that conspecifics can see the secretions.[28] However, one study suggests that gerbils can both smell and taste the secretion and that it plays an important role in thermoregulation and social behavior.[28]

Foot thumping, a rapid drumming movement of the hind legs, is another interesting behavior employed by gerbils. It is unknown exactly what the behavior is communicating but it appears to be an alarm response. It occurs most often in response to startling external stimuli but does not actually appear to result in a change in the behavior of the other individuals in the group, suggesting that it may not actually serve as an alarm signal.[9] In mixed-sex encounters, adult males may sometimes respond to threats from females by foot thumping. These episodes may last several seconds before the male resumes other investigatory or marking behaviors. Females seldom showed foot thumping behavior when encountering unfamiliar gerbils and males engaged in the behavior less when meeting unfamiliar males. Males may also engage in foot thumping after a fight.[29]

Gerbil pups produce ultrasonic vocalizations that appear to serve a distress function[30] when separated from their mothers under conditions of low temperatures.[31] Vocalizations differ between males and females when interacting, even at a very early age.[30] They eventually appear to play some role in gerbil reproductive behavior. It has been demonstrated that the male gerbil emits different ultrasonic calls during different stages of copulatory behavior. Less is known about vocalizations produced by the adult female and whether they differ significantly from the male's vocalizations.[30,32]

Lastly, audible vocalizations do not appear to be a primary method of communication among gerbils, but one will occasionally hear an adult's squeak when they are playing, fighting, or stressed. It is more common to hear the pups make similar high pitched sounds, but overall, gerbils are fairly quiet animals.

Body care

Gerbils are relatively simple to care for, although there are several environmental needs that should be addressed to allow for normal body care and grooming behavior. While gerbils tolerate a wide range of temperatures and are well adapted to regulate their body temperature, in captivity it is generally agreed that they should be maintained within a set range of temperatures and humidity. They appear to do well when provided a temperature range between 19°C and 23°C (66–73°F) and humidity of 30–50%.[10]

One method by which gerbils regulate their body temperature is by grooming. During times of heat stress they spread saliva over their body, especially areas that are hairless. When the saliva evaporates, excess heat is removed from the body.[33] In addition, when grooming, gerbils can also spread Harderian gland secretions across their face and body, darkening the pelage and increasing heat absorption from the sun. Another method by which gerbils actively maintain their body temperature is by sand bathing.[34,35] When gerbils sand bathe, they remove oils and Harderian secretions from their coat, lightening the pelage and reducing heat absorption.[35] Sand bathing also appears to serve some olfactory communicatory function as it occurs most often in highly marked areas.[9] Thus, while gerbils in captivity may not need to sand bathe in order to maintain their body temperature, providing sand bathing opportunities may be enriching by allowing them to perform a species typical behavior that has a social function.

Locomotion

Gerbils are saltatorial, meaning that they use a hopping or jumping form of locomotion.[8] Using their large hind feet and powerful hind legs, they are able to jump over 30 cm (12 in.) high.[5] They also frequently stand upright, especially when alarmed or startled. When in the erect posture, they stand on their toes and their tail serves as a support. The standing gerbil is about 12 cm (5 in.) tall and they may stand for several minutes when alert and watching for danger.[5] This alert posture may also be accompanied by tail waving.[9]

Gerbils are highly motivated to dig and digging accounts for a large proportion of their active time. If provided with the space and substrate they will dig elaborate tunnels with multiple entrance and exit holes. They will dig so vigorously as to often destroy previously dug tunnels, suggesting that their behavior does not have a goal such as the construction of a burrow of particular size or shape.[9]

As discussed earlier, gerbils live in social groups over relatively sizable territories in the wild. One study demonstrated that territories range in size from 325 to 1550 m² (355–1695 sq yds) with an average range of 91–163 m² (99–178 sq yds) per animal.[6] Thus providing gerbils with appropriate opportunity for exercise may be very important to their well-being. Options to address exercise needs include running wheels, exercise/hamster balls, and supervised out of cage time. If a wheel is used, one without slats is preferable, to avoid the potential of catching the tail.

Social behavior

Mongolian gerbils are highly social animals. In the wild they live in family units consisting of one pair of essentially monogamous breeding adults, as well as non-breeding offspring from prior litters who assist in providing for the pups.[6] This type of social structure benefits both parents and offsprings, as parental energy resources are conserved and sub-adults are able to delay the dangers of leaving the natal group to form family groups in new territory.[15] These same social behaviors are seen in captivity when the appropriate conditions are provided. However, studies to date show varying degrees of significance to captive raised offspring, depending on the test used, and the variable studied. The simple presence or absence of juvenile helpers was *not* shown to be a reliable factor in predicting the reproductive success of a family unit in captivity, although family size and density were shown to be very strong influences.[15,16,36] The predictable environment and provision of resources in captivity may make the traditional family structure less important to the survival of the group.

These family units are generally quite stable, and overt aggression is rarely seen, other than during actual or attempted hierarchy changes. Competition often erupts following the death or removal of a breeding pair member, or when a younger gerbil tries to establish the dominant breeding position. Interestingly, studies have failed to document any negative influence on the pups by such intra-family aggression.[36]

Interactions between group members are mostly limited to demonstrations of dominance relationships and sniffing of other family members.[6] According to one researcher, subordinance is shown by the subordinate animal climbing onto the dominant animal, trying to lick its face and less often, by simply following the dominant animal.[6] The dominant animal may respond by threatening the subordinate with an offensive sideways posture. The subordinate animal usually responds by rolling onto its back. Dominance may be also demonstrated by chasing and/or pushing the subordinate animal.[6] In typical family groups, the older, breeding male will be dominant most frequently, followed by younger males, older females, and young females.[6]

In encounters with unfamiliar individuals, gerbils begin by sniffing each other's faces and sometimes flanks. When taking the defensive posture, the head will be lowered and the eyes held partly closed. The individual holding their head higher than the other is taking the more offensive role. After initial contact, males may attempt more intensive investigation by sniffing the ventral scent gland and genitalia of a female. If either animal is uninterested in an interaction, they may turn their head away from or move away from the other animal. Continued unwanted investigation may provoke a threat by the uninterested individual.[37]

Threatening postures usually consist of facing or leaning over the other individual who may respond by counterthreat with a similar posture. Males may respond with a sideways posture, pushing their shoulder toward the female while turning their head away from her. This posture has also been called "sidling" and is more commonly employed by the intruder in a territory, so it may serve as a type of appeasement gesture.[9,37] Marking of the environment with the ventral scent gland also occurs frequently during these encounters, often followed by rolling over in a complete circle onto their back for a moment and then onto their belly again.

Counterthreats may also include some "boxing" where the gerbils stand on their hind legs and paw at each other with their fore paws. Afterward they may resume solitary activities or a fight may ensue. Fighting consists of both animals grasping each other with their paws and rolling over while attempting to bite the other in the throat or flank. They may stay locked together for up to 30 seconds before separating and chasing each other around the enclosure and frequently leaping into the air. If one animal eventually flees the other, it does so with its tail held vertically.[29]

In encounters with unfamiliar individuals, females tend to initiate the fights with males. Two males will sniff each other but fight much less often than mixed-sex pairs. Female–female encounters result in the same amount of fighting as male–male encounters. Thus, unlike rats and mice, but similar to the hamster, female gerbils are the more aggressive sex.[29]

Important to mention is the interaction between social grooming, chemosignaling, and temperature regulation. Self-grooming occurs significantly more often during social interactions. Social interaction elevates body temperature thus provoking the self-grooming. As mentioned earlier, grooming can serve to decrease body temperature.[28] The Harderian gland plays a critical role in this relationship. Grooming releases exocrine secretions and pheromones, which serve to increase both self-grooming and allogrooming. It has been demonstrated that gerbils have a distinct preference for grooming at 28°C (82°F). Dominant animals can displace subordinate animals from the areas with the most desirable temperature, decreasing grooming and all related activities in those subordinates.[33] Therefore the subordinate animal is at a disadvantage thermoregulatory wise and communication wise since it cannot signal as effectively with Harderian secretions.[28]

Allogrooming is most likely important to the social behavior of the gerbil as it most frequently occurs in conjunction with mutual marking behavior. One animal will lay flat on the ground, often with eyes closed, while the other grooms its head, neck, shoulders, and back. Allogrooming of the ventral surfaces occurs less frequently.[9]

Regarding the effects of captivity, one question that quickly comes to mind is whether owning a single pet gerbil results in any untoward effects on the gerbil due to its highly social nature. In other species, it has been well documented that social isolation directly affects the neuroendocrine system. Recent studies have shown that Mongolian gerbils who are isolated after weaning did indeed demonstrate an increase in aggressive behaviors, anxiety-related behaviors, and social sniffing over those that were not completely isolated.[38,39] The data suggests that ideally gerbils should be raised from weaning in pairs and that same sex pairs can live together as peacefully as mixed-sex pairs while avoiding the frequent production of offspring.

Reproductive behavior

Mongolian gerbils are continuously polyestrus, spontaneous ovulators.[40] Similar to other small rodents, female gerbils have an estrus length of 4–6 days[41] and commonly exhibit a postpartum estrus about 8–11 hours after giving birth. Reproductive behavior in gerbils is more often observed in late afternoon, unlike many other species that are sexually active at night.[40]

If the male is acceptable to the female, she will allow him to breed with her after a period of courtship. Little is known about female mate choice but several studies have demonstrated the importance of intrauterine position for both male and female gerbils when it comes to reproductive success.[42–44] Male gerbils that matured in the uterus between two males sire more offspring as adults, most likely due to higher levels of circulating androgens. Female gerbils have demonstrated an ability to recognize these males and if given the choice will preferentially choose them as mates.[44] Varying levels of protein in a male gerbil's diet have been shown to produce different odor attractiveness to the females, thus affecting her acceptance of him. Although more research is needed in these areas, it is reasonable to suspect that fitness might be reflected by a male's ability to find and ingest protein, and may be the basis for the preferential treatment by the female.[45]

Pre-copulatory behavior involves nose-to-nose sniffing followed by nose-to-anogenital sniffing. The female typically then darts away, the male chases her and when he catches up with her, she allows him to mount.[9] The female gerbil will typically stand still with forelegs and hind limbs extended as the male mounts. She lowers her head and her back is either flat or concave, exhibiting the typical posture of lordosis. The male will intromit multiple times before ejaculation and ejaculate multiple times.[46] Copulation is often followed by each animal grooming their own genitalia. The male may also display foot drumming during the post-ejaculatory intervals.[9]

Studies show that the male gerbil aggressively pursues the female during her postpartum estrus, exhibiting very persistent reproductive behavior. Prior to going into estrus, females will be harassed with copulation attempts by the males, sometimes even as they attempt to give birth. All such attempts prior to estrus are denied by the female, but during the female's 8-hour estrus period, they may copulate as frequently as once every 47 seconds, even to the point of interrupting her care of the newborn pups.[47]

Parental behavior and pup development

Once conception occurs, 4–5 pups will be born after gestating 25–26 days on average.[41]

If one closely observes the breeding female, it may be possible to pinpoint when gestation begins by watching for the small telltale vaginal plug.[40] Even so, if the female is still nursing pups from a prior litter, implantation may be delayed considerably, and the length of delay varies directly with the number of pups being nursed.[48]

Mongolian gerbils are among the few rodent species who exhibit biparental care of the young.[49] Both male and female Mongolian gerbils participate in nest building as a normal behavior, but an increase in this behavior and digging are seen during the female's pregnancy.[9] The females associate with their mate before and after parturition, though the male will often briefly leave prior to the impending birth, either voluntarily or after being forced away by the dam (*pers. obs.* A.D.F.P).

Normal maternal and paternal behavior includes: licking, crouching over, and retrieval of pups; building and rearranging nests; nursing; and bodily contact with pups.[49] If present at parturition, male gerbils may engage in the birth process, as well as in cleaning and stimulation of the pups. However, during the first 3 days after parturition, the male is more focused on his mate and attempting to copulate with her during the postpartum estrus.[47] After this period, the male's interest in the young increases and he may spend as much time with the young as does the mother.[50,51] Ultimately, the male will spend more time in the nest than the female, but females show more licking and sniffing of pups and nest building. Both parents spend equal amounts of time in body contact with the pups.[49]

Female Mongolian gerbil's are generally quiet attentive in their maternal behavior, but like many rodents, may cannibalize their offspring. Although cannibalism is much less common than in hamsters and mice, precautions should nonetheless be taken. Provide the dam with an undisturbed area to nest that is quiet, comfortable, and near nutrients, water, and extra bedding to create a low stress environment prior to, and for at least a week subsequent to parturition.[40]

Parental behavior can be affected by many variables such as age, experience, and immediate environment. Paternal care has been shown to be influenced by testosterone concentrations[50,51] and maternal care has been shown to be positively correlated with the dam's age at first breeding.[52] Paternal care during the first few days after birth has been shown to be negatively correlated with the number of males versus females in the litter and this is believed to be influenced by olfactory cues.[44]

Mongolian gerbils are altricial, born hairless with eyes and ears closed weighing about 2.5 g (0.08 oz). Gerbils are most likely to give birth at night and dystocia is uncommon.[40] During the initial hours of life, the pups do little other than sleep, suckle, and vocalize. They remain huddled close to their dam as their thermoregulatory abilities are limited. At 16–18 days of life their eyes begin to open and there is rapid improvement in their ability to locomote and thermoregulate.[53] The pups nurse for the first 3–4 weeks of life, with body weight increasing on average around 1 g/day (0.04 oz) as they continue to grow and become increasingly more independent (*pers. obs.* A.D.F.P). At about 2–3 weeks of age, they begin to partake of the solid adult herbivorous diet.[53] At this time, it is important that the food supply is located low enough for the pups to access on their own and that the dispenser has openings that are wide enough for gerbils to maneuver and access the food. Hard food may be softened by lightly wetting it with water for the growing pups.

Ingestive behavior

Gerbils are generally considered to be omnivorous. In the wild, their diet consists primarily of a variety of leaves and herbs, some grass and roots, as well as seeds and grains and much of their time is spent foraging for these foods.[6] More food is gathered than is eaten, and the excess is stored in their burrows. They are very efficient at conserving both fats and water and in the wild the majority of their water needs are acquired through their diet. Subsequently, the feces is relatively dry and they produce a very small amount of highly concentrated urine.[4,6,12]

In captivity, pelleted or block diets increase the likelihood that the animal will ingest the appropriate levels of carbohydrates, fat, protein, and other important nutrients. The pelleted diets prevent the animals from being able to selectively eat favorite items like seeds which may result in nutritional imbalances and subsequent health issues.

A variety of healthy treats can be given, although the amount should be a minor proportion (e.g., no more than 10%) of the total diet. Fresh fruits, vegetables, or other supplemental food will suit this purpose, and can also double as training aids or environmental enrichment. Due to the fact that hoarding of food is normal for gerbils, the cage should be examined daily and any items of fresh food that have become spoiled should be removed.

In addition, captive gerbils should be offered a constant source of clean, fresh water.[4,5] Automatic water suppliers or hanging bottles are excellent options for providing water. If the latter is used, the sipper tube should be made of metal or another non-breakable, non-toxic material to prevent destruction or swallowing by the gerbil. Normal daily water consumption rate in the captive gerbils should be about 4–7 ml (0.13–0.23 oz) of water for each 100 g (0.22 lbs) of gerbil body weight.[4]

Housing and enrichment

A proper environment is critical to preventing the development of problems such as stereotypic digging in the gerbil.

Gerbils are highly motivated to dig and should be provided with deep layers of appropriate bedding (compacted peat with shredded paper, moist sand, wood chips, hay, etc.) to allow for burrowing behavior, pelage health, and food storage, as well as material that can be safely chewed on for enrichment and dental health.[5,12] One study demonstrated that gerbils have a clear preference for sand and woodchip bedding.[54] Compacted peat for burrowing and shredded paper for the nesting area may be ideal.[55]

Gerbils also demonstrate a strong drive to chew and providing appropriate items to chew may serve as enrichment as well as an aid in dental health. Paper, cardboard, hay, branches, and wood sticks may all be utilized by the gerbil. Paper and cardboard should be free of ink. Empty toilet paper or paper towel rolls, paper egg containers, or cardboard boxes are all suitable materials for shredding by gerbils. Wood sticks from willow (*Salix* spp.), hazel (*Corylus avellana*), beech (*Fagus sylvatica*), birch (*Betula pendula*), maple (*Acer* spp.), and fruit trees are all believed to be safe for the gerbil to chew[5] (Figure 11.2).

As gerbils produce so little urine relative to most other rodents and mammals, less frequent cleaning of their cage is required. This is beneficial from a behavioral perspective as well, since enclosure cleaning has been shown to be highly stressful to rodents.[5] Earlier articles have recommended placing a small amount of the old bedding back in the enclosure after weekly cleaning so as to leave familiar scents in the enclosure. Alternatively, partial cleanings can be done. As these techniques have not been confirmed to reduce stress, and in mice have actually resulted in increasing stress, it is important to observe the animals for the desired response, and to alter cleaning methods if undesired behaviors arise.[5,56]

Other means of enriching the gerbil's environment include scattering the diet over the bedding to encourage foraging, exploring, and gathering behaviors. Additional enrichment can be provided by making or purchasing objects in which food or treats can be hidden. These can then be given to the gerbils to manipulate and access their contents. Special treats such as sunflower seeds or other favorites can also be offered occasionally. Any and all treats or enrichment foods should be deducted from the total daily rations so as to not contribute to obesity and associated medical problems.

Common behavior problems

Relatively speaking, Mongolian gerbils are fairly problem free. They are affected by few diseases or severe behavioral issues. That being said, some normal behavior in this species may be problematic for those who keep them in captivity and some problems may arise when an appropriate habitat is not provided.

Escaping

Mongolian gerbils are very agile, quick moving, prolific chewers and diggers, and will make sudden jumps. Housing made of soft metals, wood, and some plastics may not be escape proof if the gerbil begins chewing at corners or edges. Materials such as hard metals, wire, glass, and hard plastics are recommended. If either of the latter two is used, adequate ventilation must be ensured. Proper conditioning, appropriate physical handling/restraint, as well as secure primary and secondary enclosures will help prevent losing gerbils to escape. Any room which houses gerbils should be "escape proofed" by actions such as the following: blocking access to potential hiding places; securing open areas under sinks, behind appliances, under doors, etc. through which they could escape if they manage to get loose from their primary enclosure.

Intraspecific aggression

In general, gerbils are very social and non-aggressive animals, although there are a few exceptions. Aggression may be seen when multiple gerbils are crowded into inadequately sized quarters, when one gerbil intrudes upon another's territory, when young adult gerbils attempt to vie for breeding positions in their family, and when introducing unfamiliar adult gerbils to one another for the first time.[6]

If two sexually mature, unfamiliar Mongolian gerbils are placed together, aggression is likely to occur.[29,57] While some studies have found the subsequent fighting to be short-lived and resulting in no serious injury, others have seen serious fighting leading to injury and even death.[9,58] Fighting between unacquainted gerbils may be decreased by introducing them in a clean cage that is novel to both. However, some fighting is still likely to occur.[58]

As mentioned earlier, Mongolian gerbils are generally considered to be monogamous, forming pairs by ~8 weeks

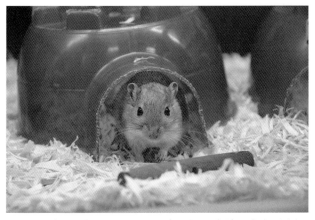

Figure 11.2 Typical pet gerbil habitat with plastic shelter and wood chew stick.

of age (sexual maturity), and mating for life. Breeding is often problematic when one member of a pair is removed or dies and replacement is attempted.[10] Success has been documented when pairing a male with two females, although some aggression may occur.[4]

Stereotypic behaviors

Gerbils in captivity have been found to develop stereotypic digging and bar-mouthing (also referred to as bar-gnawing, bar chewing, or wire gnawing). In addition, wheel running can take on a stereotypic appearance in some individuals.[59] Neither additional space, nor the presence of a substrate to dig in can completely prevent this behavior.[5] Instead, it has been demonstrated that the presence of a burrow during development is necessary to significantly reduce the behavior.[60] Whenever possible, gerbils should be allowed to construct their own system of burrows as it appears that their motivation to dig is so powerful that simply providing them with burrows is inadequate for their ideal welfare.[5,59]

Bar chewing may be prevented by not separating juvenile gerbils from their parents before the birth of the next litter. It may also help if some of the bedding from the parental cage is placed in the new cage when the juveniles are eventually moved.[5]

The provision of a wheel for gerbils should not be avoided for fear of stereotypic behavior since wheel running has been shown to have some physiological and cognitive benefits, as well as being psychologically rewarding.[10,59] When provided with an otherwise appropriate and stimulating environment, wheel running is more likely to remain at moderate levels.

Seizures

Seizures are a common problem in Mongolian gerbils, with an incidence of 20–40% due to a genetic predisposition which can intensify with inbreeding.[61,62] Although this makes them highly suited for use in human epilepsy research, it can be quite disconcerting for owners of pet gerbils, particularly if they are not aware of this predilection. The problem typically first appears in 8 to 12-week old gerbils, becoming more severe and frequent through 6 months of age.[62] Locomotor signs range from mild hypnotic behavior, catalepsy, or shaking to grand mal seizures involving full-body convulsions, collapse, and very rarely death.[62] In most cases, no permanent effects are seen and no treatment is warranted. Stress, handling, and introduction to novel environments have been shown to precipitate the seizures in susceptible animals.[61,63] Their occurrence can be reduced by habituation to human handling at a young age.[61,62,64] One study demonstrated that weekly handling beginning at 7 days of age completely prevented the development of seizures in all but one of 62 animals.[64]

Proper handling and restraint

The gerbil's natural curiosity and friendly disposition makes it fairly easy to handle. Many gerbils will approach a hand introduced into their cage and can be easily scooped into the palm of one hand while blocking access to escape jumping with the other hand. An alternative approach is to grasp the gerbil by the base of the tail with one hand and use the other hand placed under its body to lift it. Holding onto the tail may prevent escape but only the base of the tail should be held, for the skin over the end of the tail is easily pulled off resulting in a de-gloving injury.

To prevent such injuries, allow the gerbils to acclimate to humans, and use slow, gentle movements. This will often result in the gerbil readily climbing into hands that non-abruptly reach into their enclosures. These are curious animals, and can be readily conditioned for easy handling (*pers. obs.*).

Gerbils not accustomed to being handled may jump and run, but only rarely attempt to bite. Once picked up, the gerbil can be restrained by one hand with the over-the-back grip. This is done by scruffing the loose skin over their neck between your thumb and index finger while the base of the tail is held between your fourth and fifth fingers.

Summary

Much is known but much remains to be learned about the behavior of the gerbil in captivity. It's non-aggressive, social nature, as well as many unique physiological and anatomical adaptations make it an interesting and rewarding pet as well as a useful laboratory animal. As is the case with all exotic pets, a thorough understanding of an animal's normal behavior is critical to caring for it and providing it with a habitat that is most conducive to its physical and mental health and welfare.

Acknowledgments

Photos in this chapter courtesy of M. C. Tynes, copyright 2010.

References

1. McKenna MC, Bell SK. *Classification of Mammals Above the Species Level*. New York: Columbia University Press, 1998.
2. Nowak RM. *Walker's Mammals of the World, Volume II*. 6th ed. London and Baltimore: John Hopkins University Press, 1999;1344–1457.
3. Chevret P, Dobigny G. Systematices and evolution of the subfamily Gerbillinae (Mammalia, Rodentia, Muridae). *Mol Phylogenet Evol* 2005;35(3):674–688.
4. Motzel SL, Wagner JE. Mongolian gerbils: Care diseases and use in research. In: *The Laboratory Animal Medicine and Science—Series II*. V-9032. Seattle, WA: University of Washington Health Science Center for Educational Resources.

5. Waiblinger E. Comfortable quarters for gerbils in research institutions. In: Reinhardt V, Reinhardt A, eds. *Comfortable Quarters for Laboratory Animals*. 9th ed. Washington DC: Animal Welfare Institute, 2002;18–25.

6. Agren G, Zhou Q, Zhong W. Ecology and social behaviour of Mongolian gerbils, *Meriones unguiculatus*, at Xilinhot, Inner Mongolia, China. *Anim Behav* 1989;37:11–27.

7. Klaus U, Weinandy R, Gatterman R. Circadian activity rhythms and sensitivity to noise in the Mongolian gerbil (*Meriones unguiculatus*). *Chronobiol Int* 2000;17:137–145.

8. Brain PF. The laboratory gerbil. In: Poole T, ed. *The UFAW Handbook on the Care and Management of Laboratory Animals*. Oxford: Blackwell Science Publications, 1999;345–355.

9. Roper TJ, Polioudakis E. The behavior of Mongolian gerbils in a semi-natural environment with special reference to ventral marking, dominance and sociability. *Behaviour* 1977;61:207–237.

10. Wolfensohn S, Lloyd M. Section 2: species. In: Wolfensohn S, Lloyd M, eds. *Handbook of Laboratory Animal Management and Welfare*. Oxford: Blackwell Science Publications, 2003;248–255.

11. Randall JA, Thiessen DD. Seasonal activity and thermoregulation in *Meriones unguiculatus*: A gerbil's choice. *Behav Ecol Sociobiol* 1980;7:267–272.

12. Sørenson DB, Krohn T, Hansen HN et al. An ethological approach to housing requirements of golden hamsters, Mongolian gerbils and fat sand rats in the laboratory—A review. *Appl Anim Behav Sci* 2005;94:181–195.

13. Agren G, Zhou Q, Zhong W. Territoriality, cooperation and resource priority; hoarding in the Mongolian gerbil, *Meriones unguiculatus*. *Anim Behav* 1989;37:28–32.

14. Ostermeyer MC, Elwood RW. Helpers(?) at the nest in the Mongolian gerbil, *Meriones unguiculatus*. *Behaviour* 1984;91:61–77.

15. Saltzman W, Ahmed S, Fahimi A et al. Social suppression of female reproductive maturation and infanticidal behavior in cooperatively breeding Mongolian gerbils. *Horm Behav* 2006;49:527–537.

16. Silk JB. The adaptive value of sociality in mammalian groups. *Phil Trans R Soc* 2007;362(1480):539–559.

17. Sinnott J. A comparative assessment of speech sound discrimination in the Mongolian gerbil. *J Acoust Soc Am* 2001;110(4):1729–1732.

18. Maier JK, Klump GM. Resolution in azimuth sound localization in the Mongolian gerbil (*Meriones unguiculatus*). *Acoust Soc Am* 2006;119(2):1029–1036.

19. Ingle DJ. New methods for analysis of vision in the gerbil. *Behav Brain Res* 1981;3:151–173.

20. Shimozuru M, Kikusui T, Takeuchi Y et al. Discrimination of individuals by odor in male Mongolian gerbils, *Meriones unguiculatus*. *Zool Sci* 2007;24(5):427–433.

21. Brown RE, Hauschild M, Holman SD et al. Mate recognition by urine odors in the Mongolian gerbils (*Meriones unguiculatus*). *Behav Neural Biol* 1988;49:174–183.

22. Thiessen DD, Lindzey G, Blum SL et al. Social interactions and scent marking in the Mongolian gerbil (*Meriones unguiculatus*). *Anim Behav* 1970;19:505–513.

23. Arkin A, Saito TR, Takahashi K et al. Observation of marking-like behavior, marking behavior and growth of the scent gland in young Mongolian gerbils (*Meriones unguiculatus*) of an inbred strain. *Exp Anim* 1999;48(4):269–276.

24. Arkin A, Saito TR, Takahashi K et al. Age-related changes on marking, marking-like behavior and the scent gland in adult Mongolian gerbils (*Meriones unguiculatus*). *Exp Anim* 2003;52(1):17–24.

25. Yamaguchi H, Kikusui T, Takeuchi Y et al. Social stress decreases marking behavior independently of testosterone in Mongolian gerbils. *Horm Behav* 2005;47:549–555.

26. Arkin A, Saito TR, Takahashi K et al. Marking behavior is innate and not learned in the Mongolian gerbil. *Exp Anim* 2000;49(3):205–209.

27. Wallace P, Owen K, Thiessen DD. The control and function of maternal scent marking in the Mongolian gerbil. *Physiol Behav* 1973;10:463–466.

28. Thiessen DD, Clancy A, Goodwin M. Harderian gland pheromone in the Mongolian gerbil, *Meriones unguiculatus*. *J Chem Ecol* 1976;2:231–238.

29. Swanson HH. Sex differences in behaviour of the Mongolian gerbil (*Meriones unguiculatus*) in encounters between pairs of same or opposite sex. *Anim Behav* 1974;22:638–644.

30. Holman SD, Seale WT. Ontogeny of sexually dimorphic ultrasonic vocalizations in Mongolian gerbils. *Dev Psychobiol* 1991;24(2):103–115.

31. Hashimoto H. Comparison of ultrasonic vocalizations emitted by rodent pups. *Exp Anim* 2004;53(5):409–416.

32. Holman S. Sexually dimorphic ultrasonic vocalizations of Mongolian gerbils. *Behav Neural Biol* 1980;28(2):183–192.

33. Thiessen D, Graham M, Perkins J, Marcks S. Temperature regulation and social grooming in Mongolian gerbil (*Meriones unguiculatus*). *Behav Biol* 1977;19(3):279–288.

34 Pendergrass M, Thiessen D. Sandbathing is thermoregulatory in the Mongolian gerbil, *Meriones unguiculatus*. *Behav Neural Biol* 1983;37:125–133.

35. Thiessen DD, Pendergrass M. The thermoenergetics of coat colour maintenance by the Mongolian gerbil, *Meriones unguiculatus*. *J Therm Biol* 1982;7:51–56.

36. Scheibler E, Weinandy R, Gatterman R. Social factors affecting litters in families of Mongolian gerbils, *Meriones unguiculatus*. *Folia Zool* 2005;54(1–2):61–68.

37. Nyby J, Thiessen DD, Wallace P. Social inhibition of territorial marking in the Mongolian gerbil (*Meriones unguiculatus*). *Psychon Sci* 1970;21:310–312.

38. Starkey NJ, Normington G, Bridges NJ. The effects of individual housing on "anxious" behaviour in male and female gerbils. *Physiol Behav* 2007;90:545–552.

39. Shimozuru M, Kikusui T, Takeuchi Y et al. Effects of isolation-rearing on the development of social behaviors in male Mongolian gerbils (*Meriones unguiculatus*). *Physiol Behav* 2008;94(3):491–500.

40. Brower M. Practitioners guide to pocket pet and rabbit theriogenology. *Therio* 2006;66:618–623.

41. Ness RD. Rodents. In: Carpenter JW, ed. *Exotic Animal Formulary*. 3rd ed. St. Loius: Saunders Elsevier, 2005;377–406.

42. Clark MM, Galef BG. Effects of uterine position on rate of sexual development in female Mongolian gerbils. *Physiol Behav* 1988;42:15–18.

43. Clark MM, Malenfant SA, Winter DA et al. Fetal uterine position affects copulation and scent marking by adult male gerbils. *Physiol Behav* 1990;47:301–305.

44. Clark MM, Tucker L, Galef BG. Stud males and dud males: Intra-uterine position effects on the reproductive success of male gerbils. *Anim Behav* 1992;43:215–217.

45. Chen J, Zhong W, Liu W et al. Effects of dietary protein content on social behavior and some physiological properties in male Mongolian gerbils (*Meriones unguiculatus*). *Acta Theriol Sin* 2007;27:234–242.

46. Diakow C, Dewsbury DA. A comparative description of the mating behavior of female rodents. *Anim Behav* 1978;26:1091–1097.

47. Prates EJ, Gurra RF. Parental care and sexual interactions in Mongolian gerbils (*Meriones unguiculatus*) during the postpartum estrus. *Behav Proc* 2005;70:104–112.

48. Norris ML, Adams CE. Mating post-partum and length of gestation in Mongolian gerbils. *Lab Anim* 1981;15:189–191.

49. Elwood RW. Paternal and maternal behavior in the Mongolian gerbil. *Anim Behav* 1975;23:766–772.

50. Clark MM, Galef BG. Effects of experience on the parental responses of male Mongolian gerbils. *Dev Psychobiol* 2000;36:177–185.

51. Clark MM, Liu C, Galef BG. Effects of consanguinity, exposure to pregnant females and stimulation from young on male gerbils' response to pups. *Dev Psychobiol* 2001;39:257–264.

52. Clark MM, Moghaddas M, Galeg, BG. Age at first mating affects parental effort and fecundity of female Mongolian gerbils. *Anim Behav* 2002;63:1129–1134.

53. Kaplan H, Hyland SO. Behavioural development in the Mongolian gerbil (*Meriones unguiculatus*). *Anim Behav* 1972;20:147–154.

54. Pettijohn TF, Barkes BM. Surface choice and behavior in adult Mongolian gerbils. *Psychol Rec* 1978;28:299–303.

55. West CD. Gerbils. In: Benyon PH, Cooper JE, eds. *Manual of Exotic Pets*. Gloucestershire: British Small Animal Veterinary Association 1991;31–38.

56. Baumans V. Environmental enrichment for laboratory rodents and rabbits: Requirements of rodents, rabbits, and research. *ILAR J* 2005;46(2):162–170.

57. Agren G, Meyerson BJ. Influence of gonadal hormones and social housing conditions on agonistic, copulatory and related socio-sexual behavior in the Mongolian gerbil (*Meriones unguiculatus*) *Behav Process* 1977;2:265–282.

58. Norris ML, Adams CE. Aggressive behavior and reproduction in the Mongolian gerbil (*Meriones unguiculatus*) relative to age and sexual experience at pairing. *J Reprod Fertil* 1972;31:447–450.

59. Würbel H. The motivational basis of caged rodent's stereotypies. In: Mason G, Rushen J, eds. *Stereotypic Animal Behavior: Fundamentals and Applications to Welfare*. 2nd ed. Oxfordshire, UK: CABI, 2006;86–120.

60. Wiedenmayer C. Causation of the ontogenetic development of stereotypic digging in gerbils. *Anim Behav* 1997;53:461–470.

61. Thiessen DD, Lindzey G, Friend HC. Spontaneous seizures in the Mongolian gerbil. *Psychonom Sci* 1968;II:227–228.

62. Loskota WJ, Lomax P, Rich ST. The gerbil as a model for the study of the epilepsies. *Epilepsia* 1974;15:109–119.

63. Laming PR, Elwood RW, Best PM. Epileptic tendencies in relation to behavioral response to a novel environment in the Mongolian gerbil. *Behav Neural Biol* 1989;51:92–101.

64. Kaplan H, Miezejeski C. Development of seizures in the Mongolian gerbil (*Meriones unguiculatus*). *J Comp Physiol Psychol* 1972;81:267–273.

12

Hamsters

Julia Albright and Ricardo de Matos

Introduction

Hamsters are rodents of the family Cricetidae. There are over 50 species, subspecies, and varieties of hamsters. They are popular as pets and important research animals. Hamsters are known for their short gestation period, periodic pugnaciousness, ease of taming, cheek pouches, and ability to escape confinement. They are also known for storing large amounts of food in a single place. The word "hamster" is believed to be derived from the German verb "hamastra" which means "to store." Hamsters have a recent history of domestication when compared with other rodents such as mice, rats, and guinea pigs. Their small size, ease of taming, minimal care requirements, and low occurrence of spontaneous disease are positive attributes. The recently published results of the American Veterinary Medical Association survey revealed an increase in the number of hamsters kept as pets, from approximately 900,000 in 2001 to 1,250,000 in 2006.[1]

Of the many species of hamsters, four are commonly kept as pets: golden or Syrian hamster (*Mesocricetus auratus*), Siberian or Russian hamster (*Phodopus sungorus*), Roborovski hamster (*Phodopus roborovskii*), and Chinese hamster (*Cricetulus griseus*). Other hamster species used as laboratory animals, such as the European hamster (*Cricetus cricetus*), are normally not kept as pets. The most common pet hamster is the Syrian hamster. The Russian and Roborovski hamster are gaining popularity because of their docile disposition. Chinese hamsters are less commonly kept as pets because of their aggressive nature. Table 12.1 summarizes the general characteristics of common pet hamster species.

The Syrian or golden hamster is popular both as a pet and as a research animal and the one people generally associate with the word "hamster." For this reason, most of the information provided in this chapter refers primarily to this species. Syrian hamsters are indigenous to a very restricted area in northwest Syria. Most laboratory and pet hamsters are believed to have originated from three to four littermates captured near Aleppo in Syria in 1930.[2] The common fur color is golden, although there are many other color variations (Figure 12.1).

Another common pet hamster species is the Russian hamster, also known as the Siberian hamster. As the name suggests, they originated in Siberia. The body fur is gray with a white belly and a black stripe extending from the nose to the back; they can also develop a light gray winter coat. Some authors refer to the gray and the light gray Russian hamsters as two separate species: Campbell's hamster (*Phodopus campbelli*), which refers to the normal gray coloration, and winter white or Siberian hamster (*P. sungorus*), which corresponds to the light gray winter fur coloration described earlier. There are many color variations (around 40).

The Roborovski hamster, or "Robo," is the smallest member of the hamster family. They are native to the deserts of western and eastern Mongolia, China, and Russia. Their care and maintenance is similar to Russian hamsters.

Chinese hamsters originated from northern China and Mongolia, where they are found in rocky terrain, digging shallow burrows. They are good climbers. Chinese hamsters have been used as laboratory animals and pets since the early 20th century. This is the only pet hamster species for which ownership is illegal or restricted in some states in the United States (Figure 12.2).

Senses and communication

The hamster is a predominantly nocturnal rodent with small eyes. For this reason, vision is likely less important to its behavior when compared with hearing, somatic sensation, and olfaction.[3] Hamsters are generally solitary animals and encounters between adults seem to be limited to those involving either sexual or agonistic behaviors.[4]

Table 12.1   General characteristics of hamster species commonly kept as pets

Taxonomy	Common name	Life span	Physical characteristics	Behavior characteristics
Order Rodentia Family Cricetidae				
Mesocricetus auratus	Golden or Syrian hamster	18–24 months	Body weight: 140–200 g; females larger. "Wild type": dark eyes; short, soft, and smooth fur with golden brown dorsum and gray ventrum; many color variations. Hairless and long hair (teddy bear) variants also occur. Eye: black, red, or unpigmented (albinos).	Nocturnal and solitary; only meet to mate. Because they are bigger and easier to handle, may be more suitable for children compared with smaller species.
Phodopus sungorus	Russian, Siberian, Djungarian, dwarf or "furry footed" hamster	9–15 months	Smaller size (40–60 g); males larger. Gray fur with back stripe extending from nose to the back (light gray winter coat) and white ventrum; foot pads covered with fur.	Less aggressive toward cage mates. Can be housed together (two males or one male with several females) if introduced when young. Male helps raise pups.
Phodopus roborovskii	Roborovski hamster	3–3.5 years	Similar to Russian hamster but smaller (25–40 g) and with brown fur and no dorsal stripe. Only one color variation with a satin variant.	Sociable and will live in groups. Very active and small size makes handling difficult.
Cricetulus griseus	Chinese, striped-back, or gray hamster	17–20 months	Small size (40–50 g); longer and thinner than Russian hamsters; gray brown fur with dark strip down the back; two to three color variants; 1 in. tail.	Very aggressive to cage mates; house alone.

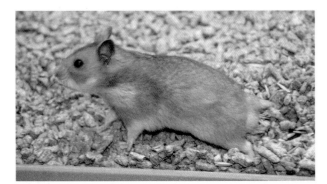

Figure 12.1   The Golden or Syrian hamster is the hamster species most commonly kept as a pet and as a research animal. (Photo courtesy of M. C. Tynes, copyright 2010.)

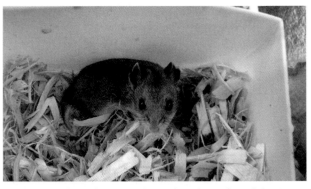

Figure 12.2   Chinese hamster with typical gray brown fur, a dark stripe down the back and a 1 in. tail. This very aggressive species should always be housed alone. (Photo courtesy of Ricardo de Matos.)

Olfactory signaling via scent marking and ultrasonic auditory communication appear to have an important role in individual recognition and reproduction.[5]

Auditory communication

Hamsters make very few audible sonic calls, mostly when hurt, frightened, handled, or fighting.[4,6] Hamsters can also produce audible sounds by repeatedly clicking their teeth together. Teeth chattering occurs more frequently in interactions between males than between females or between males and females, suggesting its use in communication in situations of agonistic tension.[4]

Adult hamsters of both sexes produce ultrasonic calls (60–170 milliseconds with a frequency range of 20–60 kHz).[4,7] These calls are used primarily in sexual contexts, mainly in the attraction and location of a sexual partner and in the facilitation of copulatory activity. Calling by male and female hamsters is strongly influenced by gonadal hormones, with females calling only when they are sexually receptive. Both female and male hamsters are stimulated to call by contact with the animals of the opposite sex or their odors.[4,8] Hamsters can quickly locate one another by mutually calling and approaching the source of another animal's call. When a male and female in estrus first meet, they produce calls. Once the female assumes the lordosis posture (ventral curvature of the spine), she does not call but the male continues to call, especially during the inter-mount intervals, to keep the female immobile. Males and females produce calls with different structures but there is no indication that hamsters can use that information. Different species of hamsters also produce calls that vary qualitatively and quantitatively, indicating a possible role of ultrasonic calls in species identity. It has also been suggested that, as for other small terrestrial mammals, ultrasonic calls assist with exploration and navigation in their environment (echolocation).[4]

Infant hamsters produce sounds that may sometimes be 100% ultrasonic or may include sonic components. These sounds are presumed to elicit maternal attention and care, as they seem to do in mice and rats.[4,9]

Chemical communication

Most of the research regarding communication in hamsters is related to chemical signaling. Flank gland secretions, vaginal secretions, and to a lesser degree Harderian gland secretions, ear gland secretions, urine, feces, and saliva communicate information used for species and individual recognition as well as sexual behavior (recognition, attraction, and copulatory behavior).[4] Scent signals are detected by the olfactory epithelium of the nasal cavity and the vomeronasal organ.[8,10]

Hamsters possess two flank glands, also known as hip or costovertebral glands. They are present in both sexes but are much more developed in the male. These sebaceous glands are darkly pigmented spots with roughened skin and coarse hairs located in the flank region.[3,4,6,11] The hamster deposits flank gland secretions by arching its back and rubbing its side against vertical surfaces, such as the wall of its cage or burrow, entrance to the tunnel or next box, etc. Flank gland secretions may also be deposited on the ground or floor of the enclosure from the animal's hind paws. Secretions from other sources (Harderian gland, ear gland) may be mixed with those of the flank gland when the animal marks vertical and horizontal surfaces.[4,12]

The Siberian hamster has similar lateral and mid-ventral scent glands[13,14] and will roll on its side or back to rub the flank glands on the substrate.[14] The mid-ventral sebaceous gland is larger in males than females.[14]

The Harderian gland (located within the orbit caudal to the eye) and the ear gland (located on the ventral surface of the pinna) also present a marked sexual dimorphism (larger in the males than females). For this reason and because secretion by these glands is androgen dependent, it is suggested that their secretions also have an important role in communication.[4,15]

Female hamster vaginal secretions contain many chemical compounds, with volume and consistency of secretions changing according to the reproductive status. Vaginal secretions are deposited in the environment by pressing their genital region against the substrate and moving forward.[4] Vaginal marking is a sexual solicitation behavior primarily directed toward males.[16] Vaginal secretions seem to be the primary olfactory stimulus that elicits ultrasonic calling from males, which will result in calling from the female and attraction in response.[17]

Hamsters scent mark in both non-social and social contexts. Non-social marking occurs with low frequency and intensity: when exploring the environment, entering or leaving the nest area, or just before or after grooming.[4,16] The most frequent and vigorous marking occurs in social contexts (territory marking and mating behavior).[3,4,6,11] Hamsters are stimulated to mark by contact with conspecifics or their odors. Odors of an individual of another hamster species are not nearly as stimulating, suggesting that flank and vaginal marking behavior also serves as a mechanism of intra-species communication. Exposure of developing pups to species-specific odors during early stages of life appears to be important for the development of odor-based species recognition and differentiation. Hamsters are also able to distinguish between individuals within the same species based on olfactory cues.[18] Golden hamsters have demonstrated an ability to recognize siblings, even when cross-fostered in different litters from birth, and olfaction is presumed to be a major factor in this familial recognition.[19]

Flank and vaginal marking are greatly influenced by sex hormone levels and reproductive state. Males are more attracted to female odors than to those of other males, and to odors of females in estrus than to odors of diestrus females. Estrus females are more attracted to male odors than to those of other females. Females mark in response to both male and female odors. When in contact with female odors, they tend to mark more using their flank glands (territory marking). When in contact with male odors, estrus females use mostly vaginal marking to attract the male.[16] When in groups, dominant hamsters mark more frequently than subordinate hamsters.[20]

It is clear then that scent marking can function simultaneously as agonistic and sexual behavior. It advertises to other animals that an individual of a particular sex and in a certain reproductive condition is occupying the area and may indicate how recently the individual has been there. Other individuals will respond in different ways depending on their sex, reproductive condition, previous experiences, and other factors. For example, scent marking of a male in breeding season will be considered agonistic behavior for other males also in breeding season (territory defense) but considered sexual behavior for females in estrus, allowing a female to localize the male (and vice versa).[4,16] Hamsters rarely mark during actual interactions with another individual (either agonistic or sexual encounters).

Scent signals are received by the main olfactory system (epithelium of the nasal cavity) and the accessory olfactory system (vomeronasal organ).[8,10] The vomeronasal organs are located on either side of the nasal septum. Several cues, including female's posture (vision), odors (olfaction), and ultrasonic calls (audition) as well as experience are factors in male hamster sexual performance. However, chemosensory input is considered to be essential for male sexual behavior.[4,8,10] Both the main and accessory olfactory systems are influential in mediating sexual behavior in male hamsters.[8,10] The vomeronasal organ appears to primarily mediate responses to relatively non-volatile components of female vaginal secretions,[21] whereas the main olfactory system primarily responds to more volatile components of the female scents.[22] The vomeronasal organ appears to have a more important role than the main olfactory system since lesions of the vomeronasal organ alone can result in deficits in sexual behavior (especially in sexually naïve males) whereas lesions of the main olfactory system alone do not.[10] Other behaviors that may be influenced by both olfactory systems include ultrasonic calling in female hamsters[23] and individual recognition.[10]

Among females, a functional olfactory system is not necessary for sexual receptivity.[24] Other female behaviors, such as maternal behavior seem to be primarily mediated via the accessory olfactory system;[25] scent-marking behavior due to perception of conspecifics odors appears to be mediated exclusively through the main olfactory system.[23]

Vision and somatic sensation

The hamster regulates its activity by the amount of light in its environment: maximum activity begins at twilight and continues into early evening; high light intensities result in cessation of movement and exploration. This behavior pattern is characteristic of animals with an all-rod retina, for which maximum acuity is achieved in dim light. Since hamster's vision is almost panoramic, visual acquisition of targets is mostly done with head and body movements instead of eye movements. Hamsters use vision to recognize and approach food.[26] Their social behavior also appears to be influenced by visual cues. The Syrian hamster has a black chest mark that some authors suggest is used as a visual threat in aggressive encounters.[27] Piloerection can occur in similar circumstances, causing an apparent size-increase which potentially serves as a visual sign.[27] As mentioned earlier, male hamster sexual performance is, in part, dependent on visual cues including the female's posture (see "Reproductive behavior").[4,8,10]

Hamsters are able to detect cliffs, find holes, and avoid barriers while running. However, despite their ability to perceive depth visually, hamsters appear to rely more on tactual information during locomotor activity, as other rodents do. Tactile information is provided by the forepaws

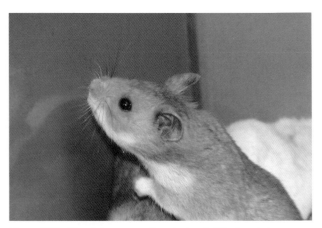

Figure 12.3 The vibrissae are an important part of the hamster's sensory system. (Photo courtesy of M. C. Tynes, copyright 2010.)

and vibrissae.[28] The vibrissae (sinus hairs, whiskers) are specialized hairs that form a highly refined vibrotactile receptor system, important for spatial orientation and communication (Figure 12.3). The hamster is unique in that it moves its cranial vibrissae in various complex patterns keyed to particular exploratory situations.[3]

Body postures

Body postures are an important means of intra-species communication and those of the Syrian hamster have been extensively studied.[4,29,30] The interactions of other solitary hamster species such as the Chinese hamster are similar. As described earlier, most interactions are agonistic or sexual because of the solitary nature of the species. Sexual body postures are described in the "Reproductive behavior" section.

Initial interactions typically involve head sniffing (Figure 12.4), presumably to gather information regarding individual identity or sexual status. The individuals may also investigate the body and genitals of the other hamster. Unless the pair consists of a male and sexually receptive female, agnostic encounters usually follow the initial sniffing interaction and may occur in either an upright (forelimbs off the ground) or standing position (bearing-weight on all four limbs). The subordinate hamster may attempt to avert attacks by lifting a paw while turning its head away from the aggressor, or assuming an upright position. Some researchers suspect hamsters use the upright position to best display the distinctly dark fur under the forelimbs as a visual threat.[31] However, others found subordinate hamsters took the upright posture more often, indicating a more defensive behavior.[29] Furthermore, some hamsters in a natural setting display the upright posture when threatened by predators.[32,33] Artificially enhancing the dark areas does not seem to affect the outcome of a fight, so the significance of these dark fur patches in the social interactions is unknown.[4]

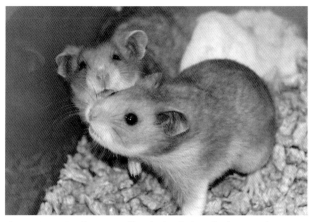

Figure 12.4   One hamster sniffing the head of another hamster during an initial interaction. (Photo courtesy of M. C. Tynes, copyright 2010.)

Fights usually begin as the aggressor knocks the other hamster off its feet, resulting in a rolling ball as both attempt to bite fur and skin of the other. This type of interaction may escalate into quick movements, accompanied by audible squeaks. The victim may try to escape using frantic, rapid movements and crash into the sides of the cage. The aggressor chases in a slower, smoother manner. The agnostic encounter often terminates with the male loser or submissive hamster arching its back upward and raising its tail, often walking off in a stiff-legged gait. Presumably, this behavior resembles a female hamster in the sexually receptive lordosis position, although in true female lordosis, the back is arched downward. In fact, the male victor may mount a male displaying this position. Females do not mount males or display the tail-up posture during a fight.[4] The tail-up posture may be used to deflect aggression in other situations, such as with a juvenile hamster placed in a new environment.[33]

Body care and housing

Syrian's hamster natural habitat is dry, rocky steppes, or brushy slopes. They live in burrows which they construct, generally one adult per burrow.[2] These deep tunnels provide them with a cool temperature and high humidity.[6] For this reason, hamsters can tolerate cold well but become heat stressed at ambient temperatures of 34°C (93°F) and usually begin dying at 36°C (97°F). Preferred temperatures are 18–26°C (65–79°F), with young maintained between 22°C and 24°C (71°F–75°F). Relative humidity should be kept at 40–70%.[13,33] The 14:10 light: dark cycle is the most often recommended and used.[13,34]

Hamsters' housing system must provide for normal physiologic and behavioral needs, including resting, nest building, grooming, exploring, climbing, hiding, digging, searching for food, hoarding, and gnawing (Figure 12.5). Hamsters prefer solid bottom cages with deep bedding. They can be housed in plastic bottom/wire top cages,

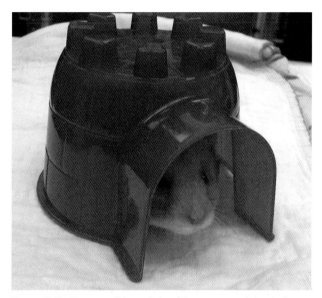

Figure 12.5   Hamster utilizing a shelter. (Photo courtesy of Ricardo de Matos.)

in totally enclosed plastic cages with tubes or in glass or plastic aquariums. Care should be taken when housing dwarf hamsters with wire cage components since these animals can get through very small gaps. Hamsters can gnaw through wood, plastic, and soft metals so cages of these materials should be avoided or checked regularly to prevent escapes. Escaped hamsters will not return to their cages, as rats and gerbils do. A secure lid must be provided. There are regulations on minimum required space for laboratory hamsters: adults must be given about 122 cm^2 (48 in.^{2}) of floor space,[35] but pet hamsters should be provided with the largest cage possible. Bedding depth requirements are not addressed by the USDA Animal Welfare Act, although hamsters should be provided with suitable substrate for burrowing and a nest or hide box should be supplied (see "Common behavior problems"). Facial tissue paper can be used as nesting material. Natural and/or synthetic fiber nesting material should be avoided, as it can wrap around the feet or teeth or be ingested and cause impaction. Pine, aspen, husks, newspaper, paper towels, and shredded paper are all acceptable dust-free substrates. However, the aromatic hydrocarbons in cedar can alter hepatic microsomal enzyme activity and irritate the respiratory tract so they should be avoided.[36] Elaborate plastic and wire housing with additional tubing is very popular and acceptable, although deep bedding, not tubing, appears to be the most important aspect to the pet hamster's environment. A water bottle is preferred to water bowl since it provides constant access to fresh and clean water as water bowls easily become soiled with bedding and food.

The hamster's natural behavior involves climbing and burrowing. In captivity, they should be provided with safe outlets for these activities, including exercise wheels (with

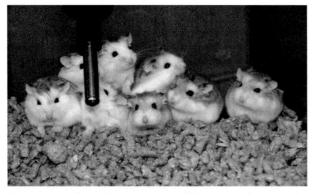

Figure 12.6 Roborovski hamsters are one of the more social species and can be housed in groups. (Photo courtesy of M. C. Tynes, copyright 2010.)

a solid running surface to avoid trauma to the limbs), ramps, and plastic or cardboard tunnels. Hamsters should also be given pieces of cardboard or soft wood to satisfy their need for gnawing and prevent incisor overgrowth.

Hamsters are fastidious in that they will utilize different areas of the cage for food storage, urination, and defecation. They produce very little waste or odor and usually do not smell if they are cleaned regularly (weekly except in the 1–2 weeks postpartum). Since the cleaning process and change of bedding induces a strong stress response in hamsters, some of the old and familiar bedding and nesting material should be kept when cleaning the cage. By providing a larger cage, the frequency of the stressful cage cleaning can be reduced.

Syrian and Chinese hamsters must be kept singly whereas the Russian and Roborovski hamsters can be housed together with others of their own species (Figure 12.6). Syrian hamsters are compatible within their own species, regardless of sex, if they have been weaned and raised together, although occasional bouts of aggression may still occur.

Behavioral thermoregulation

Syrian hamsters are capable of hibernation while the Siberian hamster exhibits daily torpor.[5] With shortened day length, temperatures below 8°C (48°F), low light intensity, and isolation, Syrian hamsters will gather food and hibernate. During this period, the hamster has a decreased body temperature, respiratory rate, and heart rate but remains sensitive to touch.[6,13] Hibernation usually lasts 2–3 days alternating with short periods of arousal to normal alertness.[6] Older hamsters start their hibernation earlier and spend more time sleeping than younger hamsters.[37]

As an adaptation to the harsh winter environment in their natural habitat, Siberian hamsters are able to decrease their body temperature to approximately 19°C (66°F) for a few hours during the day. This torpor allows the animal to conserve energy.[5]

Chinese hamsters are poorly adapted to extreme cold temperatures. Although they do not hibernate, they sleep longer during short days.[20]

In addition, under specific environmental conditions, especially cold ambient temperatures, hamsters will go into a deep sleep and may appear dead on casual observation.[6,13,34]

Social behavior

The Syrian hamster and Chinese hamster are naturally solitary species with individuals peacefully interacting only during mating and female offspring care.[38] Otherwise, adult hamster encounters in these species are agonistic. Housing adults together results in undue stress,[39,40] fighting, and injury.[41] Unlike these species of hamsters, the Siberian and Roborovski hamster can be housed in family groups (within the same species). Fighting and cannibalism are less frequent but interactions with humans may be equally pugnacious.[13]

In the predominantly solitary species, aggression is more frequent in females than males, and lactating females are more agonistic than females in other stages of estrus or pregnancy. Females tend to be dominant to males in opposite-sex pairings.[42] Body size is not a strong factor in encounter outcome. In most species, high levels of peripheral testosterone lead to aggression and dominance behaviorally, and large, darkly pigmented flank glands physically.[43,44]

Infant and juvenile Syrian hamsters are less aggressive than older hamsters, although play fighting is common. Play fighting starts around day 15 and these interactions consist of attacks directed toward the head of littermates and alternate body pinnings.[45,46] Same-sex dyads engage in play fighting more frequently than opposite-sex pairs, although there appears to be no difference in the amount of play fighting between male–male and female–female pairs.[47] Fighting peaks between days 30 and 35. At puberty, play fighting transitions to true adult aggression, in which one hamster targets the rear or ventrum instead of the opponent's head.[41] The onset of true aggression was accelerated in juvenile male Syrian hamsters subjected to repeated attacks.[48] However, juvenile females repeatedly defeated by an adult habituated both behaviorally and physiologically (cortisol) to the aggression.[49]

Reproductive behavior

Syrian hamsters achieve sexual maturity at a very young age (average 42 days).[34] Females are seasonally polyestrus with breeding quiescence in winter months in the wild (short days and restricted food).[6,13] If provided with a light cycle of 14 hours of artificial light and 10 of dark, they can reproduce in captivity throughout the year. Estrous cycles last 4 days[6,34] and begin in the evening hours. Ovulation is spontaneous and follows lordosis onset (sign of receptivity) by approximately 8 hours, occurring between 12 and 1 AM.[6,13] On the second day of the estrous cycle, female hamsters present a white, stringy, opaque postovulatory discharge, which should not be interpreted as purulent discharge due to infection. This discharge indicates that the female reached peak estrus the day before and she can be successfully mated in the evening of the third day after the detection of the postovulatory discharge (which corresponds to the first day of the next cycle since each estrous cycle lasts 4 days).[6,34]

Male–female interactions in the hamster are dependent on the female's estrous cycle, which is influenced by ovarian hormones (estrogen and progesterone).[50] Estrogen facilitates proceptivity. Estrogen priming followed by progesterone elicits the onset of sexual receptivity (lordosis). Receptivity declines with prolonged (more than 24 hours) progesterone exposure or exposure to copulatory stimuli. Within a few hours of mating, receptivity is completely lost and female hamsters develop agonistic behaviors.[50]

The proceptive period, which occurs on the day before behavioral estrus, is characterized by high levels of vaginal marking and ultrasonic calls by the female. They will also present an immobile "pre-lordosis" posture in response to male's attention. "Pre-lordosis" usually occurs 8 hours prior to the onset of lordosis. With the ultrasonic, olfactory, and visual signals characteristic of the proceptive period, the females probably exhibit "pre-lordosis" to attract the male and keep him close for successful breeding. Observation of Syrian hamsters in a semi-natural environment revealed that, during the period of proceptivity, attracted males followed females into their burrows, which the females then sealed. Testosterone may facilitate male hamsters' attraction to female odors and also inhibit the olfactory neophobia associated with an unfamiliar territory which is common in solitary species.[51] The female and male remain together through one sleep cycle. After mating, the female attacks the male and forces him out of the burrow.[50]

Using a "hand-mating" breeding technique, the female hamster in estrus is placed into the male's cage approximately 1 hour before dark. By placing the female in the male's marked cage and using an older and larger male, the likelihood of female aggressive behavior is reduced. When a receptive female is placed with a male, after a short "getting-acquainted" period (male sniffing and licking the female), the female performs a unique walk characterized by short, quick steps followed by lordosis. Females may remain immobile in this posture for 5–10 minutes at a time and even for several minutes when the male is not present.[4] Males lick and sniff the female genital region and head of the female in lordosis.[4] Mating is characterized by repeated intromissions and ejaculations and will last approximately 30 minutes.[34] If a female in estrus encounters a male that does not immediately attend to her or mount her, she will typically approach and assume the lordosis posture in front of him. If that still fails to elicit mounting, the female may emit ultrasonic calls, nuzzle, lick, bite, and in some cases mount the partner.[50] The pair should be observed when together for mating or fighting. Once mating is observed (or if fighting occurs), the female is removed from the male's cage. However, conception is sometimes improved by leaving the female with the male for 24 hours,[34,36] except for Chinese hamsters. In that species the female should be removed a maximum of 2 hours after mating.[20] Removing the female after mating minimizes fighting and allows the male to breed with other females.[34,36] This breeding scheme permits keeping one male for a "harem" of up to 12 females.[34] Alternatives to a hand-mating breeding program include monogamous pair mating (placing a prepubertal male and female together permanently; this requires a higher number of males) and group or harem mating (1–5 males placed with a larger number of females; females are removed 7–12 days after pairing and housed individually until weaning of the pups).[13]

Implantation of the fertilized ovum occurs on day 6 postcoitus.[13,34] During this time, minimal handling is essential. Pregnancy can be confirmed by the absence of estrus discharge on day 5 and 9 postmating, observation of a distended abdomen, and rapid weight gain at 10 days postmating. Pregnant females also spend less time wheel-running and more time eating and digging in the nest area. They also tend to be more aggressive. Hamster gestation is very short: on average 16 days.[13,34] Infertile matings or crowding of females may result in pseudopregnancy, which lasts 7–13 days.[13]

The reproductive life of a hamster is, in general, 10 months, with a significant decrease in reproductive capacity by 1 year of age. Once the pups are weaned, females can be re-mated within 2–3 days. During their reproductive life, a female hamster can produce 4–6 litters of pups.[34]

Siberian hamsters also present marked seasonal changes in reproductive activity (decreased during the summer and winter months). However, they breed throughout the year in laboratories and breeding facilities.[14] In this species, a female with young is usually left with the male and both parents participate in parturition and caring of the pups.[52]

Chinese hamster's aggressiveness, especially by females, creates many problems with captive breeding. Different breeding protocols are currently used, including hand-mating, artificial insemination, and monogamous mating (keeping male and female together during their entire reproductive life or separating them before the litter is born). A practical and more economical method involves placing three males in a breeding cage with three to five female littermates at weaning.[53]

The main reproductive characteristics of common pet hamster species are summarized in Table 12.2.

Table 12.2 Reproductive characteristics of common pet hamster species

Species	Sexual maturity	Gestation (days)	Litter size average (range)	Weaning (days)
Syrian (A,U)	34 days females 42 days males	15–18	11 (4–16)	20–25
Siberian (C,I)	90 to 130 days females 150 days males	18	4 (1–9)	16–18
Roborovski (Z)		20–22	3–5	
Chinese (C,Z)	90 days	20–21	4	21

Ingestive behavior

Hamsters have large well-developed cheek pouches where they can store and transport food. They are terrestrial, cursorial, diggers, and are mainly nocturnal, with limited daylight activity. In the wild, they live in burrows and are primarily granivorous. They can also eat green plant parts and shoots, roots, insects, and fruits.[2]

Young hamsters begin eating solid food at 7–10 days and should be fed a pelleted diet with a minimum of 16% protein and 4–5% fat. Mature adults do not need protein levels above 14%. Treats may include apples, raisins, and walnuts. To satisfy the foraging, food processing, and hoarding drive of hamsters, grain, seeds, peanuts, carrots, root vegetables, and pieces of apple should be distributed frequently on their bedding material in addition to the standard food ration.[54] Hamsters are coprophagic and may be seen bending their body when defecating to eat feces.[6,13] Coprophagy serves to recycle vitamins and other nutrients.[6]

Hamsters are commonly fed on the floor of the cage. If food is placed in feeders, they will remove it and pile it on the floor, with the location of the pile varying between individuals and cage environments. If the food is moved from the pile, the hamster will retrieve it and move it back.[36]

In captivity, hamsters will drink water from water bottles, bowls, and automatic systems.

Maternal behavior

Hormonal changes are associated with the initiation and maintenance of maternal behavior. The rise in pre-partum estrogen seems to be primarily associated with its onset. The increase in prolactin, possibly primed by estrogen, may be a trigger to maternal behaviors, such as licking, nursing, retrieving, and nest building, observed in the early lactation period.[55,56] Digging and gnawing will increase after mating and decline shortly before parturition. This behavior presumably reflects the expansion of burrows seen in free-ranging pregnant hamsters.[57] Four days prior to parturition, digging decreases and nest building behavior increases.[57] In a captive setting, females should be given ample deep bedding to provide an outlet for digging and nest building behavior.

Before delivery, the female becomes active, restless, and bleeds from the vulva. A 50% increase in respiratory rate and sudden jerky movements usually precede the delivery.[38] The female overtly strains and licks the genital region at parturition. Female hamsters eat the umbilical cord, birth fluids, and usually the placenta (or they may be stored in the cheek pouch or food pile to be consumed later) at the time of each pup's birth. Pups are born at 10- to 30-minute intervals, with the whole birth process taking approximately 2 hours. Generally, a female's first litter is smaller in number than subsequent litters.[13,34]

Female Syrian hamsters with pups are housed alone due to the risk of the stressed female or a non-maternal hamster killing the pups. For Siberian hamsters, females with young are usually left with the fathers and both parents participate in care of the young.[31] Male Siberian hamsters also assist mechanically during delivery, lick, and sniff the young soon after birth and open the pups' airways by clearing their nostrils.

Sensitization, or the eliciting of parental behavior by exposure to a pup, is documented in pregnant, non-pregnant, and male hamsters.[58,59] Early social exposure may be a factor in paternal care. Gibber and Terkel[60] found adult males reared with females are less likely to attack pups. A drop in peripheral cortisol seems to be associated with "midwifery" behavior in those species in which paternal offspring care occurs.[61]

Fostering is rarely successful with hamsters; both adopted and natural litters may be cannibalized by the female. Cross-fostering with other species has also not been successful due to the extreme immaturity of hamster pups (as a result of short gestation) and presence of sharp incisors. Hand-rearing is laborious and rarely successful.[13]

Baby hamsters are born hairless, with eyes and ears closed and sharp incisors. The ears open at 4–5 days and eyes open at 14–16 days.[6,34] Hair growth begins at 9 days.[13] Young start eating food and drinking water when they are 7–10 days old so care should be taken to make sure they can reach the water supply and have food available on the floor of the cage. Young are generally weaned at 3 weeks of age.[6,34] Weaning begins with the mother's building a separate nest around day 24 postparturition. The nest building continues until the pups are 29–34 days of age at which time the mother becomes intermittently aggressive to the pups but predominantly ignores her offspring. Under laboratory conditions, the female aggression ceases as the pups reach sexual maturity (approximately day 42).[38] Based on mother and offspring behavior in the laboratory, Roswell[29] suggests that under natural conditions, either the young disperse around day 35, or the mother leaves the nest around day 25.

In their natural habitat, female Chinese hamsters and her pups stay together in the burrow for approximately 22 days, after which the young begin to sleep outside the burrow.

Cannibalism of pups is a common behavior problem in hamsters and will be discussed in the next section. The female hamster, when disturbed, can also place her newborn litter in her cheek pouches and return them to the nest once considered safe. However, young may suffocate while in the cheek pouch.[13]

Common behavior problems

Most behavior problems in pet and laboratory hamsters relate to aggression or inadequate environmental enrichment.

As discussed earlier, solitary hamsters (e.g., Syrian and Chinese) are often aggressive to other hamsters and humans. Hamsters can play dead, bite, or show other aggressive behavior in response to rough handling, sudden disturbances, being around other hamsters, when caring for their pups, or when ill or in pain. Even more sociable species, such the Russian hamster, will bite in similar circumstances. Roborovski hamsters rarely bite but are difficult to handle, owing to their smaller size and extremely active temperaments.

With frequent, gentle handling, a hamster can easily become less fearful and aggressive to humans. Hamsters should initially be handled for short periods of time in their home enclosure and under dim lighting. Since hamsters are nocturnal, it has been suggested that they are more likely to be awake and amenable to handling when the lights are dim. Special food treats should simultaneously be given to allow the hamster to associate human interaction with a reward. After many repetitions, the length of handling sessions may be increased and the hamster will more readily accept being handled outside of the cage. Animals that are already showing aggression may need to be reconditioned to accept human handling. Desensitization and counterconditioning should be employed and are discussed in detail in the learning chapter (Chapter 18) of this book. The threshold level at which the hamster shows fear or aggression should be identified. In other words, does the hamster bite when seeing a hand approach, or not until physically contacted? Using desensitization and counterconditioning, the handler would slowly bring the hand to the threshold (biting) distance, give the hamster a tasty piece of food, and then remove the hand. Aggression should not be triggered. This process is repeated until the hamster appears relaxed with the hand at that distance, and then the hand may be brought closer. If a hamster does not bite until it is touched, offering a piece of food with one hand while scooping with the other hand is effective in redirecting the animal's attention as well as associating human hands with a reward.

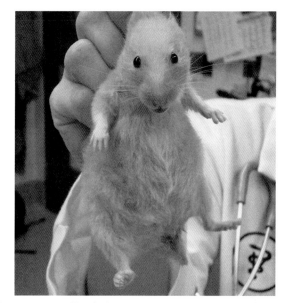

Figure 12.7   Scruffing the hamster by the skin over the neck and shoulders provides restraint for examination. (Photo courtesy of Ricardo de Matos.)

Other techniques can be used to decrease the probability of aggression or injury to a human handler. If a hamster is sleeping, it should be gently woken up by rustling the substrate near it or lightly jiggling the cage until it is awake. Once its eyes are open, it may be scooped from the substrate and cupped in the hands securely but loosely. Hamsters can also be scruffed by the abundant loose skin at the nape of the neck (neck only or whole body scruff; Figure 12.7), held in one hand with a grasp around head and shoulders, or placed in small container, or wrapped in a cloth. Young or untamed hamsters should be handled only a few inches above a secure surface to avoid trauma in case they are dropped or fall.

The propensity for intra-species aggression in Syrian and Chinese hamsters has been discussed in previous sections. These hamsters should be housed individually to prevent aggression and stress. Levels of the stress-related hormone cortisol are significantly higher in solitary hamsters housed together than those housed singly.[40]

Aggression to pups or cannibalism is common behavior problem in captive hamsters, but its prevalence in the wild is unknown and it may be an artifact of captivity. The specific causes of cannibalism have yet to be identified. However, litter abandonment and cannibalism are common during the first pregnancy and the first week postdelivery. It may occur if the nest is scant, disturbed, or too visible; if the young are abnormal, born onto wire, handled, or bite the mother while nursing; if the diet is inadequate, the litter large or small, the mother is disturbed, noises occur near the cage, or if agalactia occurs.[6,13,62,63] Females may attack and cannibalize the whole litter or nurse some while cannibalizing others.[38] Studies suggest prolactin may be involved in the switch from aggression to maternal behaviors in hamsters.[64] The most important measure to prevent pup-directed aggression is to avoid disturbing females with litters. Approximately 3 days before the expected delivery date, the pregnant female should be given a clean cage with additional nest material (such as paper tissues) and enough food and water for at least 7–10 days.[13,34] This, together with no handling of female and pups during the first 1–2 weeks postdelivery and feeding the postparturient female wheat germ, apple pieces, or a meat product, may reduce the incidence of cannibalism.[13,34]

Normal hamster behavior involves climbing, burrowing, and gnawing. In captivity, they should be provided with safe outlets for these activities, including large cages, exercise wheels, plastic tunnels, deep bedding material, and wood or cardboard for chewing. In the natural environment, Syrian hamster burrows are approximately 200 cm long and 65 cm deep.[65] The inability to perform natural behaviors such as burrowing may contribute to abnormal stereotypic behaviors. Caged rodents, including hamsters may engage in repetitive, invariant, and seemingly functionless behaviors such as bar mouthing. Hamsters in larger cages spend less time engaged in bar mouthing, or gnawing on cage bars, than those housed in smaller cages, even if the latter are provided with cardboard and twigs.[66] Bar mouthing behavior in hamsters can also be reduced by providing a running-wheel[67] or deep bedding.[68] In fact, when provided with at least 40 cm of bedding, Syrian hamsters perform little to no bar mouthing even when subjected to stressful handling.[68]

Running-wheels are popular enrichment devices for captive hamsters. Preference studies in other rodents indicate these animals prefer running-wheels to tunnels or circular tubes.[69] Some believe wheel-running is a normal substitute for walking or running, whereas others argue it is an abnormal locomotor stereotypy in hamsters housed in suboptimal caging.[20,53,70] Wheel-running is reduced in hamsters housed in large cages[20,53] with deep bedding.[68] Regardless of their motivation, hamsters do choose to spend a great deal of the night in the wheel which does not appear to compromise body condition,[71] and may improve reproductive fitness.[67]

Exercise balls are also a popular method for providing hamsters with exercise and enrichment. However, owners should use extreme caution when using these balls as it is very easy for the hamster to become lodged in small spaces, fall down a flight of stairs, be kicked or stepped on by a human, and become prey for the household dogs or cats. Reports of people forgetting about the hamster inside an exercise ball for several days are not uncommon. A hamster should only be placed in a ball if under strict supervision and away from stairs or other pets.

In summary, safe running wheels, large cages, and deep bedding should be provided for pet and laboratory hamsters as they appear to decrease stress and the incidence of many different behavior problems.

References

1. Shepherd AJ. Results of the 2006 AVMA survey of companion animal ownership in US pet-owning households. *J Am Vet Med Assoc* 2008; 232(5):695–696.
2. Clark JD. Historical perspectives and taxonomy. In: Van Hoosier GL, McPherson CW, eds. *Laboratory Hamsters*. Orlando: Academic Press, 1987;3–7.
3. Bivin WS, Olsen GH, Murray KA. Morphophysiology. In: Van Hoosier GL, McPherson CW, eds. *Laboratory Hamsters*. Orlando: Academic Press, 1987;9–41.
4. Johnston RE. Communication. In: Johnston RE, Siegel HI, eds. *The Hamster: Reproduction and Behavior*. New York: Plenum Press, 1985;121–151.
5. Newcomer CE, Fitts DA, Goldman BD et al. Experimental biology: Other research uses of Syrian hamsters. In: Van Hoosier GL, McPherson CW, eds. *Laboratory Hamsters*. Orlando: Academic Press, 1987;264–300.
6. Hrapkiewicz K, Medina L. Hamsters In: *Clinical Laboratory Animal Medicine, An Introduction*. 3rd ed. Ames: Blackwell Publishing, 2007;130–151.
7. Floody OR, Pfaff DW. Communication among hamsters by high-frequency acoustic signals: I. Physical characteristics of hamster calls. In: Van Hoosier GL, McPherson CW, eds. *Laboratory Hamsters*. Orlando: Academic Press, 1987;794–806.
8. Malsbury CW, Miceli MO, Scouten CW. Neural basis of reproductive In: Johnston RE, Siegel HI, eds. *The Hamster: Reproduction and Behavior*. New York: Plenum Press, 1985;229–259.
9. Sales G, Pye D. *Ultrasonic Communication by Animals*. London: Chapman & Hall, 1974.
10. Pfeiffer CA, Johnston RE. Hormonal and behavioral responses of male hamsters to females and female odors: Roles of olfaction, the vomeronasal system, and sexual experience. *Physiol Behav* 1994;55:138–139.
11. Field KJ, Sibold AL. Important biological features In: *The Laboratory Hamster and Gerbil*. Boca Raton: CRC Press, 1999;1–12.
12. Johnston RE. Scent marking by male hamsters: I. Effects of odors and social encounters. *Z Tierpsychol* 1975;37:75–98.
13. Wagner JE, Harkness JE. The hamster. In: *The Biology and Medicine of Rabbits and Rodents*. 4th ed. Media: Williams and Wilkins, 1995;40–50.
14. Cantrell CA, Padovan D. Other hamsters: Biology, care and use in research (check rest of title). In: Van Hoosier GL, McPherson CW, eds. *Laboratory Hamsters*. Orlando: Academic Press, 1987;369–387.
15. Payne AP, McGadey J et al. Androgenic control of the Harderian gland in the male golden hamster. *J Endocrinol* 1977;75:73–82.
16. Johnston, RE. Chemical communication in golden hamsters: From behavior to molecules and neural mechanisms. In: Dewsbury DA, ed. *Contemporary Issues in Comparative Psychology*. Sunderland: Sinauer, 1990;381–409.
17. Johnston RE, Kwan M. Vaginal scent marking: Effects on ultrasonic calling and attraction of male golden hamster. *Behav Neural Biol* 1984;42:158–168.
18. Johnston RE, Brenner D. Species specificity of scent marking in hamsters. *Behav Neural Biol* 1982;25:46–55.
19. Heth G, Todrank J, Johnson RE. Kin recognition in golden hamsters: Evidence for phenotype matching. *Anim Behav* 1998;56:409–417.
20. Bartlett P. *The Hamster Handbook*. New York: Barron's Hauppauge, 2003.
21. Clancy AN, Macrides F, Singer AG, Agosta WC. Male hamster copulatory responses to a high molecular weight fraction of vaginal discharge: Effects of vomeronasal organ removal. *Physiol Behav* 1984;33(4):653–660.
22. Johnston RE. Effects of female odors on the sexual behavior of male hamsters. *Behav Neural Biol* 1986;46(2):168–188.
23. Johnston RE. Vomeronasal and/or olfactory mediation of ultrasonic calling and scent marking by female golden hamsters. *Physiol Behav* 1992;51(3):437–448.

24. Carter CS. Olfaction and sexual receptivity in the female golden hamster. *Physiol Behav* 1973;10:47–51.

25. Marques DM. Roles of the main olfactory and vomeronasal systems in the response of the female hamster to young. *Behav Neural Biol* 1979;26(3):311–329.

26. Findlay BL, Marder K, Cordon D. Acquisition of visuomotor behavior after neonatal tectal lesions in hamster: The role of visual experience. *J Comp Physiol Psychol* 1980;94:506–518.

27. Finlay BL, Berian CA. Visual and somatosensory processes. In: Johnston RE, Siegel HI, eds. *The Hamster: Reproduction and Behavior.* New York: Plenum Press, 1985;409–433.

28. Schiffman HR. Evidence for sensory dominance: Reactions to apparent depth in rabbits, cats, rodents. *J Comp Physiol Psych* 1970;71:38–41.

29. Johnson RE. The role of dark chest patches and upright postures in the agonistic behavior of male hamsters, *Mesocricetus auratus. Behav Biol* 1976;17:161–176.

30. Floody OR, Pfaff DW. Aggressive behavior in female hamsters: The hormonal basis for fluctuations in female aggressiveness correlated with estrous state. *J Comp Physiol Psychol* 1977;91:443–464.

31. Grant EC, Mackintosh JH, Lerwill CJ. The effect of a visual stimulus on the agonistic behaviour of the golden hamster. *Z Tierpsychol* 1970;27:73–77.

32. Eibl-Eibesfeldt I. Zur ethologie des hamsters (*Cricetus cricetus* L.). *Z Tierpscyhol* 1953;10:204–254.

33. Dieterlen F. Das Verhalten des syrischen Goldhamsters (*Mesocricetus auratus* Waterhouse). *Z Tierpsychol* 1959;16:47–103.

34. Balk MW, Slater GM. The golden or Syrian hamster care and management. In: Van Hoosier GL, McPherson CW, eds. *Laboratory Hamsters.* Orlando: Academic Press, 1987;61–67.

35. Animal and Plant Health Inspection Service Web site. Animal Welfare Regulations. Available at: www.aphis.usda.gov/animal_welfare/awr. stml. Accessed Jan 1, 2009.

36. Husbandry. In: *Rodents/Committee on Rodents, Institute of Laboratory Animal Resources, Commission on Life Sciences, National Research Council (Laboratory Animal Management Series).* Washington: National Academy Press, 1996;44–84.

37. Terada A, Ibuka N. Age affects hibernation in Syrian hamsters (*Mesocricetus auratus*). *Chronobiol Int* 2000;7(5):623–630.

38. Rowell TE. The family group in golden hamsters; its formation and break-up. *Behaviour* 1960;17:81–94.

39. Zimmer R, Gatterman R. The influence of housing and rank on the activity of adrenal glands of male golden hamster. *Zeit Saugert* 1986;61:74–75.

40. Zhang J, Jia N, Wu F et al. Effects of social conditions on adult and subadult female rat-like hamsters (*Cricetulus triton*). *J Ethol* 2004;22:161–165.

41. Arnold CE, Estep DQ. Effects of housing on social preference and behaviour in male golden hamsters (*Mesocricetus auratus*). *Appl Anim Behav Sci* 1990;27:253–261.

42. Siegel HI. Aggressive behavior. In: Johnson RE, Siegel HI, eds. *The Hamster: Reproduction and Behavior.* New York: Plenum Press, 1985;261–268.

43. Drickamer LC, Vandenbergh JG. Predictors of social dominance in the adult female golden hamsters (*Mesocricetus auratus*). *Anim Behav* 1973;564–570.

44. Drickamer LC, Vandenberg JG, Colby DR. Predictors of dominance in the male golden hamster (*Mesocricetus auratus*). *Anim Behav* 1973;21:557–563.

45. Goldman L, Swanson HH. Developmental changes in pre-adult behavior in confined colonies of golden hamster. *Dev Psychobiol* 1975;8:137–150.

46. Pelis SM, Pellis VC. Play fighting in the Syrian golden hamster *Mesocricetus auratus* Waterhouse, and its relationship to serious fighting during postweaning development. *Dev Psychobiol* 1988;21:323–337.

47. Guerra RF, Vieira ML, Takase E et al. Sex differences in the play fighting activity of golden hamster infants. *Physiol Behav* 1992; 52:1–5.

48. Wommack JC, Delville Y. Repeated social stress and the development of agonistic behavior: Individual differences in coping responses in male golden hamsters. *Physiol Behav* 2003;80:303–308.

49. Taravosh-Lahn K, Delville Y. Aggressive behavior in female golden hamsters: Development and the effect of repeated social stress. *Horm Behav* 2004;46:428–435.

50. Carter CS. Female sexual behavior In: Johnston RE, Siegel HI, eds. *The Hamster: Reproduction and Behavior.* New York: Plenum Press, 1985;173–189.

51. Cornwell-Jones CA, Kovanic K. Testosterone reduces olfactory neophobia in male golden hamsters. *Physiol Behav* 1981;26:973–977.

52. Gibber JR, Piontkewitz Y, Terkel J. Response of male and female Siberian hamsters towards pups. *Behav Neural Biol* 1984;42:177–182.

53. Chang A, Diani A, Connell M. The striped or Chinese hamster biology and care. In: Van Hoosier GL, McPherson CW, eds. *Laboratory Hamsters.* Orlando: Academic Press, 1987;305–319.

54. Kuhnen G. Comfortable quarters for hamsters in research institutions. In: Reinhardt V, Reinhardt A, eds. *Comfortable Quarters for Laboratory Animals.* Washington: Animal Welfare Institute, 2007;33–37.

55. Siegel HI. Parental behavior. In: Johnson RE, Siegel HI, eds. *The Hamster: Reproduction and Behavior.* New York: Plenum Press, 1985;207–228.

56. McCarthy MM, Curran GH, Siegel HI. Evidence for the involvement of prolactin in the maternal behavior of the hamster. *Physiol Behav* 1994;55:181–184.

57. Daly M. The maternal behaviour cycle in golden hamsters. *Z Tierpsych* 1972;31:289–299.

58. Swanson LJ, Campbell CS. Induction of maternal behavior in nulliparous golden hamsters (*Mesocricetus auratus*). *Behav Neural Biol* 1979;26:364–371.

59. Siegel HI, Rosenblatt JS. Short-latency induction of maternal behavior in nulliparous golden hamsters (*Mesocricetus auratus*). *Presented at Eastern Conference on Reproductive Behavior,* Madison, Wisconsin 1978;52.

60. Gibber JR, Terkel J. Postweaning social experience on response of Siberian hamsters (*Phodus sungorus*) towards young. *J Comp Psych* 1985;99:491–493.

61. Jones JS, Wynne-Edwards KE. Paternal hamsters mechanically assist the delivery, consume amniotic fluid and placenta, remove fetal membranes, and provide parental care during the birth process. *Horm Behav* 2000;37:116–125.

62. Day CSD, Galef BD. Physiological and experiential influences on pup-induced maternal behavior in golden hamsters. *J Comp Physiol* 1977;91:1179–1189.

63. Miceli MO, Malsbury CW. Availability of a food hoard facilitates maternal behaviour in virgin female hamsters. *Physiol Behav* 1982;28:855–856.

64. Wise DA. Aggression in the female hamster: Effects of reproductive state and social isolation. *Horm Behav* 1974;5:235–250.

65. Gattermann R, Fritzsche P, Neumann K et al. Notes on the current distribution and the ecology of wild golden hamsters (*Mesocricetus auratus*). *J Zool* 2001;254:359–365.

66. Fischer K, Gebhardt-Henrich SG, Steiger A. Behaviour of golden hamsters (*Mesocricetus auratus*) kept in four different cage sizes. *Anim Welf* 2007;16:85–93.

67. Gebhardt-Henrich SG, Vonlanthen EM, Steiger A. How does the running wheel affect the behaviour and reproduction of golden hamsters kept as pets? *Appl Anim Behav Sci* 2005;95:199–203.

68. Hauzenberger AR, Gebhardt-Henrich SG, Steiger A. The influence of bedding depth on behaviour in golden hamsters (*Mesocricetus auratus*). *Appl Anim Behav Sci* 2006;100:280–294.

69. Sherwin CM. The use and perceived importance of three resources which provide caged laboratory mice the opportunity for extended locomotion. *Appl Anim Behav Sci* 1998;55:353–367.

70. Sherwin CM. Voluntary wheel running: A review and novel interpretation. *Anim Behav* 1998;56:11–27.

71. Gattermann R, Weindandy R, Fritzsche P. Running-wheel activity and body composition in golden hamsters (*Mesocricetus auratus*). *Physiol Behav* 2004;82:541–544.

13

Chinchillas

Jennifer L. Sobie

Personable and inquisitive, the domestic chinchilla has steadily increased in popularity since its introduction as a pet in the early 1960s. Averaging up to 800 g (1.8 lbs) in captivity, a chinchilla's appearance is naturally paedomorphic with a compact body, proportionally large head, very large, oblong pinnae, large, prominent eyes and, perhaps most alluring, thick, silky-soft fur (see Figure 13.1). Indeed, it is the chinchilla's fur that has historically contributed to its popularity, so much so that the wild chinchilla's very existence is threatened. Endemic to the Andean mountains, chinchillas originally enjoyed a relatively wide distribution and ranged throughout the arid high-altitude regions of South America. Their discovery and subsequent harvest for their pelts led to the decimation of their numbers and serious damage to their habitat.[1] Wild chinchillas are currently classified as endangered and in 1983 the Chinchilla Natural

Reserve was created in the Chilean mountain range. It is believed that the few remaining wild chinchillas exist in or close to that reserve.[2–4]

Natural history of the chinchilla

The chinchilla is a medium-sized rodent of the infra-order Hystricognathi (suborder Hystricomorpha, infraorder Hystricognathi, parvorder Caviomorpha, superfamily Chinchilloidea, family Chinchillidae). The two recognized species in the family Chinchillidae are *Chinchilla lanigera* (the long-tailed chinchilla) and *Chinchilla brevicaudata* (the short-tailed chinchilla). Hystricognath rodents underwent extensive radiation in the Miocene period in correlation with the emergence of grasslands,[5] and Hytricognaths such as chinchillas differ from Myomorpha rodents in that they give birth to precocial young. Gestation in *C. lanigera* is 111 days,[6] and newborn chinchillas emerge fully coated with open eyes. The average life span of chinchillas is 10 years,[6] with unverified reports of up to 27 years. This is far longer than the life span of most rodents.

Isolated from richer habitats by dispersal barriers that include the Andean mountains to the east, the Atacama Desert to the north, and the Pacific Ocean to the west, the chinchilla is a product of its environment. The relatively unique climate, terrain, and flora of the high-altitude habitat of the chinchilla have all had a profound influence on its development. For instance, the chinchilla is an opportunistic herbivore, subsisting on the woody, drought-resistant species indigenous to the area. This vegetation—including bromeliads, cacti, bahia grasses, and evergreen shrubs—is coarse and dry and low in nutrition, and requires extensive intake to meet mammalian nutritional requirements.[7] The chinchilla's digestive system is well adapted to these limitations: its teeth are all open-rooted throughout life to support extended

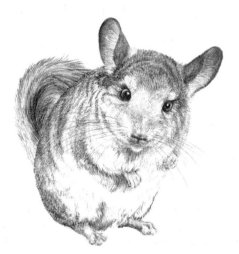

Figure 13.1 Drawing of an adult chinchilla demonstrating the appealing and child-like large head, ears and eyes. (Original artwork by the author.)

periods of grinding, its gastrointestinal tract is relatively long with a highly sacculated colon and large stomach and cecum, and it is cecotrophic to extract maximal microbiotic benefit from its food sources.[6]

High-altitude oxygen binding is another niche adaptation of the chinchilla.[8,9] Living at elevations 3,000–4,900 m (10,000–16,600 ft) above sea level, chinchillas have a greater hemoglobin oxygen affinity than other rodents. The chinchilla's limbs are also specially adapted to suit their environment. Their forelegs are quite short with grasping paws, while their hind limbs are disproportionately long and built for both bursts of strength and agility. The tibia is longer than the femur, there is almost no fibula, and the bones themselves are lightweight.[10] Coupled with hairless plantar and palmar pads, short claws, and a tail that can function as an airborne rudder, the chinchilla's limb structure facilitates flying leaps and agile scrabbles over and across rocky, sparsely vegetated terrain. The tail of *C. lanigera* is 6–8 in. in length and furred with coarse, straight, and relatively long hair; it serves as a grounding balance when the animal sits on its hindquarters and scans for predators.

Most unique to the chinchilla, however, is its coat. Luxurious, silky-soft and dense, the chinchilla's coat is created of clusters of 50–75 hairs emerging from a single follicle.[11] Human hairs, by contrast, grow one per follicle. The relatively short hairs of the coat are 2–4 cm (0.8–1.5 in.) in length and firmly adhered to skin unless molted[12] or released as a defense mechanism referred to as "fur slip."[6] The thick fur protects the chinchilla against the high-altitude hazards of hypothermia and dehydration. Typically a bluish-slate shade created of gray hairs tipped in black,[13] the coat also provides the chinchilla camouflage against the rocks of its mountain habitat.

Chinchillas are fairly large for a rodent. Although their size helps them survive in their harsh habitat, it can also make them conspicuous to predators. Natural predators include both foxes and owls.[11] As is common to other medium-to-large hystricognaths living in relatively barren environments,[14] chinchillas live in social groups as an adaptive strategy that reduces predation risk. Known as colonies, chinchilla groups can range in number from just a few individuals to several hundred, and they can range in territorial size from 1.5–113.5 ha (3.75–285 acres).[3] Scattered throughout the mountains of north-central Chile, original chinchilla colonies were estimated to have upward of 500 individuals each; today, scant decades later, few colonies have over 50 individuals.

One of the unique features of a high-altitude mountain habitat is its rocky fissures and relatively shallow earth coverage. Like other social New World hystricognath rodents,[14] chinchillas generally shelter in borrows. These burrows are often created out of the shelter of rock crevices and gaps among or below boulders, inside large bromeliads[11] and at the base of other plants. Spotorno et al.[11] describe these burrows as being a corridor that opens into a wider room. This room serves as a dormitory and probably doubles as a nest area when covered by dried hay or soft materials. Food might also be stored in the burrow. Although chinchillas are primarily nocturnal, they've been observed "sun bathing" in front of burrow entrances on bright days.

Domestication of the chinchilla

The domestic chinchilla is likely descended from a small number of long-tailed chinchillas imported to California in 1923 by Mathias F. Chapman, a mining engineer working for the Anaconda Copper Company in the Andes. The fur garment industry showed the most interest in domestication and it is probable that Chapman imported the animals for pelt ranching. Some reports have the number of Chapman's original chinchillas at 11 animals[12] or 12 animals,[11] while others place it at 13 animals.[6] The animals began attracting the attention of the pet trade in the 1960s,[12] and chinchillas are now commonly found in pet stores and animal shelters.

Sensory capabilities and communication

Data pertinent to a chinchilla's sensory capabilities in its natural environment are limited, but some general conclusions can be extrapolated from rodent data. These data suggest that chinchillas interpret their world and communicate through the four main senses of olfaction, tactile sensation, audition, and vision. Taste is secondary to olfaction, but chinchillas may accept or reject edibles based on taste.

Olfaction

A rodent's primary interpretation of its world is likely formed through olfactory stimuli; the sense of smell is commonly the most developed sensory system in rodents.[15–17] The vomeronasal organ in a chinchilla is a pair of tubular structures, approximately 6 mm in length and situated bilaterally along the base of the nasal septum.[11] Chinchillas use olfaction to make a diverse range of determinations including conspecific gender, familiarity, predation probability, spatial boundaries, and appetitive quality. The relevance of olfactory stimuli is both predisposed and learned;[18,19] this ability allows chinchillas to react to some scents without prior experience and thereby possibly avoid predation, and to learn to respond differentially to scents through experience with consequences associated with an odor.

Audition

Chinchillas have very good hearing at medium ranges and are easily able to discriminate sounds.[20–22] Their pinnae have been shown to facilitate sound localization.[23] Studies also indicate that they use a complex of perceptual sound stimuli, such as both pitch and timbre, to discriminate sounds.[24]

As prey animals, chinchillas are easily startled and distressed by loud or unpredictable sounds and noise. Data indicate that chinchillas will respond with undifferentiated avoidance to all novel sounds if they are not allowed the experience to discriminate safety stimuli from warning stimuli.[25]

It is likely that chinchillas rely on their hearing more than their vision and may even use vision mainly to help them locate the origin of sounds. This suggestion comes from data produced through studies of the structural organization of their auditory system. Examination shows that they have both a medial superior olive and a prominent lateral superior olive.[26] The medial superior olive is always large in animals with well-developed eyes and probably facilitates movement of the head and eyes in the direction of a sound in space, but prominent lateral superior olive clusters are present only in animals that rely a great deal on auditory-directed locomotion (e.g., nocturnal or echolocation species). It is thought that localization and fine auditory discrimination are dependent on the lateral superior olive.[26]

Vision

The eyes of the chinchilla are characteristic of a nocturnal rodent, having a shallow, boney orbit, large cornea, and large spherical lens. However, unique to the chinchilla and consistent with their habit of occasionally basking in the sun during the day, the iris is heavily pigmented and the pupil is a vertical slit.[27] These adaptations enhance their ability to see at night and yet adjust quickly to changes in light; however, their visual acuity is relatively poor. To facilitate navigation at night, they have abundant, strong and long (100–130 mm or 4–5 in.) vibrissae that extend beyond their bodies.[11,28]

Studies indicate that chinchillas do not rely on vision to facilitate escape or avoidance in close environments.[29] Rather, they respond to stimulation of their vibrissae[30] or an integration of these different sensory modalities.[31]

Vocalizations

Although chinchillas are shy and often retreat from observation, they are relatively vocal. In general, their vocalizations can be categorized as expressing attention seeking, interest, alarm or warning, physical distress, contentment, and aggression.[12,32,33] Categories can be distinguished thusly:

- *Attention-seeking vocalizations*—Emitted as a series of soft grunts or throaty humming that can escalate to rapid chirping.
- *Physical distress*—Expressed as a very loud and shrill single or repetitive shriek.
- *Interest*—Expressed as soft chirping emitted while exploring a novel but low-stress environment.

- *Alarm or warning*—Loud, hoarse barks, or whistle-like squeals emitted in response to possible threat or any uncertain situation.
- *Contentment*—Emitted as soft cooing.
- *Aggression*—Expressed as a low grunt that may escalate to teeth chattering. Hissing and spitting are also not uncommon aggressive threat communications.

Visual communication

As with other social species, a chinchilla's body posture reflects its emotional state and intent. Frightened chinchillas will crouch and lower their pinnae, often turning their faces away from fearful stimuli. Relaxed but inquisitive animals will direct their attention toward what interests them and begin moving toward the thing on all fours with a lively demeanor. Chinchillas also raise themselves to stand on their hind limbs, balanced on their tails, both when they are interested in something going on around them and when they are alarmed by another animal or a person. Interest can be discriminated from alarm by the direction of the chinchilla's attention—moving the head even slightly and sniffing with pinnae extended indicates interest, while direct attention toward an object without air sniffing is most often an indication of alarm. An alarmed, standing chinchilla may defend itself with a sudden release of urine directed in a stream at the perceived threat;[12] females are more likely to produce a urine stream and more likely to successfully target the object or individual considered a threat.

Body care

The atmospheric and climatic conditions of the chinchilla's native habitat are cool and dry. Accordingly, chinchillas have evolved a coat that reserves both heat and water. This coat is so remarkably dense that external parasites such as fleas and ticks cannot live on the skin of a chinchilla. However, the efficiency of the chinchilla's coat as a barrier also predisposes the animals to heatstroke at temperatures that a caregiver might consider only slightly uncomfortable. This includes temperatures as low as 30°C (80°F).[34]

Chinchillas thrive at temperatures that range from 18°C (65°F) to 24°C (75°F). Lower temperatures have been recommended as well; temperatures between 10°C (50°F) and 20°C (68°F) are reported to facilitate good coat growth.[6] Humidity should be kept below 50%.[34]

The chinchilla's coat does not require a great deal of grooming, but their environment must provide them the tools for its care. One important aspect of this care is the dust bath. Dust baths function to cleanse the heavy coat of the chinchilla; dust adheres to oils and dirt in the coat and is then spun off. Dust bathing is a natural component of grooming that is practiced in the wild, and it follows a relatively set sequence of behaviors in chinchillas.[35] The animal first thrusts its front paws forward and draws sand back toward its body; it then rubs its cheeks against the sand and, finally, rotates its body around its longitudinal axis in the direction of its cheek rub. If unable to access a dust bath for a period of days, the sequence of behaviors remain intact but the number of spins increase as a function of the days of deprivation.

Dust for dust bathing must be sufficiently fine and dry. Beach sand is not suitable.[6] Volcanic ash or pumice is an option and may be available in pet stores, but easier to obtain is dust made specifically for chinchilla dust baths such as Blue Sparkle Chinchilla Dust. A proper bathing vesicle is required as well. Because chinchillas are voracious chewers, plastic should be avoided unless the bath is removed immediately after use. A small glass aquarium, a terra cotta planter, a metal pan, or some other non-plastic bin measuring approximately 25 cm long, 18 cm wide, and 10 cm high (10 × 7 × 4 in.) will work well as a dust bath vesicle. Covered containers sold specifically for chinchilla dust bathing are becoming popular, but, again, these containers should be removed after each bath. Dust should be filled to a depth of approximately an inch. Cages can be covered during dust baths to reduce the possibility of caretakers' allergic reaction and to protect furnishings from dust. Removing the dustbin after the bath will help keep dust free of dirt and feces.[6]

Chinchillas generally require dust baths twice per week. Hot and humid weather can increase this requisite, and increased need can be determined by the appearance of the coat: greasy, damp, or sticking fur indicates the need for a dust bath. Conversely, dust baths can also dry the skin, and flaky skin or increased scratching are indications that the chinchilla is spending too much time dust bathing.

Reproductive behavior

Females are larger than males (up to 800 and 600 g respectively or 1.8 and 1.3 lbs.), but sex is most easily determined by evaluating anogenital distance. Females have a prominent urinary papilla which may be confused with the male's penis, particularly since the vaginal orifice is difficult to distinguish in the absence of estrus. However, the anus is immediately caudal to the vulva, whereas the penis is separated from the anus by a short (approximately 12 mm or 0.5 in.) stretch of bare skin.[6]

Females are relatively feisty and will not accept the male other than during estrus. In anoestrus for at least 5 months of the year, females living in the Northern Hemisphere are seasonally polyestrus between November and May and experience estrus once every 30–50 days if not pregnant.[6,36–38]

Courtship and copulation

A courting male will follow the female about on his hind legs, sniff her anogenital area, and gently nibble the fur about her head and neck. Unless the female resists his investigation, the male will mount the female *a posteriori* within a minute or so of initial investigation, clasping his forelegs around her sides just anterior to her pelvis. After a series of preliminary pelvic thrusts that serve as eliciting stimuli, the female will extend her hind legs and elevate her pelvis to expose the perineum.[36] Females will occasionally begin to hop rapidly and vigorously upon intromission; the male will generally retain his clasp and hop with her; the female will eventually come to rest and assume the coital posture long enough for the male to complete ejaculation. Copulation is completed with multiple intromissions lasting approximately 5 seconds each, and multiple ejaculations with ejaculatory intromissions lasting 8–10 seconds each.[11,36]

Non-receptive females may resist mounting or may actually aggress toward the male with the usual bipedal stance with urine squirt. Bignami and Beach[36] describe behavior in which the female leaps in the air and ejects a stream of urine mid-air, or leaps in the air and strikes the male with her hind feet, sometimes knocking him off his feet.[36] This occasionally discourages the male.

Male chinchillas produce a copulatory plug that lodges in the female's vagina after successful intromission and ejaculation. The plug is formed of gland secretions that gel when released,[39] and is usually dislodged from the female with normal activity several hours after mating.

Gestation is 105–118 days, averaging 111 days. This reproductive strategy requires less energy than shorter gestation[5] and is well suited to the chinchilla's native diet. The chinchilla placenta has a number of distinctive features that allow for an increase in the total exchange area and that help support the larger fetus at the end of gestation.[5] Wild chinchillas usually produce two litters a season. Although there may be up to six offspring—referred to as kits—litters include one or two kits each on average. Healthy domestic newborn kits generally weigh about 40–50 g (1.4–1.8 oz). As mentioned previously, kits are precocial, emerging fully furred with eyes open. They are able to walk within an hour after birth.

Parental behavior and neonatal development

Female chinchillas nurse their young for approximately 6–8 weeks; kit survival requires a minimum suckling period of 25 days.[11] The dam has three pairs of mammae, two thoracic pairs, and one inguinal pair,[39] and the coat is sparse around mammae during lactation. Kits often lie on their backs while suckling,[40] and dams stand or sit while nursing. Kits begin to take solid foods at about 1 week of age, and Quesenberry recommends that food bowls be large enough to accommodate the entire litter simultaneously to minimize fighting.[6] Older reports have indicated that dams will feed their young with small pieces of food, but this behavior may be rare in captivity. Instead, dams feed themselves, and offspring engage in opportunistic foraging (T. Wesorick, *pers. comm.*).

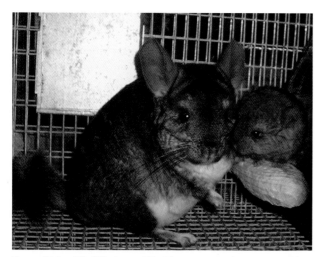

Figure 13.2   Chinchilla dam and kit. (Photo courtesy of Tracy Wesorick.)

Figure 13.2 shows a dam standing close by her kit. Both sexes make excellent and relatively tolerant parents, and for the most part the only concern regarding continued pair housing after parturition is the impregnation of the mother; female chinchillas often come into estrus within 12–24 hours of parturition. Females generally tolerate the male's presence well, and males often assist in cleansing the kits after birth. Both parents engage in kit grooming and play as the young develop, and family units often sleep huddled as a group. Adults discipline the young with a chirping or grunting vocalization if the kit pesters while the adult is sleeping or eating, but squabbles as might occur between adults under similar circumstances, involving biting or fur-pulling, are rare.

Kits are active and curious. Their play includes energetic bouncing, hopping, vertical leaping, twisting, and racing (T. Wesorick, *pers. comm.*). Although there have been no specific studies evaluating social development in kits, it has been observed that early interaction with caregivers facilitates acceptance of people. These observations are supported by an extensive literature confirming the existence of behaviorally sensitive developmental periods in a variety of species (e.g., see Ref. [41] for a discussion). Calm handling and encouragement to approach and take a small stalk of hay should begin as early as possible to help avoid later fear responses based in neophobia. The behavior of the dam—or sire if present—appears to have an influence on kit behavior; if the goal is to produce kits that interact readily and fearlessly with people, care should be taken to teach the mother to accept the presence of people. This acceptance should include people's hands reaching into the cage and people removing her from the cage and handling her. Less interactive adult chinchillas and those that appear anxious in the presence of their caregivers can be taught to accept and approach people through systematic reinforcement of movement toward people. To be most beneficial, lessons should begin with the parents before littering.

For the most part, unless kits are reared in close proximity to adults that are anxious or retreat from human handling, kits appear more tolerant of caregiver interaction than do other rodents' young such as ambulatory rat pups. Due to their inquisitive nature, kits will often approach their caregivers to sniff or nibble on a finger or hand. They might scramble up the sleeve of an extended arm or hop out the open door of the cage. Care should be taken to insure that these interactions with people are enjoyable for the animal. Kits should always be handled with calm, deliberate actions. Sudden movements, noises, the appearance of other animals, or any other potentially frightening situation should be avoided when kits are in the presence of people. The approach and presence of a person should predict fun and food.

Social behavior

There have been no published ethological studies categorizing chinchilla social behavior and development, although it is known that chinchillas coexist in large colonies. Anecdotal observations indicate that chinchillas recognize a hierarchal social structure, and young chinchillas in particular may signal deference to older social members. Such signals include high-pitched vocalizations that captive-bred young have also been heard to direct toward caregivers.

Chinchillas are also reported to engage in intraspecific mounting behavior, referred to by pet owners as "dominance mounting." This behavior appears more prevalent in situations of poor environmental enrichment and is similar in topography to copulatory mounting, but is performed in the absence of female estrus and can occur between any sex pair combination. Chinchillas that have been subject to mounting tend to avoid areas of conflict, such as preferred feeding or exercise locations, when in the presence of the mounting animal. Dominance is a poorly understood and often misinterpreted[42–44] construct that lends itself to a great deal of inappropriate behavioral counseling regarding companion animal intra- and inter-specific interactions.[45] However, the anecdotal observations of dominant and subordinate behavior in chinchillas are supported to a degree by patterns of behavior of other social burrowing herbivores for which there have been extensive ethological observations and validated analyses (e.g., see Ref. [46]).

Ingestive behavior

The chinchilla is primarily nocturnal and consumes the majority of its food between dusk and dawn.[47] However, they also display crepuscular behavior and in the wild will sometimes emerge at dusk and dawn not only to feed but to bask in the sun. They eat while sitting up on their hind limbs and grasping the food in their forepaws (see Figure 13.3).

Chinchillas require extensive intake of high-fiber, relatively low-nutrition feed. These needs are best met by

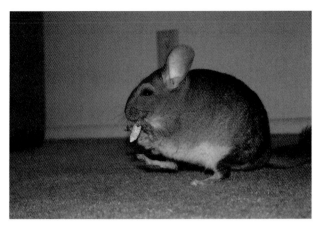

Figure 13.3 Typical posture of the chinchilla while eating. (Photo courtesy of Sylvia Gillespie, RVT.)

providing grass hay *ad libitum* and supplementing with a small amount (i.e., one to two tablespoons) of commercial chinchilla pellet diet. Commercial diets are relatively low in protein and fat and high in fiber. Quesenberry et al.[6] provide a breakdown of the accepted nutritional balance for chinchilla pellets: 16–20% protein, 2–5% fat, and 15–35% bulk fiber. It is important to note that reliance on the pelleted diet to the limitation of roughage such as grass hays has been implicated in the etiology of digestive disorders such as constipation and diarrhea in chinchillas.[12,48] Many chinchilla pet-care sources suggest feeding timothy as the primary grass source, although alfalfa has been suggested as well.[12] Alfalfa contains higher percentages of protein and calcium than other grasses.

Certain treats should be avoided, particularly those that contain high levels of rapidly fermentable starch or sugar such as corn, peas, cabbage, and broccoli,[12] and those with high levels of fat such as nuts. Appropriate treats, including sunflower seeds, fruit pieces, raisins, and grains should be limited to one or two per day. In addition, any changes in diet must be introduced gradually to allow the animal's digestive system to adjust to the change.[6] Gastric tympany has been associated with sudden changes in diet or the addition of fresh greens and fruit.[10]

Water should be freely available. Quesenberry et al.[6] suggest the use of automatic water devices, and this idea is supported by many chinchilla caregivers (T. Wesorick, *pers. comm.*). Watering bottles are difficult to adjust properly and often spill or drain improperly. Plastic is always a poor choice because it will be chewed.

Husbandry and care of chinchillas

The status of the wild *Chinchilla lanigera* is guarded at best, and captivity maximizes the likelihood of the continued existence of the species. However, an understanding and appreciation of the natural behavior of the chinchilla is essential for its well-being in the captive state (see Ref. [49]

for a general review of captivity stress as it relates to natural behavior).

Equally important as providing species-relevant care and environmental necessities is the interpretation of welfare-related communication by any captive animal. Individuals responsible for the care of chinchillas should be familiar with the social and other predispositions of chinchillas, as well as their vocal and physical communications, so as to identify the state and needs of their captive chinchillas. The reader is encouraged to refer to the chapter on welfare (Chapter 20) for more information.

Housing

Group housing

Because the chinchilla is a social animal, group housing should be considered for animals in captivity. They generally do well when housed in same-sex pairs, or as polygamous units that include one male and two or more females.[6] Many chinchilla breeders and pet owners recommend that any animal being introduced to resident animals be housed separately but in close proximity to the resident for one night to two weeks. Although there are no studies defining introduction protocol, general recommendations for introduction include:

- Use new cages. Used cages should be thoroughly cleansed and treated with a scent-reduction oxidizing agent to reduce territoriality by resident chinchillas.
- Place separate cages in the same vicinity, or place a small cage inside a larger cage. The large cage should not be the resident chinchilla's cage.
- Arrange initial greetings in a neutral territory with extensive space, such as a room. The area should include a dust bath.
- It should be apparent that animals are tolerant of each other in a spacious area before same-cage introductions are begun.
- Introduce females to males, and the introductions should be in the male's cage.

Females are the more aggressive of the sexes and may aggress toward members of either sex. This predisposition seems to be exacerbated by captivity; conflicts that extend beyond growling and teeth chattering are rarely seen in the wild.[11] This indicates that group housing should be large enough to allow animals to avoid each other when desired and should include at least as many perching and hiding areas as there are chinchillas.

Housing construction

Proper chinchilla housing should be large enough to allow the animals freedom of movement and provide opportunities to bound and climb. Quesenberry et al.[6] report that one author suggested that cage size be no smaller than

2 × 2 × 1 m (6.6 × 6.6 × 3.3 ft), and be equipped with multiple levels. It should also be considered that the chinchilla is a prey animal and is easily frightened by changes in its environment and open space. Cages should be spacious, but should also be equipped both with levels and ledges; levels should include hiding places that can be created of 10–12 cm diameter polyvinyl chloride (PVC) or clay pipe sections.[6,34] In addition, in consideration of the fact that one of the chinchilla's natural predators is the owl, cages should be elevated as high as is practical so that the animals are not in a position to be continually approached from above and unduly stressed. Overhead fans should also be avoided.

To avoid damage from chewing and facilitate easy cleaning and maximum sanitation, wood should not be used as a surface construction material. Glass and plastic are also less than ideal because they contribute to increases in humidity, and plastic may be chewed. Half-inch wire mesh floors are acceptable and will facilitate cleaning, but their use may interfere with ingestion of cecotropes. Although there have been no studies specifically evaluating flooring for cecotrophic species, experts in care of rabbits suggest that bases drilled with ¼ holes spaced 1 to 1½ in. apart are optimal. This set-up addresses both cecotroph ingestion and cleanliness (EA McBride, University of Southampton, *pers. comm.*). Litter may be spread on solid or perforated floors and can be made of hay, straw, or kiln-dried wood shavings; pine or cedar can be toxic and/or release phenols and must not be used. Cat litter may be ingested and should be avoided.

Chinchillas are nocturnal so housing should be on a normal 12-hour light/dark schedule, but their room should be quiet and kept free of psittacines or other large birds and carnivorous pets such as cats and dogs.

Enrichment

Like all animals in captivity, chinchillas have been found to exhibit environmentally induced stress responses, including stereotypical behavior such as spinning and self-mutilation such as fur-chewing. Some studies have suggested that increased endocrine activity related to non-specific stressors may be associated with the fur-chewing behavior.[50,51] Environmental stress occurs when an animal is not able to act in accordance with its motivational state.[52] Enrichment of captive animals' environment reduces indications of stress,[53,54] although it may not eliminate it; studies indicate that stereotypies and other stress behaviors sometimes remain even after welfare concerns have been addressed.[55–57] Regardless of the specific etiology of stress behavior, it is likely that enrichment of the captive chinchilla's habitat can reduce the risk of the development of such behavior.

Enrichment for any species, however, must be designed and implemented according to the species' specific environmental needs as inferred from both their natural habitat and their interactions with that habitat. Chinchillas are inquisitive and interactive with their environments. Their native environment provides them extensive opportunities to masticate, and dental growth comparisons and observations that they consume their food more slowly than other animals such as rabbits and guinea pigs[6] combine to indicate that they chew almost continuously. They commonly approach and chew novel stimuli placed in their home context. Therefore, it follows that their environment should be set up to provide them with the opportunity to interact with a variety of objects and toys designed for chewing.

In addition to satisfying their urge to chew, a variety of chew "toys" or chew "sticks" will assist the chinchilla in maintaining its teeth in a healthy state. Various sources (e.g., Refs [6, 12]) list items that are acceptable as dental chews, including cholla cactus wood chews, mineral and pumice stones, and cuttlebones. Cuttlebones can serve both as dental chews and calcium supplements. In addition to specific chews, chinchillas will benefit from access to wood branches. Most woods are safe, but one source indicates that the use of products from some tree species may be problematic.[58] For instance, although the wood of the *Prunus* genus stone-bearing fruit trees (plum, apricot, peach, etc.) is generally safe, many species produce cyanogenetic glycosides in their seeds and leaves. The leaves of some conifers, as well as those of mahogany trees may also be a problem. All yew plants are considered toxic, so use of wood from the *Taxus* sp. should be avoided. Walnut shavings induce lethargy in some laboratory animals, so should be avoided for chinchillas. The wood from many aromatic plants contain enzyme-inducing chemicals that may lead to rapid breakdown of pharmaceuticals used for therapy and can be a source of gastrointestinal irritation and diarrhea. Safe woods include bamboo, apple, pear, poplar, willow, aspen, ash, birch, elm, sycamore and dogwood, and grape vines. Any and all woods treated with insecticides, fungicides, or preservatives must be avoided.

Consideration of individual temperament

Although environmental enrichment should be of primary consideration in the care of a chinchilla or any animal in captivity, it is also important that the environment fit the specific animal housed within it. Some animals, particularly those that have been acquired from rescues, may have had little experience with enriched and changing environments. Change may be stressful for these animals. Properly socialized and handled chinchillas can be expected to gather at access doors upon the approach of caregivers—some even rattle available toys or feed bins with their teeth in their excitement—and if an animal does not approach, or retreats upon the approach of a caregiver, it should be assumed that this animal is experiencing stress of some kind. Although physical disorders such as illness or pain can contribute to reticence, if the animal is healthy but still generally anxious or prone to increasing distance from people rather than closing it, care should be taken to actively help such animals adjust to their environment. Change and handling should be kept to a minimum and approach behavior should be taught through positive reinforcement as outlined later in the section, "Retrieving chinchillas from their cages".

Play outside the cage

Chinchillas that are confident and accept and solicit interaction with their caregivers can benefit from supervised excursions outside of their cages. The area must be secure and should be indoors. Chinchillas should never be allowed out of their cage unattended, and companion animals such as cats and dogs must not be allowed access to them.

Mastication is natural and should be expected from a chinchilla whether it's secure in its cage or secure out of its cage. There are no published efficacy studies evaluating interventions designed to redirect or inhibit chewing behavior in chinchillas, but those that have been undertaken in rabbits (JL Sobie, unpublished data) indicate that behavior modification is ineffective and continuous management is necessary. Furniture, baseboards, and other relatively permanent objects should be protected with cardboard (obviously a short-term solution), enclosed with ½ in. wire mesh or, if made of a safe wood or other material, abandoned to the chinchilla's will. Wires, plants, and other small objects must be removed completely.

Chinchillas are very active and agile. They can leap almost 2 m (about 6 ft) in the air, and often ricochet off walls. They have been known to ascend the height of a refrigerator simply by propelling themselves against one side of the refrigerator to an adjacent wall and back until they reached the top. However, their bones are slender and relatively brittle, and it is not uncommon for them to fracture rear limbs, particularly the tibia. Donnelly[10] cautions that surgical repair, intramedullary fixation, and even external fixation are difficult, and fractures may result in amputation of the leg. Therefore, it's important that the environment be suitable and void of objects that could provide the chinchilla with the means to attain a height that could result in injury from a fall.

Handling

The preferred method of lifting and handling a chinchilla is to scoop it and lift it with one hand under its abdomen while securing it with the other hand at the base of its tail.[6,34] A frightened animal might be calmed by allowing it to hide its face in the crook of the handler's arm or by wrapping it loosely in a towel to obscure its vision. However, frightened animals should not be handled unless absolutely necessary. Handling of frightened animals can result in fur-slip, a defense mechanism whereby patches of fur are released during restraint. Simply handling an anxious animal without incorporating a desensitization and/or counterconditioning protocol explicitly designed to ameliorate fear and increase acceptance behavior should not be expected to habituate the animal to further handling. It is far more likely that handling will exacerbate the animal's fear and possibly condition avoidance behavior in response to the approach of people. A counterconditioning protocol is described later and more information about desensitization and counterconditioning can be found in the chapter on learning (Chapter 18).

Retrieving chinchillas from their cages

Retrieving chinchillas from large, multileveled cages can be difficult. Cage access doors should be situated so that animals can easily be retrieved without undue reaching and grabbing; chasing a chinchilla about its habitat with an extended arm is very stressful for the animal and can easily contribute to handling difficulties and stress-related physical disorders. Cage doors should be large enough to allow both a comfortable reach into the cage and access to all cage areas to facilitate cleaning as well as to remove animals when desired.

Retrieval stress can be avoided completely through conditioning by reinforcement of approach behavior and calm acceptance of handling. Most chinchillas are inquisitive and will approach a still hand; caregivers need only to say "yes" (or "good," choose a word and use it consistently) when the chinchilla approaches and then provide the chinchilla with a piece of hay or a food pellet to begin conditioning of confident approach and retrieval behavior. Soon the chinchilla will be rushing into the open hand of the caregiver. Some chinchillas are more reserved, and may initially be reticent to approach the treat at all. In these cases, the animal should first be pre-conditioned to accept the treat. In order to do this, a small bowl should be placed within tossing distance of the cage door; over the period of a few days, the cage should be periodically approached, the word "yes" spoken, and a treat tossed into the bowl. When the animal approaches the bowl upon hearing "yes," pre-conditioning has occurred and the handler can proceed to the next step of conditioning, teaching the animal to approach and move over the caregiver's extended, flat palm through a series of small steps that progressively bring the animal closer to the hand. At first, a simple shift of attention by the animal to the hand or a step or hop toward the palm should be reinforced with "yes" and a pellet; next, two steps might be required before marking the desired approach behavior with "yes" and offering a food pellet or, very occasionally, a treat. With time and patience, caregivers can teach even inhibited or fearful chinchillas to step onto their hand. Every interaction, including mealtime, should progress so that approach behavior is reinforced with "yes" and food.

Nips and bites

Chinchillas tend to investigate their surroundings orally, and a chinchilla can be expected to nibble on any person transporting it. Nibbling should not be disciplined in any way and instead should be anticipated and redirected to a suitable object such as a stalk of hay. Frightened chinchillas may resort to biting, but biting must be addressed through proper conditioning and stress reduction rather than discipline of any sort.

Counterconditioning avoidance or fear reactions

Avoidance or escape-directed responses that are not related to guarding food or chew items should be interpreted as expressions of fear or anxiety. Fear of common procedures such as handling must be counterconditioned. Counterconditioning protocols associate feared stimuli and experiences with food or preferred activities to change the predictive qualities of the stimuli from threat to pleasure. At the same time, responses that indicate a reduction in fear such as approach or acquisition of food can be operantly reinforced.

Handling fear can best be counterconditioned by first conditioning hand-approach behavior as described earlier in the section on, "Retrieving chinchillas from the cage." As the chinchilla's approach behavior increases, actual handling can be introduced gradually. The first steps in conditioning a chinchilla to accept handling, entail a simple touch of the handler's fingers at the base of the tail, a "yes," and delivery of a pellet. Actual holding of the tail base can then gradually be reintroduced. Once the animal stands relatively quietly while awaiting the "yes" and a treat when its tail is held, it can be introduced to having a hand placed beneath it while having its tail held, and then to being lifted by its abdomen for scant seconds. Each successful trial wherein the chinchilla is released and fed before attempting to escape provides a building block for the next trial.

Counterconditioning steps are initially time consuming, but they are worth it when measured in ease of handling and reductions in stress-related physical disorders and fur-slip. Readers can learn more about modifying animal behavior by reading Chapter 18, *From Parrots to Pigs to Pythons: Universal Principles and Procedures of Learning.*

References

1. Jiménez JE. The extirpation and current status of wild chinchillas (*Chinchilla lanigera* and *C. brevicaudata*). *Biol Conserv* 1996;77:1–6.
2. Deane A. A summary of transect data for endangered *Chinchilla lanigera*. *Field notes*. Available at: www.wildchinchillas.org/. Accessed Sep 13, 2009.
3. Jiménez JE. Conservation of the last wild chinchilla (*Chinchilla lanigera*) archipelago: A metapopulation approach. *Vida Silvestre Neotropical* 1995;4:89–97.
4. Deane A. Small mammal tracks: Field observations in north-central Chile. *Field notes*. Available at: www.wildchinchillas.org/. Accessed Sep 13, 2009.
5. Rodrigues RF, Carter AM, Ambrosio CE, dos Santos TC, Miglino MA. The subplacenta of the red-rumped agouti (*Dasyprocta leporina L*). *Reprod Biol Endocrinol* 2006. Available at: http://www.rbej.com/content/4/1/31. Accessed Sep 13, 2009.
6. Quesenberry KE, Donnelly TM, Hillyer EV. Biology, husbandry, and clinical techniques of Guinea pigs and chinchillas. In: Quesenberry KE, Carpenter JW, eds. *Ferrets, Rabbits and Rodents: Clinical Medicine and Surgery*. 2nd ed. St. Louis, MO: Saunders. 2003;232–244.
7. Deane A. Use of line-intercept methods to quantify vegetation characteristics of endangered long-tailed chinchillas (*Chinchilla lanigera*). *Field notes*. Available at: www.wildchinchillas.org/. Accessed Sep 13, 2009.
8. Hall FG. Minimal utilizable oxygen and the oxygen dissociation curve of blood of rodents. *J Appl Physiol* 1966;21:375–378.
9. Ostojic H, Cifuentes V, Monge C. Hemoglobin affinity in Andean rodents. *Biol Res* 2002;35:27–30.
10. Donnelly TM. Disease problems of chinchillas. In: Quesenberry KE, Carpenter JW, eds. *Ferrets, Rabbits and Rodents: Clinical Medicine and Surgery*. 2nd ed. St. Louis, MO: Saunders, 2003;255–263.
11. Spotorno AE, Zuleta CA, Valladares JP, Deane AL, Jiménez JE. *Chinchilla laniger. Mammalian Species No. 758*. No publication location given: American Society of Mammalogists, 2004;1–9.
12. Alderton D. *Chinchillas*. Neptune City, NJ: T.F.H Publications, 2007.
13. Kopack H. *Chinchilla chinchilla*. Available at: http://animaldiversity.ummz.umich.edu/site/accounts/information/Chinchilla_chinchilla.html. Accessed Sep 13, 2009.
14. Ebenspergera LA, Blumstein DT, Sociality in New World hystricognath rodents is linked to predators and burrow digging. *Behav Ecol* 2006;17:410–417.
15. Crawley JN. *What's Wrong with my Mouse? Behavioral Phenotyping of Transgenic and Knockout Mice*. New York, NY: Wiley-Liss, 2000.
16. Doty RL. Odor-guided behavior in mammals. *Experientia* 1986;42:257–271.
17. Farbman AI. The cellular basis of olfaction. *Endeavour* 1994;18:2–8.
18. Johnson BA, Leon M. Spatial coding in the olfactory bulb: The role of early experience. In: Blass EM, ed. *Developmental Psychobiology, Developmental Neurobiology and Behavioral Ecology: Mechanisms and Early Principals*. New York: Kluwer Academic/Plenum Publishers, 2001;53–80.
19. Leon M, Johnson BA, Olfactory coding in the mammalian olfactory bulb. *Brain Res Rev* 2003;42:23–32.
20. Bowe CA, Miller JD, Green L. Qualities and locations of stimuli and responses affecting discrimination learning of chinchillas (*Chinchilla laniger*) and pigeons (*Columba livid*). *J Comp Psychol* 1987;101(2):132–138.
21. Heffner RS, Heffner HE. Behavioral hearing range of the chinchilla. *Hear Res* 1991;52:13–16.
22. Ohlemiller KK, Jones LB, Heidbreder AF, Clark WW, Miller JD. Voicing judgements by chinchillas trained with a reward paradigm. *Behav Brain Res* 1999;100:185–195.
23. Heffner RS, Koay G, Heffner HE. Sound localization in chinchillas, III: Effect of pinna removal. *Hear Res* 1996;99:13–21.
24. Shofner WP, Yost WA, Whitmer WM. Pitch perception in chinchillas (*Chinchilla laniger*): Stimulus generalization using rippled noise. *J Comp Psychol* 2007;121:428–439.
25. Luz GA. Conditioning the chinchilla to make avoidance responses to novel sounds. *J Comp Physiol Psychol* 1969;68:348–354.
26. Harrison JM, Irving R. Visual and nonvisual auditory systems in mammals. Anatomical evidence indicates two kinds of auditory pathways and suggests two kinds of hearing in mammals. *Science* 1966;154:738–743.
27. Peiffer RL, Johnson PT. Clinical ocular findings in a colony of chinchillas (*Chinchilla laniger*). *Lab Anim* 1980;14:331–335.

28. Walker EP. *Mammals of the World.* 3rd ed. Baltimore, MD: Johns Hopkins University Press, 1968.

29. Dyer RS, Hammond MA, Weldon DA, Booker TC. Influence of enucleation upon two-way avoidance behavior of rats, hamsters, chinchillas and BALB/cJ mice. *Physiol Behav* 1975;14:211–216.

30. Wilcox HN. Histology of the skin and hair of the adult chinchilla. *Anat Rec* 1950;108:385–397.

31. Sparks DL. Translation of sensory signals into commands for control of saccadic eye movements: Role of primate superior colliculus. *Physiol Rev* 1986;66:118–171.

32. Eisenberg JF. The function and motivational basis of hystricomorph vocalizations. *Symp Zool Soc London* 1974;34:211–247.

33. Morris D. *The Mammals: A Guide to the Living Species.* New York and Evanston: Harper & Row Publishers, 1965.

34. Ritchey L, Cogswell EC, Beeman R. *The Joy of Chinchillas.* Menlo Park, CA: Authors, 2004.

35. Stern JJ, Merari A. The bathing behavior of the chinchilla: Effects of deprivation. *Psychon Sci* 1969;14(3):115.

36. Bignami G, Beach FA. Mating behavior in the chinchilla. *Anim Behav* 1968;16:45–53.

37. Weir BJ. Aspects of reproduction in the chinchilla. *J Reprod Fertil* 1966;12:410–411.

38. Weir BJ. The induction of ovulation and oestrous in the chinchilla. *J Reprod Ferti* 1973;33:61–68.

39. Weir BJ. Reproductive characteristic of hystricomorph rodents. *Symp Zool Soc London* 1974;34:265–301.

40. Weir BJ. Chinchilla. In: Hafez ESE, ed. *Reproduction and Breeding Techniques for Laboratory Animals.* Philadelphia: Lea & Febiger, 1970;209–223.

41. Bateson P. How do sensitive periods arise and what are they for? *Anim Behav* 1979;27:470–486.

42. Bernstein IS. Dominance: The baby and the bathwater. *Behav Brain Sci* 1981;4:419–457.

43. Rowell TE. The concept of social dominance. *Behav Biol* 1974;11:131–151.

44. Van Hooff J, Wensing J. Dominance and its behavioral measures in a captive wolf pack. In: Frank H, ed. *Man and Wolf: Advances, Issues and Problems in Captive Wolf Research.* Dordrecht, Netherlands: Dr. W. Junk Publishers, 1987:219–252.

45. Friedman SG, Brinker B. The struggle for dominance: Fact or fiction? A bird's eye view. *Orig Flying Mach*, 2001;6:17–20.

46. Adams N, Boice R. A longitudinal study of dominance in an outdoor colony of domestic rats. *J Comp Psychol* 1983;97:24–33.

47. Wolf P, Schröder A, Wenger A, Kamphues J. The nutrition of the chinchilla as a companion animal—basic data, influences and dependences. *J Anim Physiol Anim Nutr* 2003;87:129–133.

48. Cousens PJ. The chinchilla in veterinary practice. *J Sm Anim Pract* 1963;4:199–205.

49. Jordan B. Science-based assessment of animal welfare: Wild and captive animals. *Rev Sci Tech* 2005;24(2):515–528.

50. Tisljar M, Janić D, Grabarević Z et al. Stress-induced Cushing's syndrome in fur-chewing chinchillas. *Acta Vet Hung* 2002;50(2):133–142.

51. Vanjonack WJ, Johnson HD. Relationship of thyroid and adrenal function to "fur-chewing" in the chinchilla. *Comp Biochem Physio A Comp Physiol* 1973;45(1):115–120.

52. Jensen P, Toates FM. Stress as a state of motivational systems. *Appl Anim Behav Sci* 1997;54:235–343.

53. Morgan KN, Tromborg CT. Sources of stress in captivity. *Appl Anim Behav Sci* 2007;102(3–4):262–302.

54. Cooper JJ, Mason GJ. The identification of abnormal behaviour and behavioural problems in stabled horses and their relationship to horse welfare: A comparative review. *Equine Vet J Suppl* 1998;(27):5–9.

55. Cooper JJ, Nicol CJ. Stereotypic behaviour in wild caught and laboratory bred bank voles, *Clethrionomys glareolus. Anim Welf* 1996;5:245–257.

56. Gillham SR, Dodman NH, Shuster L et al. The effect of diet on cribbing behaviour and plasma beta-endorphin in horses. *Appl Anim Behav Sci* 1994; 41:147–153.

57. Mason GJ. Stereotypies and suffering. *Behav Proc.* 1991;25:103–111.

14

Prairie dogs

Debra M. Shier

Natural history

Prairie dogs (*Cynomys* spp.) were originally described by Lewis and Clark in 1804.[1] Prairie dogs are diurnal colonial burrowing mammals that live throughout the western grasslands of North America. They were named prairie "dogs" because their frequent bark vocalization reminded early settlers of a domestic dog's bark.[2,3] In reality, *prairie dogs* are rodents that belong to the squirrel family *Sciuridae*, which also includes flying squirrels, chipmunks, tree squirrels, marmots, and ground squirrels. Prairie dogs are most closely related to ground squirrels and are thought to have diverged from ground squirrels 2–3 million years ago.[4] They are larger bodied than ground squirrels, have larger teeth with higher crowns, and broader skulls.[5]

Taxonomists currently recognize five species of prairie dogs in the genus *Cynomys*.[5,6] Adults of all species are pear shaped weighing 600–1500 g (2–3 pounds), have brown fur, stand about 30–35 cm (12–14 in.) tall, and typically live in large colonies. Their front legs are short and muscular for digging out burrows. Each forefoot has four toes with long claws and a half thumb-like inner toe. The hind feet have five toes with short claws. Morphological features that distinguish the species are the length and color of hairs at the distal end of the tail, presence of a black or brown line above each eye, and vocalization characteristics. Because the geographic range overlap of the five species is minimal, locality alone is diagnostic for identification.[7]

Mammalogists recognize two subgroups within the genus *Cynomys*.[6] The black-tailed subgroup consists of the Mexican (*C. mexicanus*) and black-tailed (*C. ludovicianus*) prairie dogs. These species have long (7–10 cm or 2.7–4 in.) black-tipped tails, live at low elevations (700–2200 m or 2300–7200 ft above sea level) in low growing vegetation and do not hibernate. The white-tailed group contains Gunnison's (*C. gunnisoni*), Utah (*C. parvidens*), and white-tailed prairie dogs (*C. leucurus*). These animals have short

(3–7 cm or 1.2–2.8 in.) white or gray-tipped tails, live at high elevations (1500–3000 m or 4900–9800 ft above sea level) with some medium to tall shrubs and hibernate for an average of 4 months.

Prairie dogs were once found throughout the prairies and historic estimates put their numbers between 3 and 5 billion in the early 1900s. Since that time their numbers and distribution in the wild have declined by an estimated 98% due to conservation of grasslands for agriculture, hunting, poisoning, and sylvatic plague. The capture for the exotic pet trade also reduces the numbers of prairie dogs in the wild, but currently has much smaller impacts on the decline of the species. Today, all five species of prairie dogs are rare and of conservation concern.[8] The two species that have been listed are Mexican prairie dogs (endangered) and Utah prairie dogs (threatened). Gunnison's prairie dog is currently a candidate for listing. A petition was submitted to list white-tailed prairie dogs and is pending. The United States Fish and Wildlife Service concluded in 2000 that the black-tailed prairie dog warranted listing as threatened but that listing was precluded due to the agency's logistic constraints. In 2004 that listing was reversed and the protection for black-tailed prairie dogs remains uncertain.

Of the five species, the black-tailed prairie dog is the most conspicuous, the most common, and the most likely to be found in zoos or as pets.[7] Thus, the remainder of this chapter refers specifically to the behavior and habits of the black-tailed prairie dog.

Black-tailed prairie dogs are collected from the wild for the exotic pet trade in the United States, Canada, Europe, and Japan. If captured when young, prairie dogs make excellent pets. With lots of love and gentle handling, they seem to "imprint" on their human owners. They are easily house-trained and respond with a jump-yip call when the owner sneezes or returns from a short absence (*pers. obs.*).[9] They like to be groomed by their owners and will groom in return. Some even sleep with their owners and will come when called by name.

To capture wild pups, newly emergent young are removed from their underground burrows each spring at first emergence with a large vacuum truck, water trapping truck, or wire mesh live traps. Prairie dogs are difficult to breed in captivity,[10] but it has been successful on several occasions. Removing them from the wild is a far more common method of supplying the market demand.

In 2003 several prairie dogs in captivity acquired monkey pox from a Gambian pouched rat imported from Ghana.[11] Subsequently a few humans were also infected. This led the Center for Disease Control (CDC) to institute a ban on the sale, trade, and/or transport of prairie dogs within the United States. The disease was never introduced to any wild populations. On September 8, 2008 the CDC rescinded the ban making it once again legal to capture, sell, and transport prairie dogs.[12] Although the federal ban has been lifted, several States still have their own ban on prairie dogs in place.

Prairie dogs are also very susceptible to sylvatic plague. Sylvatic plague is caused by a bacterium (*Yersinia pestis*) carried by fleas from other infected mammals[13] and is thought to have been brought to the United States at the turn of the 20th century via commercial ships from China.[13] Plague moves quickly through prairie dog colonies killing nearly 100% of the inhabitants in less than 14 days. It is rarely transferred to humans from prairie dogs because prairie dog fleas tend to be highly host-specific and therefore avoid humans.[13]

A final zoonotic disease found in prairie dogs is tularemia. Tularemia was documented in a single large captive group of prairie dogs in Texas in 2002.[14] Japan banned importation of prairie dogs in response to this event. As with any wild animal brought into captivity, there are risks associated with having a prairie dog as an exotic pet.

These incidents highlight the importance of standardizing exotic animal husbandry practices to reduce the risk of disease transfer between animals, species, and to humans from infected wild-caught animals. Because there are no regulations in place to ensure proper animal husbandry in the exotic pet trade, it is important to acquire these animals, particularly prairie dogs, from a reputable dealer.

Senses and communication

Prairie dogs have elaborate communication systems. They use everything from loud vocalizations to drumming of their feet to body posturing to produce a signal. The most well-known vocalization for a prairie dog, and the one after which it was named "dog," is the "bark." Bark vocalizations (Figure 14.1) are brief and repetitious ranging from one or two per second to as few as 10 or 20 barks per minute,[3,15,16] last from just a few seconds to over an hour and may be accompanied by tail flicking.[10,16] In general, barks are used in response to the presence of a mammalian or aerial

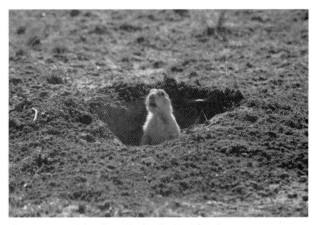

Figure 14.1 Adult male prairie dog "barking" from burrow entrance.

predator,[7] or to other prairie dogs within or between coteries which are seeking interactions that would interfere with the caller's current activity.[3] When a predator is detected, adult prairie dogs typically run to their burrow entrance and begin barking. Sonograms show that the barks produced upon the detection of a predator vary in duration, harshness, harmonics, and number of syllables.[3] Bark calls by the same individual at different times also differ. Barks to other prairie dogs appear to be a signal used to repel the other individual. For example, if two prairie dogs are interacting and a third attempts to make contact, one of the prairie dogs in the initial interaction may bark. The communicator may be foraging, gathering nest material, or engaged in any activity with which contact interaction would interfere and it barks in order to avoid further social involvement. Barks are also used between coteries as a territorial signal. When territorial boundaries are challenged, prairie dogs often bark to repel the potential intruder. Barks grouped into brief bursts are called chitters or chatter barks.[3,16] Chitter barks are most often produced when a female is signaling that she is unreceptive. For example, if a male approaches his mate and attempts to kiss, greet, or sniff her anal region and the action is not wanted, the female may run to her burrow and chitter bark.[3] If the male approaches again, or merely looks at her, she may resume barking. The "rasp" or "snarl" is a prolonged very harsh vocalization associated with fighting.[3,16] It is usually produced just before a prairie dog is about to attack. The "scream" is a clear, high pitched, and always prolonged vocalization. Most often, screams are produced by prairie dogs that are hurt, caught in live traps, when being handled, or when caught or chased by a predator. The "yip" also termed the "jump yip" or "yahoo" is the most prominent display of the species.[17] It combines a leap, arch of the back, and raising of the arms with a vocalization. Jump-yips are performed in very diverse circumstances. Some researchers describe jump-yips as an "all clear" call used after an individual is startled, participated in a territorial dispute, when it is about to emerge from the burrow, or when a predator has left the area.[17] However, jump-yip calls are also used in the presence of snakes.[18,19] Adult prairie dogs interacting with snakes are typically confrontational, often biting, kicking substrate at or otherwise harassing snakes. During these interactions, the engaged prairie dog will often give a series of jump-yip calls (*pers. obs.*) that appear to be directed to the snake and signal the interaction will persist.[18] These displays may also direct the attention of other coterie members to the snake. The "tooth chatter" is a non-vocal noise produced by repeatedly striking the incisors together.[3,16] Tooth chattering is usually produced in an agonistic context with the chattering individual oriented toward the source of trouble.

Prairie dogs also use their feet for communication. Because prairie dogs spend a great deal of their lives underground, it is not surprising that they can produce low frequency signals via foot drumming.[18] Prairie dogs shift their weight onto their front feet and pick up their back feet and repeatedly strike them on the ground to drum (Shier, unpublished data). Foot drumming produces both auditory and seismic vibrations.[20] Very little is known about prairie dog foot drumming except that it has only been documented during above-ground interactions with snakes. Prairie dogs can detect these low frequency signals with their excellent hearing. Hearing ranges in prairie dogs extend from very low frequency (4 Hz) to high frequency sound (26 kHz); they are most sensitive to low frequency sound.[21]

Unlike foot drumming which appears to be a signal specific to the presence of a snake, body posturing is common in prairie dogs and produced in many contexts. In fact, some people suggest that if you can read your prairie dogs body language, you'll know just how he or she "feels."[9] If a prairie dog approaches someone or something with a horizontal tail, it is investigating the object or individual with indecisiveness or uncertainty. If, however, a prairie dog's tail is vertical, the prairie dog is calm and approachable. For adult prairie dogs, a flicking, quivering, arched, or frizzed tail generally indicates excitement, though the type of excitement varies. Frizzed tails are usually a sign that the prairie dog is escalating toward aggression and will bite while arched tails indicate that the interaction may turn to play or aggression.[15,22]

Prairie dogs emerge from their burrows at sunrise and forage above ground most of the day. Thus, their vision is similar to other diurnal species. Prairie dogs have a plethora of cones and paucity of rod photoreceptors in their retinas (9:1 ratio).[15,22,23] In general, cones are used for color vision, while rods are more sensitive to light and allow for night vision. Therefore prairie dogs become disoriented if out of their burrow past sunset. Their eyes are located high on the sides of their skull, typical of prey species.[24] Eye placement at the sides allows for heightened peripheral vision which yields a large visual field for predator detection.[24] However, lateral eye placement also means that prairie dogs have poor depth perception.[9] This must

be considered when housing prairie dogs in captivity or treating them in a veterinary clinic. If their captive environment includes a multi-level cage, the floor of the upper levels must be continuous aside from burrow entrances to ensure that prairie dogs do not fall and injure themselves. When seen in the veterinary clinic, care must be taken to ensure that prairie dogs are not left alone on examination tables.

Finally, like most mammals, the olfactory senses are well developed in prairie dogs. They have glands in their mouth and anus that are used in intraspecific identification, social bonding, and perhaps scent sharing. The mouth corner apocrine glands appear to be well developed in Scuirids.[25] During a "kiss" greeting (Figure 14.2), the prairie dog tilts its head at a 45° or 90° angle, opens its jaws, and touches the open mouth of another prairie dog which responds in kind.[10] This is often accompanied by tail wagging and its frequently following by allogrooming.[10]

Prairie dogs also have three secretory glands located in the opening of the anus used for intraspecific identification.[22] The perianal glands look like small pinkish tubes that will protrude when the prairie dog is excited. The odor is mildly offensive and secretions are waxy in nature. During interactions, both prairie dogs assume a crouching position. One animal then turns around, everts the three perianal gland duct nipples through the anal orifice, and present them to the second animal. The second animal smells the nipples, and then the positions are reversed and the activity is repeated.[22] Males that have not been neutered will have a stronger odor (*pers. obs.*). Once altered, the smell will decrease and not be offensive. Young pups usually scent more often, but this decreases over the first year of life.

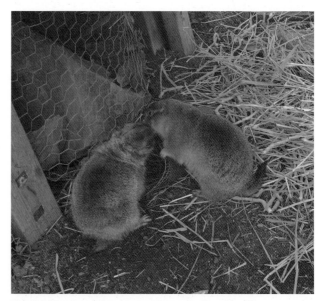

Figure 14.2 Two prairie dogs greeting each other with a "kiss."

Histochemistry indicates that black-tailed prairie dogs secrete neutral lipids and proteins from the holocrine element of their perianal glands.[26] It is possible that the lipids also serve as a carrier for more volatile apocrine secretions.[26]

Body care

Prairie dogs groom themselves and other family members (allogrooming) in order to remove ectoparasites as well as for social bonding.[7] A prairie dog's pelage is dry and odorless. Prairie dogs undergo a molt of their entire pelage twice a year with the first molt beginning in late spring and the second molt in late summer to early fall. The molt may last 2–3 weeks during which the heaviest shedding is in the first week or two and then shedding tapers off.[6,7] The summer pelage is short, sleek, and darker in color. The undercoat is dark gray. In winter the fur is fluffier and lighter in color. The skin is dry and not oily. It is not necessary to shampoo prairie dogs in captivity, but if necessary, a warm damp cloth can be used to clean their face and body pelage.

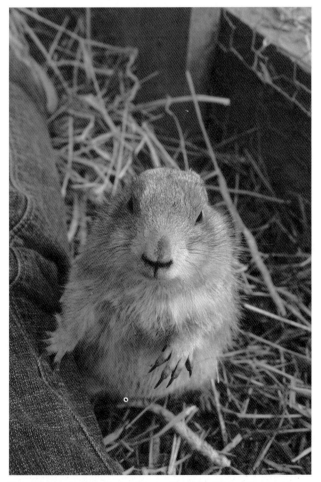

Figure 14.3 A prairie dog's nails are adapted for digging. They are long, sharp, and slightly curved.

A prairie dog's nails are adapted for digging. They are long, thick, and slightly curved (Figure 14.3). The nails on the front feet are longer than those on the back feet. In captivity, the ideal housing environment includes a space for digging. Occasional digging can help to keep the nails worn down. If the animals are being housed in an indoor cage, which is recommended in most environments, a space for digging may not be feasible. In this case, it is possible to blunt approximately 1/16 in. off the tips[9] if they become too sharp.

Prairie dog incisors also grow continually and are worn down by constant gnawing, chewing, and grinding in the wild. Thus, in captivity it is important to provide toys (wood, leather, chewing logs, cardboard) and coarse foods (hays, hard pellets) to help wear the teeth down.[9] Bird toys work well as long as they do not include pieces with high calcium content. If the diet lacks coarse foods, incisors can become overgrown. A small cuticle clipper can be used to trim off the excess incisor.

Locomotion

Prairie dogs are semifossorial rodents. They dig elaborate burrow systems which have different chambers for sleeping, mating, defecation, and urination, and a separate natal burrow for raising young.[7] They travel in and out of their burrows multiple times during the day and submerge at or around dusk, remaining underground until morning. Thus, prairie dog morphology is adapted for digging. Their primary mode of location occurs in a quadrapedal posture which allows them to run low to the ground. However, they also spend a great deal of time in a bipedal "sit" or stance, in order to forage, rest, or scan for predators (Figure 14.4). Thus, captive housing for prairie dogs must have sufficient space to allow for the animals to stand fully upright (33–38 cm or 13–15 in.; Figure 14.5) and ideal housing would also provide animals with a burrow for play and nest chamber for sleeping. For little pups, a standard

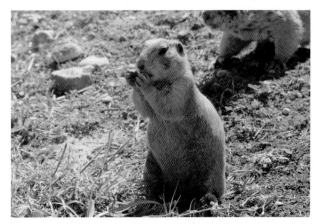

Figure 14.4 Prairie dog feeding in a bipedal stance. (Photo courtesy of M. C. Tynes, copyright 2010.)

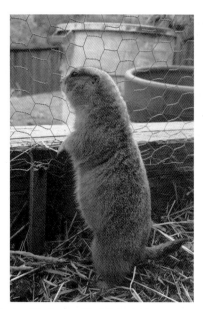

Figure 14.5 A prairie dog standing fully upright.

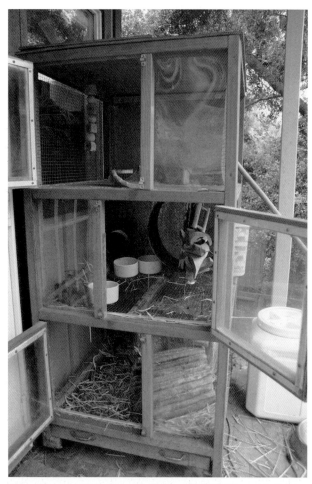

Figure 14.6 A multi-level cage to house prairie dogs. This cage includes an insulated nest box on the first level, an exercise wheel and toys on the second level, and a third level for eating and looking out. All levels are connected with enclosed PVC or wire mesh burrows.

15–20 gallon aquarium with a secure lid is ideal. The solid glass sides will keep the air warm and allow it to see its new surroundings. For adults a much larger cage is required. Two- or three-story cages are well suited for housing adult prairie dogs, especially if housing multiple adults together (Figure 14.6). More than one floor will allow animals to avoid interactions with cage mates. Due to the size of their feet, the wire spacing on the cage floor must be no larger than 1.3 by 1.3 cm (1/2 × 1/2 in.). Larger mesh can result in smaller animals getting a foot or leg caught.

Social behavior

Prairie dogs are highly social animals that live in colonies (also called towns or villages) which can span hundreds of miles. They live in territorial family groups called coteries which are usually comprised of 1–4 females and their offspring and 1 breeding adult male.[7] Coterie size can vary from 1 to as many as 29 individuals with an average of 11.[27] Large coteries sometimes contain two breeding males that are close kin (father and son or two full brothers). Occasionally, yearling males will delay dispersal and remain in the home coterie foregoing reproduction for an additional year. Females typically remain in the natal family groups their entire lives. Thus, families contain females of close kin (mothers, daughters, sisters, grandmothers, aunts, nieces, and cousins).[7]

Within the family groups, interactions are frequent and most often amicable including "kiss" greetings, play, and allogrooming[7] (Figure 14.7). These friendly interactions disappear at the onset of the breeding season during which males fight for access to females and females defend natal burrows. Once pups emerge in the late spring, sociable interactions return. Pups remain near burrow entrances at emergence, forage, and play. They are often seen initiating play with coterie adults, most often mothers and fathers.

In contrast to the interactions between family members, interactions between family groups are infrequent and usually aggressive and involve territorial disputes. During

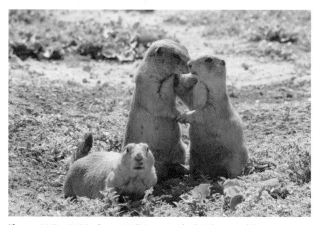

Figure 14.7 Prairie dogs socializing outside their burrow. (Photo courtesy of M. C. Tynes, copyright 2010.)

a dispute, animals will stare, chatter their teeth, chase, approach with a flared tail and if it escalates, a full out battle will ensue, usually between the breeding males of the respective coteries. Territories range in size from 0.05 to 1.0 ha (0.12–2.50 ac).[7]

Social behavior is key to the fitness of wild prairie dogs.[27] For prairie dogs, the single most important benefit of colonial living is a lower risk of predation.[7] While individual prairie dogs spend less time scanning for predators in large colonies, the collective time spent scanning by all colony members is greater than on small colonies.[7] Consequently, individuals in large colonies detect enemies more quickly and more often than do individuals that live alone or in small colonies. With such well-developed antipredator defenses, prairie dogs can live up to 5 or 6 years in the wild.[7] In a captive and thus predator-free environment, prairie dogs can live up to 10 or 12 years.[9] Colonial living also has its costs. Prairie dogs in large colonies harbor more fleas, lice, and ticks and therefore are more likely to contract diseases such as sylvatic plague.[7,13,28] But, the antipredator benefits of group living outweigh these costs.[7]

Intrasexual dominance hierarchies are present in wild prairie dogs. In both sexes, the hierarchies appear to be related to body weight. For males, the heaviest males typically initiate, and win aggressive encounters with lighter males.[7] Likewise, reproductive females with a higher body mass have been shown to dominate females with a smaller body mass in behavioral interactions.[7] These dominant interactions appear in captive prairie dogs in the context of a feeding order.[10] During food presentation tests in captivity, alpha individuals approached and began feeding first in all cases. Beta individuals showed a delayed response followed by the omega prairie dog which initiated feeding after a long delay.[10] While a feeding order may be present, aggressive contacts were not observed in adequately fed prairie dogs.

Reproductive behavior

Unlike other times of the year, the mating season usually fosters intense fighting among males and defense of natal burrows by females. This is because a female prairie dog is sexually receptive for an estimated 5 hours on only 1 day of each year.[7] To gain access to receptive females, a male must be able to out-compete other males and protect females from solicitations by other males. About 98% of matings occur underground.[7] A typical mating sequence involves a male and female submerging underground into the same burrow, emerging, and submerging again multiple times. Most of these visits underground together last for 3 minutes or less but at least one usually lasts substantially longer, around 30–40 minutes.[7] Above-ground males fight and chase other breeding males out of the coterie. Breeding males can give a unique mating call in response to the receptive female and takes several mouthfuls of grass into the burrow before submerging with her. Typically on

the first day after mating, females select a nursery burrow which she fills with nesting material and defends vigorously for the next 11 weeks of pregnancy and lactation. Most females mate with only one male during the short period of sexual receptivity, but some mate with two or three different males during this period. Multiple paternity occurs when two or more males each sire at least one offspring of a single female's litter. Between 5% and 10% of prairie dog litters show multiple paternity.[7] Most females (84%) mate with the resident breeding male in their home coterie, 11% mate with a breeding male from another coterie, and 4% mate exclusively with breeding males from other coteries.[7] The timing of matings each year determines the timing of reproductive events. Mating usually occurs from February through early March. Females are thus typically pregnant by February or through mid-April and the period of nursing offspring begins in mid-to-late March and extends into May. Juveniles first emerge from their natal burrows in mid-May through early June. Females can be reproductive as yearlings,[27] but the majority of prairie dogs of both sexes do not produce litters until year two.[7]

Maternal behavior

After copulation the average length of gestation is 33–38 days.[7] Pregnant females spend most of their days foraging during this period; they emerge early in the morning, spend the entire day foraging, and are usually among the last to submerge for the night. On the day of parturition, pregnant females typically are the last to emerge for the day (typically 4–5 hours after all other individuals) and she visits the nursery burrow for long periods 1–2 times a day for the first few days after giving birth. The number of pups born ranges from 1 to 8 per litter.[7] Pups nurse for an average of 41 days. When a female is pregnant, the first visual sign is that the fur circling the nipples becomes white (D. Shier, unpublished data). As the pregnancy progresses, the remainder of the fur will continue to change color until the entire belly is white. The female gives birth underground in the nursery burrow that she has been defending during most of her pregnancy. Pups typically weigh 3–4 g (0.1–0.14 oz) at birth, are blind, deaf, and furless. They are completely dependent upon their mother for food, warmth, and nurturing. Pups are typically translucent pink at birth (Figure 14.8). Pigmentation will color the back, head, face, and tail as the pup matures (D. Shier, unpublished data). The markings are a dark gray. The pigment designates where the darker fur will grow later in the pups development. The fur will start to show on or around day 14 and the pup will look as if he/she is covered with a fine fuzz of suede. The eyes remain closed (Figure 14.9). At 24 days, the fuzz continues coming in and begins to develop into actual fur. Their eyes will not open until 38–39 days. During the first few weeks underground, pups depend primarily on their mother's milk for nourishment, but they also eat plants brought underground by

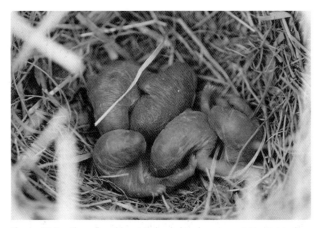

Figure 14.8 Three-day old prairie dog babies born in captivity. Prairie dogs are born furless, blind, and deaf. Note that the toe nails are present by day 3.

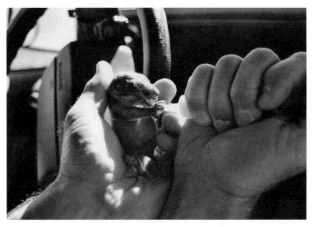

Figure 14.9 Feeding "Cherry," a 2-week old prairie dog, goat's milk from a syringe.

the mother. When the eyes open, a new freedom is experienced. The pups can see their siblings and mom and they begin to explore their surroundings. The mother will cease lactation after approximately 41 days (D. Shier, unpublished data). With sight, and weaning imminent, the babies are initiated into life above ground. The babies are now old enough to begin foraging on their own.

During the first week after emergence, pups continue to nurse and litters begin to mix.[7] In fact, coterie females will allonurse the newly emergent young of their kin.[7] Alloparenting takes many forms in prairie dogs. Adult male and female coterie members enhance juvenile survivorship by antipredator calling, allogrooming, playing with young, defending the coterie from predators, and maintaining burrows.[7] It takes a whole family group to raise and protect prairie dog pups, not just the mother.

Ingestive behavior

Prairie dogs are herbivorous rodents that occasionally ingest insects.[7] During spring and summer, they feed primarily on wheat grass, buffalo grass, scarlet globe mallow, and rabbit brush. In winter when grasses are few, they switch their diet to prickly pear, cactus, thistle, and roots. It is during this time that they use up the fat reserves they accumulated during the late summer and early fall. This cycle of weight gain and loss is normal in wild prairie dogs and weight can fluctuate from 600 g (1.3 pounds) in February to a whopping 1500 g (3.3 pounds) by the end of August! This pattern of weight change can also be seen in captive prairie dogs despite being maintained on a regular diet (*pers. obs.*). Wild prairie dogs inhabit grasslands that vary from mixed grass to short grass prairies and desert grasslands, thus they get their water requirements from vegetation and dew.

In captivity prairie dogs thrive on a diet that is low in protein (13%), low in fat, and at least 60% fiber.[9] The most well-accepted diet for captive prairie dogs consists of timothy, brome, fescue and oat hays (not alfalfa), washed and dried grass (free of fertilizers and pesticides), commercial prairie dog pellets, and water. If a prairie dog diet is not available, a pelleted chinchilla diet or a low-calcium rabbit pellet may be combined with a vegetable mix with a ratio of 1.5–2:1 calcium to phosphorous as a supplement. The hay should be offered free choice and comprise 70% of the diet while the pellets should be rationed at ¼–⅓ cup per pet daily to minimize obesity (Mark Burgess, DVM, *pers. comm.*). Obesity and bowel upsets are common among prairie dogs fed with a wide variety of items (Mark Burgess, DVM, *pers. comm.*). Avoid mixes which contain seeds and nuts, dried fruits, yogurt, cabbage, sweets (e.g., fruit, corn, baby carrots, tomatoes), and high protein items. Fresh vegetables, mostly leafy greens, are suggested and may be added to the diet (up to 10–15%) of the total food intake daily.

Neutering male prairie dogs

A male prairie dog should be neutered if he is to be an enjoyable pet.[9] If you fail to neuter the first fall of the year of his birth, the surgery should be scheduled the following late spring. During breeding season or "rut," males exhibit hormonally controlled behavior such as extreme, unpredictable biting, and increased urinating. Due to the extremely brief period of the female's fertility, the urge to compete and mate is powerful and pronounced. Males may kill each other when attempting to gain access to fertile females. Captivity is not a safe place to keep an intact male. Anyone trying to hold or restrain the unneutered male prairie dog during January through February will likely receive a serious bite. The once-friendly, sweet, and loveable prairie dog may learn aggression and even if the male is neutered after rut, the learned behavior is likely to remain.[9]

Physical changes during rut are descended testicles, engorged vasculature in the scrotum, a heavier scented musky odor, and increased dribbling of urine and/or secretions from the penis. Behavioral changes may include aggressiveness, unpredictable behavior, biting, and tooth chattering. The physical changes will subside with the arrival of spring.

Even if males are neutered, they can go through a "pseudo" rut, during which their behavior changes drastically. During the spring, summer, and fall, neutered male prairie dogs are loving, cuddly creatures, but, for a few months of every year, they can be "moody" and aggressive. Isolation is recommended during this period if housing constraints do not allow cage mates to retreat when necessary.

Common behavior problems: Diagnosis and treatment

Perhaps the biggest complaint among prairie dog owners is chewing (Figure 14.10). Prairie dogs are busy curious animals. Their instinctive need to chew, dig, and move objects can be extremely destructive. If allowed to roam freely in a room, they will inevitably find and gnaw on electrical cords, precious wood sculptures, rugs, window screens, furniture, etc. To prevent destruction of property and ensure a long healthy life for a captive prairie dog, it is important to prairie dog proof your home.[9] Check each room thoroughly for risks. Keep electrical cords off of the floor and unplug them, move cleansers to higher shelves, keep doors securely latched, and ensure that no open spaces 2 in. larger or more are available for a prairie dog to access and get trapped. It is critical for prairie dogs to be supervised at all times when allowed free play. If destructive behavior occurs during supervised activity, distraction is often an effective training tool. Calling the name of the prairie dog, disrupting the activity, and providing an acceptable toy such as a cardboard box, tube, old T-shirt, or newspaper can keep it busy and curtail the unwanted chewing.

Aggression toward non-family members is another common complaint. Prairie dogs can be highly "protective" of family members. Thus, any unfamiliar person who comes into the home may be considered a "threat." The same prairie dogs that want to cuddle into the nook of your arm and sleep with you at night may lunge and bite to protect you from your sister who is unfamiliar to them. It is important to keep prairie dogs in their home cage when entertaining visitors.

In captivity, keeping prairie dogs in small groups is ideal. If two pups are housed together the sex of the individuals does not matter. Aggression can come into play when you add another prairie dog at a later time or when a male is not neutered. If neutered, two or more adult males can be housed together without difficulty. Usually, it is recommended to house two females with one male or all females or all males.[9] Regardless of gender, it is important not to overcrowd your cage. Overcrowding sets up an environment for aggression. Two prairie dogs of each sex can coexist in a single cage if they are given adequate space and the males are raised together as juveniles or are neutered. With each

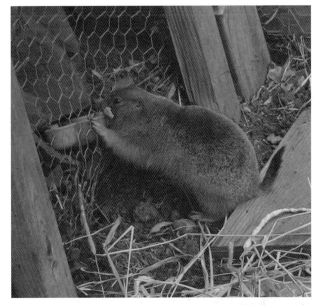

Figure 14.10 Prairie dogs can be extremely destructive if left unattended. It is important to provide acceptable toys to explore and chew while in a safe environment for play and exploration.

addition, it is important to be prepared with a second cage and to introduce new animals over an extended period of time.[9] Housing prairie dogs individually and in isolation is not recommended. According to some sources, isolated prairie dogs can become depressed, aggressive, and die prematurely.[9] Due to the highly social nature of the prairie dog, individual housing does not meet with the recommended "Five Freedoms" (see Chapter 20) and is likely to result in poor welfare.

Acknowledgments

Except where otherwise noted, all photos in this chapter are courtesy of the author.

References

1. Moulton GE, ed. *The Definitive Journals of Lewis and Clark.* Vol. 3. Up the Missouri to Fort Mandan. Lincoln Nebraska: Bison Books, 2002.
2. Clark TW. The hard life of the prairie dog. *Natl Geogr* 1979;156: 270–281.
3. Smith WJ, Smith SL, Oppenheimer EC et al. Vocalizations of the black-tailed prairie dog, *Cynomys ludovicianus. Anim Behav* 1977;25:152–164.
4. Bryant MD. Phylogeny of nearctic Sciuridae. *Am Midl Nat* 1945;33:257–390.
5. Hall ER. *The Mammals of North America.* New York: John Wiley and Sons, 1981.
6. Hollister N. A systematic account of the prairie dogs. *North Am Fauna* 1916;40:1–37.
7. Hoogland JL. *The Black-Tailed Prairie Dog: Social Life of a Burrowing Mammal.* Chicago, IL: University of Chicago Press, 1995.
8. Hoogland JL, ed. *Conservation of the Black-Tailed Prairie Dog.* Washington: Island Press, 2006.

9. Stoica K, Callis B, Watson L. *Bringing a Prairie Dog Pup into Your Home.* Canton, OH: Karen Stoica, 2001.

10. Anthony A. Behavior patterns in a laboratory colony of prairie dogs. *Cynomys ludovicianus. J Mammal* 1955;36(1):69–78.

11. Reed KD, Melski JW, Graham MB et al. The detection of monkeypoxin humans in the Western Hemisphere. *N Engl J Med* 2004;350(4): 342–350.

12. Chao PL. Control of communicable diseases: Restrictions on African rodents, prairie dogs, and certain other animals. *Fed Regis* 2008;73(174):51919.

13. Cully JF, Biggins DE, Seery DB. Conservation of prairie dogs in areas with plague. In: Hoogland JL, ed. *Conservation of the Black-Tailed Prairie Dog.* Washington: Island Press 2006:157–168.

14. Avashia SB, Petersen JM, Lindley CM et al. First reported prairie dog-to-human tularemia transmission, Texas, 2002. *Emerging Infect Dis* 2004;10(3):483–486.

15. King JA. *Social Behavior, Social Organization, and Population Dynamics in a Black-tailed Prairie Dog Town in the Black Hills of South Dakota.* Contributions from the Laboratory of Vertebrate Biology: The University of Michigan, 1955.

16. Waring GH. Sound communication of black-tailed, white-tailed and gunnison's prairie dogs. *Am Midl Nat* 1970;83(1):167–185.

118. Owings DH, Owings SC. Snake-directed behavior by black-tailed prairie dogs (*Cynomys ludovicianus*). *Z Tierpsychol* 1979;49:35–54.

19. Owings DH, Loughry WJ. Variation in snake-elicited jump-yipping by black-tailed prairie dogs: Ontogeny and snake-specificity. *Z Tierpsychol* 1985;70:177–200.

20. Randall JA. Evolution and function of drumming as communication in mammals. *Am Zool* 2001;41:1143–1156.

21. Heffner RS, Heffner HE, Contos C et al. Hearing in prairie dogs: Transition between surface and subterranean rodents. *Hear Res* 1994;73(2):185–189.

22. Smith R. Natural history of the prairie dog in Kansas. *Misc Publ Mus Nat Hist, Univ Kansas* 1967;49:1–39.

23. Jacobs GH, Yolton RL. Some characteristics of the eye and the electroretinogram of the prairie dog. *Exp Neurol* 1972;37(3):538–549.

24. Walls GL. *The Vertebrate Eye and its Adaptive Radiation.* Bloomfield Hills, Michigan: Cranbrook Institute of Science, 1942.

25. Steiner AL. Greeting behavior in some Sciuridae from an ontogenetic evolutionary and socio behavioral perspective. *Nat Can (Quebec)* 1975;102(6):737–751.

26. Jones TR, Plakke RK. The histology and histochemistry of the peri anal scent gland of the reproductively quiescent black-tailed prairie dog *Cynomys-ludovicianus. J Mammal* 1981;62(2):362–368.

27. Shier DM. Effect of family support on the success of translocated black-tailed prairie dogs. *Conserv Biol* 2006;20(6):1780–1790.

28. Hoogland JL. Aggression ecto parasitism and other possible costs of prairie dog sciuridae *Cynomys*-spp coloniality. *Behaviour* 1979;69(1–2):1–35.

15

South American camelids

Marcelo Alfredo Aba, Carolina Bianchi, and Verónica Cavilla

The Camelidae family: Origin

The Camelidae belong to the order Artiodactyla (even number of digits), suborder Tylopoda (ruminants with a pad or callus on each foot), and share similar features of a small head and long neck. They originated in western North America in the late Eocene, 40–45 million years before present (b.p.), and underwent millions of years of evolution before the appearance of the current species.[1,2] The earliest camel and common ancestor of the family, *Protylopus petersoni*, looked a little like today's guanaco and stood 30 cm (11.8 in.) at the shoulder. This ancient species had four toes and a full set of 44 teeth with no gaps between them. An early descendant of *P. petersoni*, *Pebrotherium wilsoni*, was similar in size to a sheep (60 cm or 23.6 in.) and had two toes on each foot. These ancestral camelids had remarkably elongated limbs matched by a long and powerful neck that made them much more efficient runners than contemporary ruminants. Possibly, this morphologic characteristic was an adaptation to their natural habitat on the extensive savannas of the high open plains of North America.[1] Major changes in morphology, feeding behavior, and locomotor adaptations followed and by the early Miocene (12–25 million years b.p.), primitive ancestors of the family were divided into four groups: *Titanotylopus*, *Paracamelus*, *Megatylopus*, and *Hemiauchenia*.[1]

About 3 million years b.p. (late Pliocene) camelids first migrated to Eurasia via the Bering Land Bridge. *Paracamelus* reached the Old World, spread rapidly into Europe, east Africa, and China, and developed into the two present day species of Old World camelids, of the genus *Camelus*: *Camelus bactrianus* and *Camelus dromedarius*. By the beginning of the Pleistocene, the *Hemiauchenia* line had emigrated through the Panamanian Land Bridge into the east Andes and pampas of South America. Finally, by events that are not fully understood, the long-limbed flatland-adapted *Hemiauchenia* line further evolved into the four species of the New World camelids or South American Camelids (SACs).[1,3] Toward the end of the Pleistocene, during the Ice Age (10–12 thousands years ago), all North American camelids became extinct.[1]

Domestication

According to fossil records, the domestication process of SACs is dated from 4000 to 5000 years ago in the Andes.[1,2,4] A remarkable increase in the camelid population occurred around this period, suggesting the establishment of a predominately herding economy. Although, it has long been accepted that the Peruvian Central Andes was the heartland of camelid domestication,[2,5] recent research indicates that similar developments occurred in parallel in the region of the South–Central Andes of southern Peru, northern Chile, and northwestern Argentina.[6]

The origins of the domestic species are highly debated. There are different evolutionary models of llama and alpaca ancestry according to morphological changes and behavior.[2] Based on unique shared behavioral traits and data from Telarmachay and other Andean archeological sites, some authors suggest that the llama is descended from the guanaco and the alpaca from the vicuña with subsequent hybridization between the two domestic forms producing the *huarizo*.[2] Other authors have supported the idea that both domestic camelids descend from the guanaco, and the vicuña was never domesticated.[2,7–9] Finally, other hypothesis[2,10] attribute llama ancestry to the guanaco and considering some similarity in morphological and behavioral traits it postulates that the alpaca is a mixture resulting from the hybridization between captured vicuñas and domestic llamas.

Recent genetic research has supported the idea that the llama descends from the guanaco and the alpaca is the domesticated vicuña.[11,12] Nevertheless, all members of the Camelidae family have 37 pairs of chromosomes and the karyotypes show a notable similarity. Moreover, all four species of SACs can interbreed and produce fertile offspring.[4,13]

Taxonomy

Today, the genus *Lama* includes two domesticated species: *Lama glama* (llama) and *Lama pacos* (alpaca); and two wild species: *Lama guanicoe* (guanaco) and *Lama vicugna* (vicuña). However, there is no full consensus concerning the taxonomic classification of SACs: most European scientists place the four species within the genus *Lama*, whereas North and South American researchers place the vicuña into the separate genus *Vicugna*.[1,2] Based on a study by Miller[14] that reports some peculiarities of vicuña incisors as well as some recent genetic studies, further division of the genus *Vicugna* into two genera has been suggested.[11] Moreover, many genetic and morphological characteristics of alpacas are similar to that of the vicuña. Thus, definitive taxonomic classification needs to be discussed and would require additional morphological and biochemical studies.[11,12]

Importance to man

The Inca Empire's culture and economy was supported by the llama. They were used to obtain food, fiber, and pelts, and carried food as well as burdens for buildings, temples, irrigation projects, military expansion, and silver and gold mining. It is interesting to note that the limits of the powerful Inca Empire closely conformed to the range and ecological limitations of the llama.[5,15]

When the Spanish arrived in the 1530s they found vast herds of llamas and alpacas, numbering in the tens of millions of animals. In order to obtain fiber and meat, the natives hunted vicuñas in the Andean highlands, as well as guanacos in Patagonia. These activities were regulated by the Inca society (vicuña) and Tehuelche and Ona tribes (guanaco), which practiced various forms of wildlife conservation and management.[1]

South American Camelid numbers drastically declined during the century following the Spanish invasion of the Central Andes.[16] Uncontrolled slaughter, disruption of the Incan social order, and the introduction of sheep were responsible for the collapse.

Habitat

Today, the guanaco occupies the most diverse habitat types. Its distribution extends from northern Peru to central Chile, across Patagonia. Meanwhile, llamas, alpacas, and vicuñas are limited to the *puna*, that is the dry Andean highlands of Peru, western Bolivia, northern Chile, and northwestern Argentina. The puna, covering an estimated 25 million hectares (61.7 million acres), is a very high altitude grassland (between 3500 and 4800 m above sea level [11,482–15,748 ft]) where, consequently, the atmospheric pressure is also low. It is a cold, dry, and often windy environment. The average rainfall in this region is between 500 and 900 mm (19.7–35.4 in.), with precipitation occurring mainly in the summer (December–April). Typical mean annual temperatures range from 4.6°C to 5.5°C (40.3–41.9°F), and temperatures at night often drop below 0°C (32°F). The ecosystem is very sensitive to perturbation and easily damaged.[1] Plants, even if well adapted, grow very slowly and spread out only gradually. Grasses usually grow in tufts and are largely of the genera *Festuca*, *Stipa*, and *Calamagrostis*. In the moist areas, richer in humus, there is a mixture of *Poa*, *Muhlembergia*, and *Distichia* grasses.[17]

Due to this harsh environment, agriculture is not a profitable alternative in these areas. Meanwhile, SACs have demonstrated a formidable capacity for adaptation being able to efficiently transform poor quality grasses into a source of stored protein for the inhabitants of the puna. They are well adapted to their respective habitats and are often the only livestock that can survive and reproduce under the prevailing environmental conditions.

As a result, raising SACs has been an essential resource for humans for many years. Today, for some 300,000 peasant families in South America, the raising of SACs is their major source of income.[18] Llamas are still used as pack animals by some high Andean communities. Llama and alpaca meat continues to be almost the only source of animal protein available to the inhabitants of the puna. The coarser and stronger llama fiber is mainly used for carpets and coarser textiles, while the finer and softer alpaca fiber is preferred by the textile industry and artisan producers.[19,20] The guanaco fiber has a small diameter; the fibers are short and produced in low quantities. In part because the species has not yet been domesticated, the guanaco is of little commercial importance. The vicuña, still an endangered species, is considered to have a great economic potential in the Andean nations. Protected by governments, the number of vicuñas is slowly increasing, and some attempts at production in semi-captivity are currently being carried out. More recently llamas and alpacas have become popular livestock species in North America where they may be kept as companion animals, pack animals, show animals, and/or for their fiber (Figure 15.1).

Camelid social activity

Camelids are highly social animals communicating with an intricate set of signals that, similar to real language, serves multiple vital functions. Almost all studies on social organization and behavior of SACs have been done

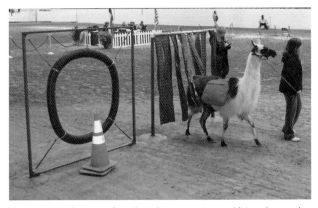

Figure 15.1 Llamas are friendly and easy to train. In addition, they can be used as pack animals. (Photo courtesy of V.V. Tynes, DVM.)

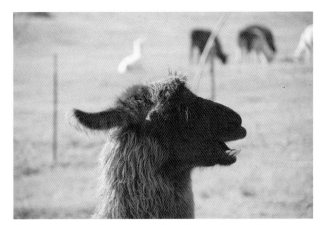

Figure 15.2 Young llama showing signs of aggressiveness. (Photo courtesy of V.V. Tynes, DVM.)

on populations of wild species in South America. However, llamas and alpacas closely resemble their ancestors in nearly all aspects of morphology and behavior. Thus, understanding wild camelid behavioral and social organization will aid in the care and effective handling of the domesticated forms in such a way as to minimize stress for both animals and humans. Moreover, knowing the normal behavior of an individual makes it possible to evaluate behavioral changes that could indicate pain and incipient illness.[21] When llamas and alpacas become accustomed to handling they are usually submissive and friendly. Conversely, wild species often require chemical immobilization to be controlled.

Communication

Camelid communication includes visual, auditory, and chemical signals. All of them are involved in the transmission of social information. An amazing feature of their communication signals is their subtlety. In addition, according to the social context some signals could have more than one connotation.

Visual signals

South American Camelids communicate moods or feelings to each other, humans, and other animals by a series of displays, postures, and positions of the body, neck, tail, and ears that encodes an authentic body language as a whole. These expressions allow SACs to communicate over long distances. These signals can be differentiated by two types of communication: inter- and intra-group. Generally, body and neck postures are important for inter-group communication between adult males during advertisement and defense of their territories, while ears and tail positions are especially used for conflict between members within the group.[22] Ears and tail adopt variable positions depending on the message that an animal is trying to transmit. Thus, ears can vary from vertical to forward, above horizontal, horizontal, below horizontal, and flattened on the neck.

Tail positions include normal (flat against the perineum), below horizontal, horizontal, above horizontal, vertical, and forward curl.[23]

Thus, the combination of variable positions of ears, tail, body, and neck can suggest different moods and welfare states. A normal and contented animal will display ears in a vertical position and the tail usually lying down flat against the perineum. During alertness, alarm, or special interest, the ears are turned forward and the tail rises to horizontal or as much as 45° above horizontal. A submissive adult llama holds their ears in a vertical to above horizontal position, the tail fully curved forward over the back with the head and neck toward the ground and the front limbs slightly bent. Submissive vicuñas and juvenile llamas usually keep the head curved back over the body.[23]

On the other hand, aggressive animals will adopt variable positions of the ears in conjunction with various tail and neck postures.[22,23] In general, the lower the ears are, the higher the level of aggression (Figure 15.2). Consequently, the dominant individual of an interacting pair is invariably the individual with the lowest ear position.[24] In contrast to ear position, the higher the tail, the higher the level of aggression.

Other forms of visual signals used to express different degrees of aggression include:

- *Spitting*—When animals feel threatened they may spew their stomach contents as a defensive action.
- *Kicking*—By arching a rear limb forward and outward with a quick jab directly backward.
- *Biting*—A defensive action usually restricted to intact males that bite with their formidable saber-like canine teeth. However, SACs hardly ever kick or bite unless provoked.

Auditory signals

Although SACs are only slightly vocal, they have a repertoire of sounds known as *humming* that function to provide auditory contact between individuals in a variety of circumstances. *Humming* is low in tone and hard to hear (for humans), and according to the volume and tone it might express different moods or feelings. During contact between herd members and especially between the mother and her newborn, a soft auditory contact call is produced. A deeper tone is used to communicate tension, discomfort, or pain between adults. Babies desiring to nurse make a higher pitched sound with an inflection at the end. Some louder forms are used by infants, mothers, or group members upon separation or reunion and became a more whistle-like distress hum when a young animal is frightened or becomes separated from its mother.[22,23]

In an aggressive social interaction, the most common sounds that can be heard include snorting, clicking, and grumbling usually accompanied by ear and tail threat displays. Screaming indicates extreme fright and is made by an animal generally when it is restrained, captured, or sheared. Animals perceiving danger emit a particular alarm call consisting of a high-pitched, rhythmic braying sound. Orgling is a rhythmic, expiratory, guttural grunting sound emitted by a male while copulating or chasing a female.[22,25]

Chemical signals

Dung piling behavior

The four species of SACs routinely defecate and urinate using dung piles.[22,26] This behavior serves an important role for intra-group orientation, helping to keep members of a family group together within their territorial boundaries. In addition, it is essential for inter-group communication between dominant males, as it is performed by territorial males as a part of their territory defense process, serving as a display to the male's opponent. Dung piles situated close to the sources of water and in the path are usually of communal use and bigger than those situated in sleeping territories that are used only for the members of a family group.[27] There are two interesting consequences of dung piling behavior: it can improve the environment by increasing the availability of highly preferred and high-producing forage types around the dung piles, and it can aid in reducing the dissemination of some infectious and parasitic diseases. Thus, this behavior can be useful to those managing SACs because the behavior helps to maintain the barn in a more sanitary condition.

Flehmen behavior often occurs in close proximity to a dung pile. The animal, usually the male, raises the nose in a vertical position into the air with the mouth slightly open in order to pick up and decode the scent message (pheromones) in the vomero-nasal organ. Males when detecting an estrus female exhibit this behavior after smelling her urine. Flehmen may also be exhibited by female llamas after sniffing the ground.[21,26]

Glands

South American Camelids have metatarsal scent glands, one inside and one outside of each cannon bone on the lower rear limbs, associated with hairless patches. They are often referred to as "chestnuts." Usually, animals rub the gland on the opposite rear limb. Although the function of these glands has not yet been elucidated, it has been reported that in the cervids they produce an alarm pheromone when animals are frightened. Additional scent glands, the interdigital glands, are found on all four feet. Their function is unknown but it is most likely that they are associated with individual and group identification.

Body care in SACs

South American Camelids are amazingly clean and quite odorless. They usually define different zones within their territory assigning them different uses. Some of these areas become important for normal body care by the animal. As previously described, dung piling is one behavior that contributes to the maintenance of a clean environment.

Rolling places

Rolling places are large circular depressions on the ground where no grass grows due to repeated rolling by camelids (Figure 15.3). These sites and the rolling behavior appear to play a role in maintaining coat cleanliness and self-comfort. Camelids appear to use rolling places in order to maintain the insulative properties of their fiber and for eliminating parasites. They usually roll over on their side, sit up, and roll back down again several times before pausing. After a short break, they start to roll on the other side. Apparently,

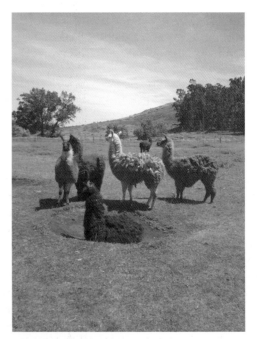

Figure 15.3   Characteristic rolling place used by a group of llamas in Tandil, Buenos Aires province, Argentina.

this behavior powders their peculiar coat creating an air mattress affect that insulates the fiber and helps to maintain a healthy, fluffy coat of wool. One disadvantage of rolling places is their possible role as a source of external parasites.[27]

Sebaceous glands secretion

Sebum, produced by the *sebaceous glands* associated with each hair follicle, also contributes to the maintenance of the hair fiber in high-quality condition. The combination of sebum with sweat covers and protects the skin and fiber, enhancing water repellency, inhibiting microorganism penetration, and dehydration via the skin.[21,26]

Reproductive behavior

South American Camelids are induced ovulators, requiring copulation to trigger the ovulatory process.[15,28] Ovulation has been reported to occur within 36 hours after copulation in llamas and alpacas.[29] Unlike other ruminant species, non-pregnant female camelids show continuous sexual acceptance (estrus) during several days (even weeks), interrupted by short periods (2 days) of non-acceptance.[30] Thus, the sexual behavior of females in the presence of the male may involve immediate acceptance, slow acceptance, or refusal. Immediate acceptance is manifested when the female adopts the copulation position of sternal recumbency when approached by the male or after a short chase of 1–2 minutes. Slow acceptance is more apparent in yearlings than in adult females.[31] Occasionally, some females in heat mount other females or females may mount a male during mating or seat themselves next to a mating couple.[28] Females refuse males by spitting, attempting to escape, kicking, and in some cases vocalizing.[32] This behavior is indicative of a non-estrus female while eventual acceptance of the male is typical of non-pregnant females. However, on some occasions even pregnant females will allow breeding if the male is particularly persistent.

When males are introduced to a herd, they will attempt to mate with the first receptive female they encounter. If many males are introduced together, dominance hierarchies are usually established quickly before breeding activity begins. This behavior consists mainly of males challenging each other and is characterized by spitting, neck wrestling, and jumping at each other[30] (Figure 15.4). The initiation of breeding activity is marked by the pursuit of females by males. Mating behavior is divided into two phases: courting and copulation. During the courting phase the male attempts to mount the standing female to encourage her to assume the sternal position. The length of the courtship may be influenced by the level of the libido of the individual males and may only last a few seconds or up to 10 minutes, but attempts longer than 4 minutes usually result in mating not taking place.[30] Copulation takes place in a recumbent position with the female resting on her sternum and with

her hind legs forward, her front legs extended or bent back at the knee, and the pelvis elevated[30,33] (Figure 15.5).

During copulation, the male lies prone upon the back of the female. The head of the male is above and slightly behind that of the female. His forelegs rest on her back, his elbows hold her at the shoulders, and his forefeet are off the ground.[28,30,34] Camelids are the only ungulates to pair in the recumbent position. Intromission of the penis is achieved only after considerable time is spent searching and probing: first around the perineal area for the vulva and then in traversing the vagina and cervix.[33] During copulation, males show their excitement with trembling ears, tail flipping up and down, nostrils dilating, and constantly vocalizing making a guttural sound (orgling).[28,35] Females assume a very passive attitude and in some instances may change position and lie in lateral recumbency.[30,35]

It is impossible to ascertain exactly when ejaculation occurs. There is no tail flagging, as in the stallion, or pelvic thrust, as in the bull.[15,34] In camelids, ejaculation is continuous and prolonged and semen is deposited directly into

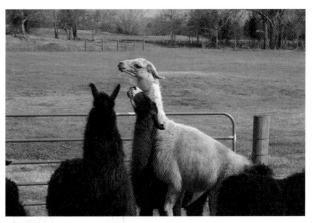

Figure 15.4 Two llamas displaying neck wrestling in order to establish dominance. (Photo courtesy of V.V. Tynes, DVM.)

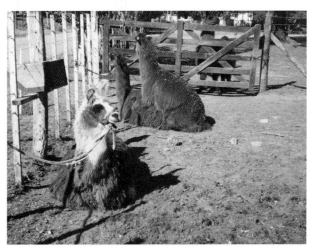

Figure 15.5 A pair of llamas copulating and a receptive female sitting nearby.

the uterine horns.[33,34] The male determines the length of copulation which lasts from 3 to 65 minutes, with an average time of 20–30 minutes.[30]

The beginning of the reproductive season seems to vary depending on the environment and management system. In their natural habitat, breeding in all four species of camelids appears to be seasonal and is confined to the warmer, rainy months from November to April.[33]

Sexual activity is particularly intense during the first week following the introduction of males into a herd of non-pregnant females. More than 70% of the females are mated at least once during this time. Thereafter, the continuous association of males and females inhibits the sexual activity of the males in spite of the presence of estrus females.[15,36,37] Although the physiological basis for the decline remains unknown (fatigue, boredom, etc.), it has been shown that if the males are allowed to rest for 4–5 days, keeping them separated from females, they will resume normal sexual activity when returned to the female group. Replacing them with new males at frequent intervals or moving them between female groups seem to be alternatives to aid in maintaining high levels of libido and overall high fertility rates.[15,38]

Maternal behavior

The signs of impending parturition in female camelids are observed the day before, or more commonly, some hours before birth. They are nervous, restless, and isolate themselves from the rest of the herd. Immediately before delivery, females stop feeding, urinate, or adopt the position to urinate frequently. They lie down and get up repeatedly and vocalize while exhibiting abdominal straining.[39,40] They often assume a lateral lying position with their legs to the side. At the moment of the delivery, females adopt the labor position, which is similar to that of urinating. This has the advantage that the young is born more quickly and the umbilical cord is broken when the newborn falls.[41]

Parturition occurs mainly in the morning, between 07:00 and 13:00 hours. It is considered an adaptation to the hard environment in their natural habitat where temperatures below zero are reached at night. If the newborns are not dried off and have not suckled and walked before dusk they will have less chance of survival.[40,42]

Immediately postpartum the female is very calm and patient. Female camelids are considered very good mothers because they defend their crias vigorously and rejection of their own cria is extremely rare.[40] The first movements of the newborn are uncoordinated with repeated lateral movements and attempts to stand. The time to standing varies between individuals and is usually between 5 and 60 minutes.[39] Once the neonate is standing it tries to find the udder, and about 1 hour after birth the cria starts to suckle. Usually the initial encounters with the udder are not successful. The cria may change teats until it receives

colostrum and success seems to be expressed by the cria raising its tail.[40]

Females verify by smell that the neonate is their own and reject strange crias by spitting and threatening. When the neonate has been resting for long periods, the mother will begin to nose it in order to stimulate suckling. However the offspring usually starts to suck each time without any stimulation. The period of nursing is determined by the mother, with her moving apart from and pushing away her cria when she is ready for suckling to stop.[40]

Social organization and behavior

Intra-species

Camelids are considered territorial, gregarious, and highly social, typically living in groups of many animals.[43] The main difference between vicuñas and guanacos is that the latter species is more variable and flexible in their behavior and geographical distribution than the vicuña (Figure 15.6).

A free population of camelids in a defined area is usually divided into the following three social groups: (1) the family group formed by an adult male with a variable number of females and their offspring, (2) the group of single males with a variable numbers of individuals including juveniles and adults, and (3) solitary males that may be looking for females with which to form a new family group or very old males that were rejected from other groups.[44,45]

The family group is the most stable and well-defined social unit. It includes an adult male and various females with or without their offspring. Crias must be younger than 12 and 15 months old in order to be accepted into the group for vicuñas and guanacos, respectively. A linear social hierarchy exists within the family group, with the adult male being dominant over the females and adult females dominating over the crias.[1] The group size can vary according to the time of the year. It can change depending on

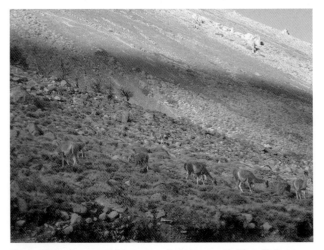

Figure 15.6 A group of 15 guanacos in their natural habitat: Chubut Province, Argentina.

the number of parturitions due to the isolation of adult females with their crias at the beginning of the autumn, and their subsequent return to the group during the spring.[44] Similarly, the number of individuals forming the group varies according to the different species of camelids and the region. For vicuñas, the family group size oscillates between five and seven individuals per group, while for guanacos, three to twelve animals per group is typical.[46]

Additionally, two types of family groups seem to exist. The main family group is comprised of a dominant adult male followed by at least five females. Secondary groups are made up of a younger male with less experience and one to five mature females. Usually, the young male belonged to a family group until he reached sexual maturity and became interested in fighting with the dominant male of the main group for a couple of females to form his own family group. These secondary groups tend to stay some meters apart from the main group but continue to follow it from some distance. Eventually, the young male will be the dominant adult of a main group.[44]

The adult males defend their territory against the intrusion of non-group members, and regulate the size and density of the family group. For the more sedentary vicuñas, the territory consists of a feeding area where the groups spend most of the time and a sleeping area, usually located on higher terrain where the animals spend the night. Guanacos groups are much more spread out and fragmented.[1]

The male social group is made up of animals older than 1 year that have left their natal family group. Males stay in this group until they reach the age to be able to defend their own territory. They usually move together and meet in specific areas where they share daily activities with great synchronization between group members. Occasionally, females are observed to move between the single male groups until they settle with one male. This kind of group varies in size between two and fifty or even a hundred individuals depending on the region they inhabit.[44]

Solitary males are generally juveniles that have recently reached puberty. Frequently, they stay in a group of males until the rainy season when reproductive activity begins and they then travel alone trying to find a group of females so they can build their own family group. Solitary, aged males may try to incorporate themselves into a group of males but some of them finally obtain their own territory.[44]

In addition, it is possible to observe transitional groups. It is common for many family groups to stay together during the winter until the reproductive season starts. Also, during some periods it is possible to see groups of females with their offspring but without the dominant male.[44] Males, especially guanaco males, can sometimes be seen alone on hilltops or other elevated areas, watching for other invading males and predators. In this way, they defend and protect their own territories.[24] The presence of mobile family groups has also been reported. These groups are composed of females associated with a male that does not yet have an established territory. These groups are most frequently seen during early summer when juvenile females have been expelled from their family groups.[1]

Members of the same group of camelids are highly synchronized in their activities. It has been observed that vicuñas spend 65–75% of their time grazing. Female vicuñas spend more time grazing than males and less time being alert. The groups of single males and the family groups with more than eight individuals move frequently, and the time they spend being alert means less time they can spend grazing. Males eat less and spend more time alert, especially as the family group they defend increases in the number of females and offspring. Dominant males vocalize more often and this behavior allows them to alert the group about a possible danger like the presence of dogs, other predators, or human beings.[47]

While a limited amount of information is available about the social behavior of domestic camelids in captivity, it appears that, in spite of the manipulations of man, most of the behavioral repertoire of the wild species remains unchanged and the behavior of the domestic species is similar to the wild species.[1,4] Social organization of llamas and alpacas seems to be similar to that observed in guanacos and vicuñas, respectively. In herds composed of males and females, a social hierarchy is established with a single dominant male who controls the access of other males to the females, food, and water. The dominant male uses the same attack and threat mechanisms as the wild species in defense of their territory.[4]

Play behavior

Play behavior is still not well defined in SACs. However, it is considered to be a key component in learning about the establishment of social relationships between individuals and may contribute to the development of the locomotor and nervous systems. Camelid play can be divided into locomotor, sexual, and aggressive play. Locomotor play behavior consists of short runs, fast stops, turns, and jumps. Aggressive or attack play behaviors are expressed by spitting, biting, kicking, and neck wrestling and sexual play by attempting to mount. Play behavior is most often observed between crias and juvenile animals when they are relaxed and secure, and it can be practiced alone or in groups of several juveniles.[39]

Inter-species

Some studies on the social behavior of llamas refer to their relationship to other species. It is well known that llamas are being used as guard animals (in the United States and experimentally in other countries) to protect sheep from predators such as dogs and coyotes.[24,48] Llamas are typically aggressive toward dogs and appear to readily bond with sheep and aggressively protect them when confined with them away from other llamas. Good guardian llamas must be curious and aggressive toward dogs but stay close to the sheep in order to be able to defend all of them. It has been observed that usually the more dominant the llamas are in their own groups, the better guardians they are for sheep. In addition, it was reported that heavier llamas displayed a higher level of aggression toward dogs than smaller llamas. This aggressiveness has been correlated with the age and the weight of the animals. It has been suggested that larger llamas may be more self-confident against a predator and might also be more intimidating to a predator.[24]

In relation to humans, llamas and alpacas are generally very docile and easily handled, responding very well to human contact.[23] In our opinion, domestic camelids are curious, peaceful, and intelligent animals making them excellent pets, companions, and pack animals. They are easy to train, learn readily and retain many learned behaviors. Llamas are used as pack animals because of their surefootedness and ease of handling, and have become the animals of choice for many activities. However, it has been reported that some male llamas become aggressive toward humans, when they are around 2 years old. Many owners have suggested that castration and training by an experienced llama handler improves the behavior of these animals.[49]

Locomotion

Camelids are digitigrade; they walk on their phalanges instead of on their toes like other ruminants.[50] This feature, in addition to the soft plantar surfaces of their feet, allows them to minimize the damage caused to the environment,[47] and enables them to have better contact with the ground and a greater surface area with which to support their weight. These anatomical features insure them exceptional stability and a surefooted walk even in very rugged environments.[50]

South American Camelids have several different types of gaits: they can walk, gallop, trot, and stot (or pronk). They are also unique among mammals in the employment of a natural lateral pacing gait.[50] During the pace, the ipsilateral front and hind legs move forward together in unison, with a period of suspension between the movements of each limb pair during which all four feet are off the ground. The pace prevents the fore and hind legs on the same side from interfering with each other during fast locomotion, allowing a longer stride length, and hence a faster and more efficient mode of locomotion than the trot.[51]

Three distinct types of pace gait can be distinguished in these species: a slow pace, where the animal may be supported by four legs during some part of the locomotory cycle; a medium pace, where the animal is only ever supported by two legs; and a fast pace, where there are times during the cycle when no legs are on the ground.[51] Although the pace is the more adapted gait for living in open and flat habitats, there are two major disadvantages: the lateral stability and maneuverability are considerably

reduced. Anatomical adaptations have evolved in SACs to compensate for such difficulties: wide, splay toed feet, strong ligaments supporting the feet, placement of the limbs close to the midline of the body, and the low forward placement of the neck, with the weight of the neck and head tending to counterbalance the side to side body sway during pacing.[1]

Feeding behavior

Feeding behavior can be defined as the process by which animals ingest the food required to satisfy organic needs while refusing non-alimentary or toxic compounds.[52] Most reports about camelid feeding behavior study preferences for the particular vegetation that constitutes their diet and how they differ from other domestic ruminant species in their natural environment.

Most camelids mainly feed on the herbaceous stratum. They are considered "adaptable mixed feeders" for their ability to alternate dietary preferences between grasses and forbs or between grazing and browsing according to vegetation availability.[53] Vicuñas and alpacas are both strictly grazers although some differences between both species were observed. While vicuñas eat mainly forbs and grasses,[54] alpacas, when environmental conditions allow them the choice, prefer grasses, followed by sedges and reeds. Apparently, forbs do not constitute a large proportion of the diet of alpacas, most likely because they are very unpalatable to them. During the dry season, when food availability decreases, alpacas increase their ingestion of seeds, suggesting that seeds are important in providing energy during this period.[55]

Guanacos and llamas are both grazers and browsers. Guanacos have a great preference for grasses and forbs but they avoid high shrubs with a large proportion of ligneous tissues such as *Fanerophytes*. Also, guanacos reject coarse grasses (*Sporobulus, Stipa*) and *Astralagous*, the only forb always avoided and known to have a toxic effect on livestock. In their habitat, the population of guanacos is positively correlated with the intensity of favorite vegetal species.[56] *Poa* and *Festuca* are the most preferred species of available grasses.[53,56,57] However, when the availability of *Poa* and other palatable grasses and forbs diminishes during winter, they prefer short shrubs such as *Hyalis*.[53,56] Llamas are considered primarily grazer herbivores, having a high preference for large quantities of coarse bunchgrasses such as *Festuca* and *Stipa*, but they will also browse available shrubs and trees. Similar to the alpacas, llamas consume very few forbs but select diets with mostly tall grasses, while alpacas select both tall and short grasses.[58] Regarding *Astragalus*, the same avoidance behavior observed in guanacos has been noted in llamas and alpacas from Peru, where it is reported that these species are less affected by *Astragalus* than other domestic ruminants. Fowler[59] suggests that this avoidance behavior derives from a process of co-evolution with the native flora, since it has not been observed in camelids transferred to new environments.[53]

The time that camelids spend feeding varies considerably with the region where the animals live and the distance they have to cover to find forage in quantity and quality. The distance walked by animals during the feeding period is more in poor areas where it is difficult to find food than under extensive or intensive management where food is more available. Thus, when the vegetation is dominated by species of low value, the time spent feeding (looking for food and eating) increases. Consequently, animals assign shorter total times to ruminating and resting.[60] It seems that camelids eat faster during the morning trying to graze the most accessible forages first, as has been observed in sheep and cattle. In addition, rumination occurs more often at night in llamas than in sheep.[52]

The dromedary camel is well known for being able to go for long distances without needing to drink water. However this is not the case for SACs. Vicuñas are obligate drinkers. While adapted to live in arid environments, they must drink water once or twice daily during the dry season.[1] It has been observed that the distribution of vicuña populations depends on the availability of water, often being located around 1.6 km (1 mile) from the source of water.[47] Conversely, guanacos are periodic drinkers, requiring only occasional, free, or vegetational water. Guanacos can live in arid areas during the dry season, drinking water from brackish saline lagoons and ocean tide pools or being provided the water of plant moisture.[1]

Handling and restraint

Llamas and alpacas are very docile animals, and easy to work with. Some peculiarities of their behavior can aid in their handling. One of the most important aspects to be considered is that camelids are very social animals with a strong herding instinct so it is much easier to move them in groups of many animals. Moving a single individual may be very difficult and stressful for the animal. Moving several animals together will facilitate many procedures.

To enclose several camelids, use a small catch pen associated with a pasture. Feeding the animals in the area will encourage them to become accustomed to entering. It is relatively easy to restrict the movement of one or many llamas or alpacas with ropes, poles, or even humans with outstretched arms. Once in a restricted area, the llama may be slowly approached and one arm placed around the chest and neck while the opposite hand grasps the tail. It may be difficult to hold an adult llama in this manner unless it can be quickly pushed against a wall or fence.[23] Untrained alpacas are best controlled by pulling the head and neck close to the chest of the animal with one hand while the other hand rests on the top of the shoulders. Alternatively, the tail may be grasped by the second hand.[23]

Although camelids are very docile animals they are very sensitive to sudden movements. Sudden gestures may be interpreted as frightening and animals may react to them by screaming and in some cases spitting or kicking.

Most of the physical examination can be performed by manual restraint. However, a chute is sometimes necessary to safely perform a complete examination, especially of the reproductive tract.[23] While camelids can be trained to stand in a chute, if one is unavailable, genital examinations can also be performed in sternal recumbency with the legs up underneath the body. An assistant is needed to apply light pressure to the camelids shoulder to ensure that she remains in this position for the examination.

Wild camelids can be tamed if reared in close association with humans and handled regularly during maturation. Such animals may then be handled and restrained in a manner similar to that used for llamas or alpacas, but one should be aware that they are more easily frightened or excited. More vigorous manual restraint is needed to control wild guanacos and vicuñas. Most of these animals will not tolerate being tied and will fight if placed in a chute designed for the domestic species. A less traumatic and stressful method of restraint is intramuscular chemical sedation.[23]

Acknowledgments

Except where otherwise noted, photos in this chapter are courtesy of the authors.

References

1. Franklin WL. Biology, ecology, and relationship to man of the South American camelids. In: Mares MA, Genoways HH, eds. *Mammalian Biology in South America.* Spec. Publ. Ser., Vol. 6. Pittsburgh, PA: Pymatuning Laboratory of Ecology, and University of Pittsburgh, 1982a;457–489.
2. Wheeler JC. Evolution and origin of the domestic camelids. *Alpaca Registry J* Vol. III. Available at: www.alpacaregistry.net/journal/win98j-11.html. Accessed Winter–Spring, 1998.
3. Fowler ME. General biology and ecology. In: Fowler ME, ed. *Medicine and Surgery of South American Camelids.* Ames, IA: Iowa State University Press, 1989a;3–8.
4. Wheeler JC. Origen, Evolución y Status Actual. In: Fernández-Baca S, ed. *Avances y perspectivas del conocimiento de los Camélidos Sud Americanos.* Santiago, Chile: Oficina Recional de la FAO para América Latina y el Caribe, 1991;11–48.
5. Murra JV. Herds and herders in the Inca state. In: Leeds A, Vayda AP, eds. *Man, Culture and Animals.* Washington, DC: Publication No. 78 of the American Association for the Advancement of Science, 1965;185–215.
6. Mengoni Goñalons GL, Yacobaccio HD. The domestication of South American camelids. In: Zeder MA, Bradley DG, Emshwiller E, Smith BD, eds. *Documenting Domestication: New Genetic and Archaeological Paradigms.* 2006;228–242.
7. Thomas O. Notes on some ungulate mammals. *Proc Zool Soc Lond* 1891;384–389.
8. Piccinini, M, Kleinschmidt T et al. Primary structure and oxygen-binding properties of the hemoglobin from guanaco (*Lama guanicoe*), tylopoda. *Biol Chem Hoppe Seyler* 1990;371:641–648.

9. Gentry A, Clutton-Brock J, Groves C. The naming of wild animal species and their domestic derivatives. *J Archaeol Sci* 2004;31:645–651.

10. Hemmer H, 1990. *Domestication: The Decline of Environmental Appreciation.* Cambridge, UK: Cambridge University Press, 1990;217.

11. Kadwell M, Fernandez M, Stanley H et al. Genetic analysis reveals the wild ancestors of the llama and the alpaca. *Proc R Soc B* 2001;268:2575–2584.

12. Marín JC, Zapata B, González BA et al. Sistemática, taxonomía y domesticación de alpacas y llamas: nueva evidencia cromosómica y molecular. *Rev Chil Hist Nat* 2007;80(2):121–140.

13. Sumar J. Studies on reproductive pathology in the alpacas. *Master of Science Thesis*, Swedish University of Agricultural Sciences, Uppsala 1983;9–103.

14. Miller GS. A second instance of the development of rodent-like incisors in an artiodactyls, in *Proceedings*. United States Museum 1924;66:1–4.

15. Aba MA. Studies on the reproductive endocrinology of llamas and alpacas. *Acta Vet. Scand. Master of Science Thesis*, Swedish University of Agricultural Sciences, Uppsala, Sweden, 1995.

16. Flores-Ochoa JA. Aspectos mágicos del pastoreo: Enqa, Enquaychu, Illa y Khuya Rumi. In: Flores-Ochoa JA, ed. *Pastores de Puna Uywmichiq Punarunakuna.* Lima: Instituto de Estudios Peruanos, 1977;211–237.

17. Tosi JA. *Zonas de vida natural en el Perú. Boletín Técnico.* Zona Andina: Instituto Interamericano de Ciencias Agrícolas de la Organización de los Estados Americanos, 1960;5:1–271.

18. Aba MA. Hormonal interrelationships in reproduction of female llamas and alpacas. *Doctoral Thesis.* Swedish University of Agricultural Sciences, Uppsala, Sweden, 1998.

19. Sumar J. South American camelids raising and reproduction in the high Andes. In: Örnas AH, ed. *Camels in Development: Sustainable Production in African Drylands.* Uppsala: Scandinavian Institute of African Studies, 1988;81–93.

20. Frank EN. Mejoramiento genético en camélidos sudamericanos domésticos. Una propuesta para la población argentina. *Actas del Segundo Seminario Internacional de Camélidos Sudamericanos Domésticos* 1997;51–74.

21. Fowler ME. Llama and alpaca behavior—An aid to diseases diagnosis. In: *Proceedings.* Current veterinary care and management of llamas and alpacas. International camelid heath conference for veterinarians. The Ohio State University. March 2006;21–25.

22. Franklin WL. Lama language—Modes of communication in the South American camelids. *Llama World* 1982b;3:6–11.

23. Fowler ME. Restraint and handling. In: Fowler ME, ed. *Medicine and Surgery of South American Camelids.* Ames, IA: Iowa State University Press, 1989b;24–34.

24. Cavalcanti SMC, Knowlton FF. Evaluation of physical and behavioral traits of llamas associated with aggressiveness towards sheep-threatening canids. *Appl Anim Behav Sci* 1998; 61:143–158.

25. Tillman A. *Speechless Brothers: The History and Care of Llamas.* Seattle: Early Winters Press, 1981.

26. Franklin WL. Territorial marking behavior by the South American vicuña. In: D Müller-Schwarze, RM Silverstein, eds. *Chemical Signals: Vertebrates and Aquatic Invertebrates.* New York: Plenum Press, 1980;53–66.

27. Canedi AA, Pasini PS. Repoblamiento y bioecología de la vicuña silvestre en la provincia de Jujuy, Argentina. In: Boyazoglu J, ed. *Programa de las Naciones Unidas para el medio ambiente.* Organización de las Naciones Unidas para la Agricultura y la Alimentación. 1996;7–23.

28. Novoa C. Reproduction in camelidae. Review. *J Reprod Fertil* 1970;22:3–20.

29. Ratto M, Huanca W, Singh J, Adams GP. Comparison of the effect of natural mating, LH, and GnRH on interval to ovulation and luteal function in llamas. *Anim Reprod Sci* 2006;91:299–306.

30. England BG, Foote WC, Cardozo AG et al. Oestrous and mating behaviour in the llama (*Lama glama*). *Anim Behav* 1971;19:722–726.

31. Bravo W. Female reproduction. In: *The Reproductive Process of South American Camelids.* Library of Congress Cataloging—Publication Data. United States of America. 2002a;1–31.

32. Pollard JC, Littlejohn RP, Scott IC. The effects of mating on sexual receptivity of female alpacas. *Anim Reprod Sci* 1994;34:289–297.

33. Brown BW. A review on reproduction in South American camelids. *Anim Reprod Sci* 2000;58:169–195.

34. Bravo W. Male reproduction. In: *The Reproductive Process of South American Camelids.* Library of Congress Cataloging—Publication Data. United States of America. 2002b;49–64.

35. Vaughan JL, Tibary A. Reproduction in female South American camelids: A review and clinical observations. *Small Ruminant Res* 2006;61:259–281.

36. Fernandez-Baca S, Novoa C. Comportamiento sexual de la alpaca hembra en empadre a campo. *Memorias de la Asociación Latinoamericana de Producción Animal* 1968;3:7–20.

37. Fernandez-Baca S, Sumar J, Novoa C. Comportamiento sexual de la alpaca macho, frente a la renovación de las hembras. *Revista de Investigaciones Pecuarias* 1972;1:115–128.

38. Novoa C, Sumar J, Leyva V et al. Incremento reproductivo en alpacas de explotaciones comerciales mediante método de empadre alternativo. *Revista de Investigaciones Pecuarias* 1973;2:191–193.

39. Sarasqueta DV. Cría y Reproducción de guanacos en cautividad Lama guanicoe. Comunicación Técnica No. 110. Recursos Naturales—Fauna. Centro Regional Patagonia Norte. INTA EEA Bariloche. 2001;20–44.

40. Bravo W. Maternal behavior and neonatology. In: *The Reproductive Process of South American Camelids.* Library of Congress Cataloging—Publication Data. United States of America. 2002c;33–39.

41. Güttler E. Investigations on the physiology and pathology of reproduction for the improvement of llama breeding in the Andes of Argentina. *Anim Res Develop* 1987;25:109–126.

42. Knight TW, Death AF, Wyeth TK. Photoperiodic control of the time of parturition in alpacas (*Lama pacos*). *Anim Reprod Sci* 1995;39:259–265.

43. Lucherini M. Group size, spatial segregation and activity of wild sympatric vicuñas *Vicugna vicugna* and guanacos *Lama guanicoe*. *Small Ruminant Res* 1996;20:193–198.

44. Marchetti B, Arregui Oltremari J, Peters H. Estrategias para el manejo y aprovechamiento racional del guanaco (*Lama guanicoe*). Documento Técnico No. 9. Programa de las Naciones Unidas para el medio ambiente. Organización de las Naciones Unidas para la Agricultura y la Alimentación. 1992;25–30.

45. Sosa RA, Sarasola JH. Habitat use and social structure of an isolated population of guanacos (*Lama guanicoe*) in the Monte Desert, Argentina. *Eur J Wildl Res* 2005;51:207–209.

46. Cajal JL, Bonaventura SM. Densidad Poblacional y dinámica de los grupos familiares de guanacos y vicuñas en la reserva de biosfera San Guillermo. In: Cajal, JL, Fernández García J, Tecchi R, eds. *Bases para la conservación y manejo de la puna y cordillera frontal de Argentina. El rol de las reservas de la biosfera.* Uruguay: Fundación para la conservación de las Especies y del Medio Ambiente. UNESCO, 1998;167–174.

47. Vilá B. La importancia de la etología en la conservación y manejo de las vicuñas. *Etología* 1999;7:63–68.

48. Markham D, Hilton P, Tompkins J et al. Guard llamas—An alternative for effective predator management. *Int Llama Assoc Educat Bull* 1995;1–4.

49. Grossman JL, Kutzler MA. Effects of castration in male llamas (*Lama glama*) on human-directed aggression. *Theriogenology* 2007; 68:511.

50. Ault JS, Anderson DE. *Structure and Maintenance of the Foot of South American Camelids*. Columbus, Ohio: Ohio State University. College of Veterinary Medicine, 2003. http://www.rmla.com/foot.htm.

51. Janis CM, Theodor JM, Boisvert B. Locomotor evolution in camels revisited: A quantitative analysis of pedal anatomy and the acquisition of the pacing gait. *J Vertebrate Paleont* 2002;22:110–121.

52. Baumont R, Doreau M, Ingrand S, Veissier I. Feeding and mastication behavior in ruminants. In: Bels V, ed. *Feeding in Domestic Vertebrates from Structure to Behaviour*. Paris, France: National Museum of Natural History, 2006;241–262.

53. Puig S, Videla F, Monge S et al. Seasonal variations in guanaco diet (*Lama guanicoe* Müller 1976) and food availability in Northern Patagonia, Argentina. *J Arid Environ* 1996;34:215–224.

54. Fowler M. Feeding and nutrition. In: *Medicine and Surgery of South American Camelids*. 1st ed. United States of America: Ames Iowa State University, 1989c;9–23.

55. Reiner RJ, Bryant FC. Botanical composition and nutritional quality of alpaca diets in two Andean Rageland Communities. *J Range Manage* 1986;39(5):424–427.

56. Puig S, Videla F, Cona MI. Diet and abundance of the guanaco (*Lama guanicoe* Müller 1976) in four habitats of Northern Patagonia, Argentina. *J Arid Environ* 1997;36:343–357.

57. Bahamonde N, Martin S, Sbriller AP. Diet of guanaco and red deer in Neuquen Province, Argentina. *J Range Manage* 1986;39(1):22–24.

58. Pfister JA, San Martin F, Rosales L et al. Grazing behaviour of llamas, alpacas and sheep in the Andes of Peru. *Appl Anim Behav Sci* 1989;23:237–246.

59. Fowler M. Toxicology. In: Fowler ME, ed. *Medicine and Surgery of South American Camelids*. Ames, IA: Iowa State University Press, 1989d;366–382.

60. Raggi LA, Jiliberto E, Urquieta B. Feeding and foraging behaviour of alpaca in northern Chile. *J Arid Environ* 1994;26:73–77.

16

Hedgehogs

Valarie V. Tynes

History

Hedgehogs belong to the order Insectivora and are considered a relatively primitive mammal. They are widely distributed throughout the Old World and exist in a variety of habitats. It is likely that their benign nature, secretive, nocturnal habits, and their ability to adapt to a wide variety of densely populated human habitats has contributed to their universal appeal. They are the subject of much mythology and folklore and have been immortalized in children's stories (Beatrix Potter's, Mrs. Tiggy-winkle). Yet, due to their nocturnal habits very little is known about the behavior of most species of hedgehogs. The behavior of the European hedgehog has been studied more than any other species of hedgehog and it appears that behaviorally, most spiny hedgehogs are similar and, with some caution, much can be extrapolated from one species to another. While not domesticated, hedgehogs are readily tamed and people often keep European hedgehogs as pets. The African hedgehog has recently gained popularity as a pet in the United States.

This chapter will cover primarily what is known regarding the behavior of the two species of spiny hedgehogs most commonly kept as pets, *Erinaceus europaeus* and *Atelerix albiventris*. Both species are members of the subfamily Erinaceinae and are members of two of the most numerous and widespread genera.

Of the genus *Erinaceus*, *E. europaeus* has been most studied. *E. europaeus*, often referred to as the western European hedgehog or brown breasted hedgehog, is distributed across western and central Europe, into northern Europe, Britain, Ireland, Sicily, Sardinia, and Corsica. In the late 1800s, it was introduced to New Zealand where it now thrives. The head and body length of *E. europaeus* averages 200–300 mm (7.8–11.8 in.) and they weigh about 600–700 g (21–24.7 oz) during the summer. Their weights can increase dramatically in preparation for hibernation, 900–1000 g (31.7–35.3 oz) is common but some males may weigh as much as 1200 g (42 oz). *E. europaeus* prefers grassland, scrub, or cultivated areas as habitat.[1] They tend to avoid thick forests, although they will use forest edge habitat[2] and they are common visitors to suburban gardens.[3] The European hedgehog has been known to live for 7–8 years both in the wild and captivity.[1]

There are four species of *Atelerix* distributed across the continent of Africa. *Atelerix albiventris*, the hedgehog most commonly seen in the pet trade in the United States, has been referred to as the West African, white-bellied, central African, African pygmy, and four-toed hedgehog. It is unique from others in its genera for its lack of a hallux, or big toe, on its hind feet. It is patchily distributed across central Africa from Ethiopia to the Zambezi River, through Nigeria and down into Tanzania and Kenya.[1,4] *A. albiventris* inhabit grassland, scrub, savannah, and suburban gardens. Similar to the European hedgehogs, they are unlikely to be found in dense forests, wetlands, or areas that are extremely dry.[1]

A. albiventris is notably smaller than the European hedgehogs with a head and body length ranging from 140 to 210 mm (5.5–8.2 in.) and a weight range of 200–500 g (7–17.6 oz).[5,6] In captivity weights of 675–900 g (23.8–31.7 oz) are not uncommon.[7] In the wild, their spines are mostly white with a dark brown or black band around the middle. The face, legs, and tail are covered with a dark brown or grayish brown fur and the underside is usually white.[1] In recent years, captive-bred African hedgehogs have been bred in a variety of colors including pure white.

A. albiventris has slightly larger ears, longer, thinner legs, smaller paws, and less powerful claws than the European hedgehog.[8] They have a slightly wider center part of the forehead spines and their spines are generally shorter.[7] They typically have two pairs of pectoral mammae and may have an additional odd number of mammae on the abdomen.[9]

Although limited research has been done on *A. albiventris* in the wild, one study suggested that it may be uncommon for them to live for more than 2 years.[5] In captivity, it has been suggested that they may live up to 8 years[10] but more recently, the high incidence of malignant neoplasia in hedgehogs over 3 years of age, suggests that 4 to 5 year life spans may be more realistic.[11]

Senses and communication

Hedgehogs are nocturnal, so vision is the least important of their senses. Tactile signals from the whiskers probably aid them in moving through the brush and foraging for food in the dark, but their senses of smell and hearing are likely most important to their survival.

Vision

The hedgehog has moderately sized eyes and their visual acuity appears to be fair to good. Their retina contains only rods suggesting that they lack color vision.[12] However, one researcher found that some rods contain cone-type nuclei and he was able to train hedgehogs to discriminate between certain colors. With good lighting, they may be able to discriminate yellow from shades of gray and blue.[3,13]

Olfaction

Hedgehogs have well-developed olfactory lobes and the excellent sense of smell that feature suggests.[13] Their sense of smell plays an important role in many aspects of their behavior including foraging for food, detecting predators, navigating, sexual behavior, and maternal behavior. Their long snout with its moist tip also contributes to their olfactory acuity. A hedgehog foraging for food walks with its nose to the ground sniffing almost continuously.

Several researchers have attempted to determine the exact degree of hedgehog olfactory capabilities with some confounding results, in part due to the fact that hedgehogs were almost impossible to train! In one study, an attempt to train hedgehogs to associate a food reward with an odor resulted in three hedgehogs that required 1500–2000 trials to learn the task (even then they behaved unreliably) and one hedgehog that never learned even after 4000 trials![14] Nevertheless, one researcher determined that hedgehogs could detect crushed beetles at a range of 1 m (3.2 ft) with a 41% success rate and a dog at up to 11 m (36 ft) with a 42% success rate.[15]

The hedgehog also has a well-developed Jacobson's organ (vomeronasal organ).[3] The vomeronasal chemosensory system plays an important role in the behavior and physiology of a variety of species. It communicates directly with the central nervous system, separately from the nasal olfactory organ, via the accessory olfactory bulb. It is capable of detecting large molecules with low volatility, such as steroids, and remains in constant contact with the environment.[16] In other species it has been found to be involved with many aspects of reproduction, including sexual maturation, control of female cycling, hormone levels, courtship, mating, and maternal behavior, to name a few. Although, the Jacobson's organ is involved in the hedgehogs' unique behavior of "self-anointing," little is known of its actual function in the hedgehog.

No pheromones have yet been identified in the hedgehog.[3] Nevertheless, it is reasonable to expect that odor cues play an important role in their social and sexual behavior. Although, no one as yet understands exactly how odor cues are involved with hedgehog behavior, the numerous sources for odors suggest that they are of some importance. Numerous glands have been identified in several different species of hedgehogs. These include sebaceous glands, lubricating glands in the vagina, sexual accessory glands, a proctodeal gland, and eccrine sweat glands.[3] Hopefully, the role of these glands in the behavior of the hedgehog will be further elaborated in the future.

Audition

Hedgehogs have hearing that is especially sensitive to high frequencies (7.6–84 kHz). This capability makes them well adapted to hearing insects move about in soil and leaf litter. It also plays an important role in predator detection. Hedgehogs will flinch their head rapidly downward, bringing their spines over their face in response to any loud, high frequency sounds. If the high frequencies are also at a very high volume, they may cause the hedgehog to roll up completely. Lower frequency sounds, even when they are very loud, do not necessarily elicit the same response.[17]

Vocalizations

A wide variety of vocalizations have been reported in different species of hedgehogs. The sounds that have been most documented in *Erinaceus* and *Atelerix* include: snorting, spitting, huffing, or puffing, screaming and the high pitched twitters, whistles, and squeaks produced by nestling hedgehogs.

The most commonly heard sounds produced by hedgehogs will be the snorting, hissing, huffing, and puffing sounds that are most likely aggressive or warning sounds. These are produced by sharp exhalations through the nostrils and have been compared by some to the spitting of a frightened cat.[18,19] These are likely to be heard when the hedgehog is startled by a person or predator and sometimes when two hedgehogs meet. These sounds may become louder and more snort-like in response to a stronger stimulus.[19]

The scream is a loud call associated with extreme distress.[19,20] Screams have been reported to occur when two male hedgehogs fight and once when a hedgehog was held by all four feet. In both cases, the screams continued for a while after the fight stopped and the restrained hedgehog was released.[19]

When separated from their dam, most infant hedgehogs will vocalize. This has been described as a high pitched squeal or whistle that may be heard as far as 3 m away (almost 10 ft).[9] Once the dam retrieves the young, vocalization stops.

A vocalization that has been described as a quack has been documented in European hedgehogs. The quack has been heard when two hedgehogs meet and once when one was being lifted and returned to its box. It has also been reported to occur occasionally during courtship. One author suggested that it reflected a heightened level of excitement[21] but it may also be associated with a disturbance that bothered the hedgehog or something causing pain.[3,18]

Two unique vocalizations have been documented in *A. albiventris* and no other hedgehog thus far. One vocalization has been described as a twitter and is a high frequency sound made with the mouth closed. It is barely audible at a distance of 20 cm (7.9 in.) and rarely heard from as far away as 2 m (6.5 ft). This sound is made by both sexes of adult animals and is often accompanied by sniffing. It has usually been documented when hedgehogs were in unfamiliar surroundings, picked up, or lowered to the ground.[19]

The other vocalization that may be unique to *albiventris* is a bird-like call heard during courtship and called "the serenade."[19] It has been described as varying from a whistle to a coarse squawk. Females responded typically, with hisses, snorts, and evasive maneuvers. In virtually all incidents where adult males were placed with females the serenade was heard. It was never heard to be produced by a female, or a male in the absence of a female or situations other than courtship behavior. It was always reliably produced after the male sniffed the female hindquarters and discontinued when the females trail was lost or courtship ceased. The serenade is a relatively loud vocalization that can be heard as far away as 30 m (98 ft) or more.[19]

Taste

The hedgehogs taste sensitivity has been noted to be similar to other insectivores such as the opossum. They demonstrate a slight aversion to formic acid solutions and quinine with stronger solutions being completely rejected. They even have a "sweet-tooth." Sucrose is highly preferred except at the highest concentrations. They show less of a preference for saccharin and have a surprisingly high tolerance of and a slight preference for sodium chloride.[22]

Ingestive behavior

The hedgehog belongs to the order Insectivora but many of the species within the order appear to be more omnivorous than most other insectivores. The hedgehogs have a stronger jaw, blunter teeth, and a longer gut than the other insectivores and they have no cecum. It may in fact be more appropriate to describe them as predators, foraging for a diet made up of a huge variety of invertebrates, small vertebrates, and even carrion. Plant material is sometimes eaten but makes up a very small portion of the overall diet.[7,20] Studies of wild European hedgehogs demonstrate that they spend at least half of their time, probably more, foraging.[3] When foraging, hedgehogs walk slowly, often with their nose to the ground. They may pause occasionally to sniff the air and will dart forward rapidly to seize prey in their mouth, once it is identified. Hedgehogs can move surprisingly fast in an attempt to catch prey but many fast-moving species will be able to escape. Since hedgehogs lack canine teeth, when they do catch larger, vertebrate prey, they must gnaw and bite persistently in order to ingest them. They have been known to hold down prey with their body and their fore paws in order to eat them.[3] They have also been seen to grab and shake prey, such as mice and lizards, similarly to a dog.[13]

Hedgehogs primarily use their sense of smell to locate prey but they may also locate prey by hearing movement amongst the leaf litter on the ground. They will dig into litter, soil, and rotting wood for prey but do not appear to dig very deeply.[20]

Most dietary studies of the spiny hedgehogs have examined the diets of the European hedgehogs, *E. europaeus* and *E. concolor* and found them to be similar. These studies demonstrated that in the wild, European hedgehogs feed almost entirely on invertebrates, including beetles, caterpillars, earthworms, earwigs, mollusks, flies, centipedes, etc. It is generally believed that any plant material consumed is eaten by accident during foraging and it appears that most plant material is not digested at all.[3] However, in a study of hedgehogs in New Zealand, while it was demonstrated that their diet consisted primarily of snails and slugs, there was also evidence that the tender buds and leaves of clover were selectively eaten. This study also reported the apparent capture and eating of frogs and the eating of carrion.[23]

Hedgehogs do appear to be somewhat opportunistic in their feeding behavior. All of the studies reveal that the quantities of different food items taken varies considerably by region and season with hedgehogs consuming whichever foods are most readily available.[3] However, hedgehogs are not at all unselective. They appear to have definite dietary preferences and aversions.

Little research has been done on the natural diet of the African genus *Atelerix* in the wild but it appears that their diets are similar to the European hedgehogs.[3] The studies that have been done reveal that their diet is also quite varied and may consist of snails, centipedes, insects, some small vertebrates such as snakes, lizards, and frogs, beetles, ants, termites, grasshoppers, moths, earthworms, slugs, small rodents, eggs and chicks of ground nesting birds, crabs, vegetables, fruit, and fungi.[3,19]

African hedgehogs have thrived and reproduced on a variety of different diets in captivity, including, a mixture of ground beef, canned ZuPreem, milk, hard boiled eggs, pureed beef, and vegetable baby foods, apples and ripe bananas without peel; a mixture of commercial cat food, supplemented with small mice, crickets, and mealworms; and a mixture of commercial dry dog or cat chow, commercial cooked meat mixture (Bird of Prey Diet), a small amount of fruit and vegetables, crickets, and mealworms.[9,24,25]

A common problem of captive hedgehogs is obesity. This is complicated by the fact that their exact nutrient requirements are unknown. Hedgehogs are known to possess chitinases, so it appears that in the wild, the chitin from insects probably provides the necessary dietary fiber.[26] The typical diet of dog or cat food contains less fiber than needed and may contribute to the high incidence of obesity in captive hedgehogs. It is highly likely that the decreased activity associated with captivity also contributes to this problem.

In the wild, hedgehogs may travel 1–2 km (0.6–1.2 miles) per night foraging for food and searching for mates.[27] It has been demonstrated that in captivity hedgehogs do maintain similar feeding rhythms to those in the wild. One study found that the period of maximum feeding activity is between 1900 and 2200 hours with a second smaller peak of activity at about 0300 hours. No hedgehogs in this study fed before 1800 or after 0700 hours. In general they fed for short periods of time, feeding longer during the early evening feeding periods than during later feeding periods. The smaller the animal, the shorter the feeding periods and the more frequently they fed. The animals in this study increased their body weight by 20–50% in 9 weeks[28] demonstrating how easily hedgehogs can gain weight in captivity. The decreased amount of energy expended to eat food provided in a dish, as opposed to having to forage over 1–2 km, combined with the plentiful food presented in captivity likely leads to a calorie surplus and consequent obesity. Since dietary fat often decreases as fiber content increases, simply as a result of nutrient dilution, higher fiber diets are recommended for captive hedgehogs.[26] Captive hedgehogs should be weighed regularly so as to monitor obesity and make husbandry changes as needed to prevent extreme obesity. It is not uncommon to see hedgehogs so obese that they can no longer roll up in a ball!

Water consumption

In the wild, it is believed that hedgehogs acquire their water requirements from the insects they eat as well as the occasional consumption of droplets of water from dew, rain, or what is exuded from low growing plants.[3]

In captivity, since feeding a diet composed primarily of insects is uncommon, drinking water should be provided at all times. Many but not all hedgehogs will learn to drink from water bottles with sipper tubes.[25] Alternatively, heavy crock-style water bowls can be offered. These should be shallow enough to prevent accidental drowning and cleaned frequently as hedgehogs tend to foul them with shavings or other cage bedding materials.

Elimination behavior

Captive hedgehogs will leave their nest to defecate at any time of the day or night. One report[9] described a tendency for captive hedgehogs to eliminate in one corner of the enclosure, a tendency also noted by the author. The animals never soiled their nest box or water. Defecation occurred most often in the early evening. Animals commonly lifted their tail and placed their vent against the cage wall, leaving feces smeared about 25 mm (0.98 in.) above the floor.[9]

Body care

One interesting and unique aspect of the hedgehog family is their covering of short, sharp spines that have replaced most of the hair on their crown and back. Unlike porcupines, hedgehog spines do not break off readily and they do not bend easily. Their structure is uniquely designed to absorb shock and may be why hedgehogs appear to have evolved with little fear of heights or falling. A falling hedgehog may simply curl up and erect its spines to cushion the blow of landing.[3] One researcher noted that hedgehogs have been known to drop from heights purposely if that is the easiest method for getting down.[29] As adults, hedgehogs appear to gradually and continuously replace molting spines. However, some researchers have noted more intensive losses associated with a flush of new growth, so in certain situations, hedgehogs may undergo partial molts.[3] Nevertheless, any hedgehog noted to be losing large numbers of spines should be given a careful physical examination to rule out parasite infestation or disease.

Self-grooming usually occurs immediately after awakening and consists of a few shakes and then some licking or combing of the spines with the long rear claws. Later in the evening, after exercise, hedgehogs may also stop to groom, using their hind claws to groom their hair and flattened spines. Afterward, they may erect their spines and shake.[21] Hedgehogs are able to reach much of their body with their mouths but do not appear to spend a lot of time on personal hygiene. In fact, wild hedgehogs often carry a large number of ectoparasites and do not appear to make much effort to remove them, even when attached ticks are within easy reach.[3]

Self-anointing

Self-anointing is a behavior unique to the spiny hedgehogs and has been observed in several species.[3] The behavior is usually elicited when the animal encounters a substance with a strong smell, taste, or both. When encountering the stimulating object, the hedgehog sniffs, licks, and chews the material until it works up a frothy saliva. It then stretches its head and bends its body so as to be able to apply the foamy saliva to its spines. This can continue for quite some time as the hedgehog applies the saliva to both sides of its body and even stretches its back legs forward so it can apply the saliva to the posterior spines as well. While self-anointing, the hedgehog may seem highly absorbed in the behavior and difficult to distract. It appears to be in a state of high olfactory arousal, reminiscent of a cat encountering catnip.[3]

Many substances have been observed to elicit self-anointing including: toad skin, tobacco, perfumes and cosmetics, varnish, glue, leather and polish, wool, nylon, fish, egg, coffee, cream, a variety of different plants, dog urine and feces, and even other hedgehogs, to name a few. The substance may be one that is consumed, such as fish, slugs, or worms. It does not necessarily have to be novel.[15,20,30,31] The hedgehog in Figure 16.1 routinely self-anoints when presented with cilantro leaves which it also consumes.

The purpose of self-anointing behavior remains a mystery although many theories about its purpose exist. It has been suggested that when seen in captivity, it may be a displacement activity[20] but the fact that it has been observed in the wild, and in captive hedgehogs under such a wide variety of conditions, makes this unlikely.[32] Other purposes that have been hypothesized include camouflaging the hedgehogs' own smell to hide from predators,[32] to make the hedgehog unpalatable to predators,[33] to get rid of ectoparasites and groom the spines,[3] or as a form of sexual signaling.[32] However, none of these explanations can completely resolve the mystery.

The self-anointed hedgehog has been noted to have a very strong odor and could be noticed as far as 5–10 m (16.4–32.8 ft) away.[32] One study using a dog to find hedgehogs found that hedgehogs were always detected at a distance of about 12.5 m (41 ft) whether they had recently self-anointed or not. Hypothesizing that it might be an antipredator behavior, one researcher demonstrated that spines with toad venom on them caused uncomfortable skin irritations when jabbed onto the arms of volunteers.[33] While this might be effective, it does not explain the function of all of the other more innocuous substances that hedgehogs will also use to self-anoint. Self-anointing is not a very effective grooming behavior. Hedgehogs are usually much dirtier after self-anointing. It does not appear to be an effective way to remove ectoparasites. High ectoparasite burdens are common in wild hedgehogs and captive hedgehogs with no ectoparasites commonly self-anoint. There are far better ways to remove ectoparasites such as rolling in mud or sand. Long-eared hedgehogs (*Hemiechinus auritus*) often sand-bathe and have a much smaller ectoparasite load than other wild hedgehog species.[34] It is unlikely to be related in any way to sexual behavior since subadult and even neonatal hedgehogs as young as 15 days have been observed self-anointing.[20,24,33]

There is evidence that the foamy saliva comes into contact with the oral openings of the nasopalatine ducts leading to the Jacobson's organ. Anointed spines do provide an extremely large surface area, making them an excellent means of dispersing odor. These facts support the explanation that the act of self-anointing most likely serves as some form of personal scent marking. Potentially it could play a role in many different socio/sexual behaviors.[3] It may convey information during sexual encounters that serve to make one mate more acceptable to the other.[32] It may help to leave odor trails around a home range so that hedgehogs may avoid each other. It might also support interactions between a mother and her young. An anointed, separated, nestling may be more likely to be found by its mother and returned to the nest.[32] Further research is needed in order for us to fully understand the significance of this unusual behavior.

Hibernation and nest-building behavior

Due to the fact that in the wild hedgehogs must spend their daytime hours safely hidden, nest building is an

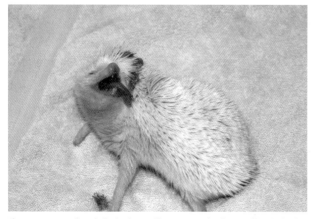

Figure 16.1 A female hedgehog self-anointing after being offered a leaf of cilantro.

important part of their behavioral repertoire. In addition, the building of an adequate nest is critical to the European hedgehog's survival during winter hibernation and to the successful rearing of a litter of young by any female hedgehog. In the wild, hedgehogs build most of their nests at ground level under brambles or other vegetation that contribute to the support of the "roof." Nests can also be found in rock crevices, hollow tree trunks, under the floors of old buildings, and even barn attics. A relatively few hedgehogs may dig shallow burrows but they are more likely to take over an abandoned rabbit burrow.[35] The hedgehog builds it nest by picking up material such as leaves, twigs, or hay in its mouth and arranging them in a pile. Once the pile is large enough to fill the space under some ground vegetation, the hedgehog enters the center of the pile and rotates it body several times until the leaves are compacted into firm walls.[36] Hedgehog nests may vary in their degree of sturdiness and permanence depending on whether they are summer nests, winter nests for hibernation, winter nests in extremely cold latitudes or more temperate latitudes, or if they are for raising young.[21,36,37]

The captive hedgehog attempting to make a nest without benefit of supporting vegetation performs similar maneuvers. He/she will pile the available materials one upon the other and walk around in a circle in the middle of the pile forming a slight cup shape. If the pile is high and stable enough, the hedgehog may also walk into the middle of the pile and turn around repeatedly making a nest within the pile of material. Captive hedgehogs will use a variety of materials provided for nest making. They will tear newspapers or paper towels by standing on them, grasping an edge in their mouth and twisting their head from side to side until a piece of the paper tears loose. They will repeat this as needed and use the pieces to form their nest.[21]

If simply provided with a few soft materials, captive hedgehog will often choose to sleep on top of them and typically, they turn around several times before lying down.[21] When not hibernating, hedgehogs usually sleep lying on their sides, only partially curled up with their head and legs extended.[3]

The nest-building behavior of the African hedgehogs has apparently not been well documented but it is likely that they use similar motor patterns to form nests appropriate to the environmental conditions and with whatever materials are typical to the area. There is no indication that A. albiventris hibernates[19] so their nests may not be as elaborate or robust as the nests of hedgehogs in less temperate climates.

Cold temperatures require that an animal expend more energy staying warm and this obviously requires an increase in calorie consumption. Since food availability is also usually decreased when temperatures drop, hibernation is the adaptation that allows an animal to survive this challenging period. Most species of hedgehogs, when exposed to lowered temperatures, will hibernate or enter torpor.

In fact low ambient temperatures appear to be the most important factor for inducing torpor in E. europaeus but decreasing food availability may also play a role. Photoperiod changes alone are usually insufficient.[38] Hibernation and energetics in the European hedgehog are well documented elsewhere so will not be covered in detail here.[3]

When housing A. albiventris, temperatures should not be allowed to fall below 25°C (75°F) as it may lead to an increased susceptibility to respiratory infections. At temperatures under 18°C (65°F) animals are likely to enter torpor, further increasing their chance of illness.[25]

Locomotion

Hedgehogs usually amble along with a waddling walk or trot, with their spines directed backward (Figure 16.2). Dimelow noted that when his captive hedgehogs were allowed out to exercise they walked at a human pace and so were easily followed. He also noted a tendency for them to explore while staying at the base of walls as is common for rodents.[21] Hedgehogs are capable of moving rapidly and have been known to run up to 2 m/sec (6.5 ft/sec). Hedgehogs can also climb and are able swimmers.[39] However, the smaller feet and less developed claws of the African hedgehogs make them poorer climbers than their European relatives.[7]

Defensive behavior

The spines of the hedgehog are just one important feature of its defensive behavior. Each spine is erected by its own erector muscle (smooth muscle) which originates in deeper layers of striated muscle. When a hedgehog is first confronted with a threat, it erects its spines and freezes momentarily. The erected spines interlock and bristle in different direction, forming an imposing, impenetrable layer of points. If the threat is not too close, the hedgehog may try to flee, otherwise it will remain frozen, crouch down,

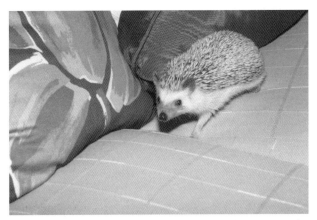

Figure 16.2 A relaxed hedgehog explores when allowed exercise outside of its cage.

and pull its forehead muscle, the fronto-dorsalis, down over its forehead so as to cover its face with bristling spines (see Figure 16.3). This reflex action is likely to also occur in response to any high pitched noise and can happen quite rapidly (less than 0.01 seconds).[17] In this position, the hedgehog may also huff and flinch, bucking its back upward to jab at the perceived predator. Many researchers have referred to this as "boxing."[3] Nestling and juvenile hedgehogs are especially likely to utilize this form of defensive behavior before they are capable of rolling up completely.

If the threat escalates to actual physical contact, then the hedgehog will bring its legs inward, under its body and curl its head ventrally. The dorsal skin and associated muscles are flexible and loose. The dermal muscle, known as the panniculosus carnosus, is thickened around the edge to form a special circular muscle called the orbicularis. When the hedgehog rolls up, these muscles drop down over the face and rump and the orbicularis muscle is contracted like a purse string to seal the hedgehogs' soft underside, face and feet inside the spiny ball[40] (see Figure 16.4). Several specialized modifications to the intervertebral disks and vertebral processes also contribute to making this feat

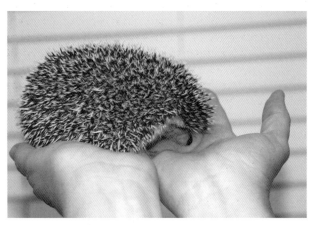

Figure 16.3 A defensive hedgehog with erected spines and its fronto-dorsalis muscle pulled over its face.

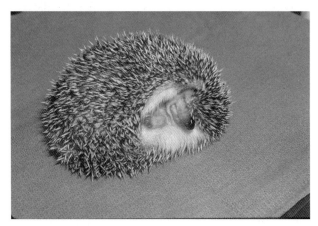

Figure 16.4 A defensive hedgehog rolled-up into a ball.

possible. The behavior is primarily voluntary with mostly striated muscle involved, but the presence of the smooth muscle and the rapidity with which the hedgehog flinches in response to sound suggests that there may be an involuntary component to the behavior as well.[40]

Social behavior

Hedgehogs are primarily solitary animals that spend their evenings foraging and looking for mates and their days sleeping underground or in nests constructed in protected cavities. They have large, overlapping home ranges and thus far, there has been no evidence to suggest that they defend an exclusive territory.[27,41–44] No territorial behaviors such as scent marking with feces, urine, or scent glands have ever been observed.[3,41] Agonistic interactions between females have never been observed in the wild.[3,43] When adult male hedgehogs encounter each other, they are likely to behave aggressively; snorting, "boxing," and attempting to bite each other's spines and skin. However, other reports of hedgehogs encountering each other in the wild noted that the hedgehogs simply sat nose-to-nose and snorted at each other.[21] When hedgehogs are still young (under 3–4 months of age) meetings are more likely to result in nosing, licking, and trying to crawl under each other while snorting occasionally. Until sexual maturity, captive hedgehogs have even been seen sleeping on their sides next to one another.[21] The defensive behavior of curling up in a ball is not seen when hedgehogs encounter conspecifics.[21]

Most studies of European hedgehogs find that the home ranges of reproductively active males are significantly larger than those of females and subadults, and tend to overlap the home ranges of several females.[27,42,43] Home ranges, defined by most as the area familiar to the individual and used most regularly, vary greatly in size. Male home ranges as large as 32–40 ha (79–99 acres) have been documented. This is about three times the documented home range of females and younger males, whose home ranges are about 10–12 ha (25–30 acres).[27,41] In general, adult males travel widely in an apparent attempt to cross the home ranges of as many females as possible, with some males traveling upward of 1–2 km (0.6–1.2 miles) nightly.[41] The record is 3.14 km (1.9 mi) in a single night![27] Adult females average about 1 km (0.6 mi) per night.[27]

Males are apparently capable of covering these great distances because they walk faster than females. The average speed of the male hedgehog is 3.73 m/min (12.24 ft/min). The female's average speed is 2.19 m/min (7.19 ft/min).[41] Males have been seen on occasion to travel at speeds greater than 30 m/min (98 ft). In one study, a male hedgehog was observed to cross a 60 m (65.6 yds) fairway in about 1 minute and this did not appear to be in response to a fearful stimulus.[41]

Hedgehogs in the wild utilize different nests each night, rarely using the same nest twice.[27,41] On only a few occasions have they been seen sharing nests.[43] However, one researcher housed *A. albiventris* (adults, juveniles, and young) together without aggression and noted that the animals frequently slept together with their bodies touching[9] (see Figure 16.5). In a study of captive European hedgehogs, some nest sharing was common and attempts to return individuals to their own nests were ineffective as they would soon return to sharing a nest with their cagemate![36]

It has been suggested that the hedgehog social structure might be most closely compared to the cat.[3] They have overlapping home ranges that they do not defend. They cohabitate; probably using individual olfactory cues and a system of mutual avoidance.

Some authors have suggested that hedgehogs can be safely housed in groups as long as no more than one male is in the group.[24,25] Another author successfully housed hedgehogs at a density of 1 animal per 5 square meter (54 sq ft) using groups of three females to one male. He did, however, report that on occasion, injuries due to fights did occur.[45] In a study of rehabilitated group-housed hedgehogs awaiting release, it was reported that 8 of 13 had cuts, abrasions, abscesses, or evidence of recently healed injuries that were believed to be due to bite wounds. The report, however, did not include the details of housing so the population density of the captive hedgehogs in this case is unknown.[46]

Those wishing to house multiple captive hedgehogs should simply be aware that aggression between conspecifics can be a problem. Population densities of European hedgehogs during the summer have been documented at one to three animals per hectare (1–3/2.4 acre).[27,37,41] Without more research into the housing of captive hedgehogs it is impossible to know exactly how much space is needed for group-housed animals to avoid confrontation. Using the feline example again, it should simply be recommended that a group of captive hedgehogs should be given as much space as possible. Making the environment rich in resources such as shelters, feeding stations, water bottles, and exercise wheels may allow the animals to avoid

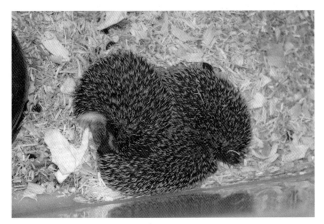

Figure 16.5 Three sibling hedgehogs sleeping together.

each other if and when they so desire, and thus decrease the likelihood of intraspecific aggression.

Housing

Hedgehogs have been kept in a variety of types and sizes of housing including wire mesh pens, glass aquariums, pet carriers, and metal rabbit cages.[45] The most important criteria, after space, is that the pens be made of smooth materials in which the animal cannot get its toes or limbs caught. Housing must be constructed such that hedgehogs cannot climb out. If housed outdoors, walls should be buried about 1 foot (30 cm) underground to prevent hedgehogs from burrowing out.

Bedding material should be soft and absorbent but cloth or towels should be avoided since loose strings can be dangerous if ingested or caught on toes or toenails. Newspapers and wood shavings are both good choices. Abundant nesting material should be available. While hedgehogs will use the newspapers and wood shavings for nests, facial tissues and paper towels are also safe materials that can be added to the enclosure for nest building.

Cage accessories should include heavy crockery dishes for food and water (or sipper bottles for water), shelters for sleeping, and an exercise wheel. Shelters can be any material that can be sanitized, such as plastic, or cardboard boxes that can be disposed of when soiled. Typical rodent exercise wheels with metal bars on the running surface should be avoided because the feet of hedgehogs can fall through and be injured. Large plastic wheels with more solid running surfaces are now available and make excellent wheels for hedgehogs (see Figure 16.6).

Environmental temperatures should be maintained between 25°C and 30°C (75–85°F).[24,25]

Reproductive behavior

European hedgehogs reach sexual maturity on average at about 9–11 months of age.[30] However, body weight may be the best predictor of sexual maturity. In one study of captive, European hedgehogs, most females did not become pregnant while weighing less than 600 g (21.1 oz) and most weighed more than 700 g (24.7 oz) before becoming pregnant for the first time.[47] Sexual maturity in most African hedgehog species occurs much earlier, between 61 and 68 days in both males and females.[13] Sexually mature adult's weights range between 205 and 224 g (7.2–7.9 oz).[24] However, one study of *A. albiventris* in the wild found that weights varied widely amongst adults so may not be a good way to estimate age in this species.[19]

In the Northern Hemisphere, European hedgehog females come out of anestrus in late March. The peak of male spermatogenesis occurs from April to late August.[45] Sexual behavior is first seen in late April and it peaks in mid-May and again in late June/early July.[41,43]

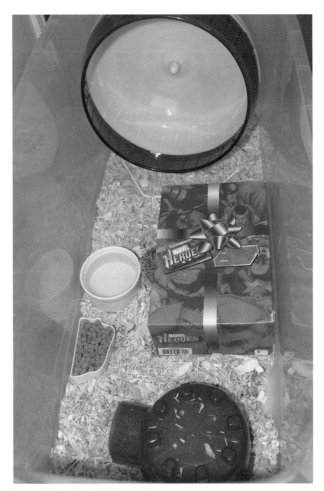

Figure 16.6 A suitable habitat for a pet hedgehog.

African hedgehogs appear to be sexually active throughout the year.[24,25] More recently, it has been suggested that, similar to other insectivores, *A. albiventris* appears to be an induced ovulator.[48]

All species of hedgehogs that have been studied have been determined to be promiscuous and polygamous.[42,43] Courtship can be a noisy and lengthy affair, often lasting for over an hour[49] but does not always result in copulation so some mate selection appears to be at work.[42] European hedgehog males have been observed to court several different females, some repeatedly (although not on the same night), and some females were seen to be courted by as many as 10 different males. However, in one study of European hedgehogs, only 5 of 76 observed courtships ended in copulation.[42] A female may on occasion copulate with more than one male before a vaginal plug forms so some sperm competition may also occur. Due to the presence of the vaginal plug, mate guarding is not necessary and has never been observed in hedgehogs.[3]

When a male hedgehog approaches a female, he begins circling her, sniffing, and snorting. She may act as if frightened and lower her spines over her forehead, erect her spines, and snort loudly. She may even occasionally butt him while snorting almost continuously. He may shove and butt at her, sometimes with his mouth open and tongue extended as if gaping or demonstrating flehmen. Both hedgehogs may then circle each other, snorting loudly, squealing, and nipping at each other's spines. They may also urinate and defecate.[3,24]

If and when courtship results in copulation, the female stops and presses her belly to the ground exposing her genitalia. The female may also raise her head and arch her back into the classic position of "lordosis." The male then mounts from behind using his forepaws to grasp her spines and often grasps the spines over her neck with his teeth. The male may remain mounted for 1–4 minutes, copulating multiple times; each copulation consisting of 10–11 rapid thrusts.[3]

It has not been well documented how long hedgehogs remain capable of reproducing. One report of captive African hedgehogs found that after 2 years females stopped reproducing. However, one wild caught female remained reproductively active for 33 months.[24]

Maternal behavior

Female hedgehogs are very attentive mothers but males do not participate in the rearing of the youngsters at all.[3] In fact, females should be separated from the males near the time of parturition as males have been known to eat newborn hedgehogs.[50,51] However, many captive female hedgehogs will cannibalize their entire litter if disturbed during or shortly after parturition.[24,25] In captivity, the mortality rates of captive born hedgehogs may be as high as 25%. Mortality rates of newborns in the wild are not that much better: it has been calculated that 20% of wild-born hedgehogs may die before weaning.[52] Nevertheless, when breeding hedgehogs in captivity, it has been recommended that the dam and newborn litter should not be disturbed prior to about 7 days post-parturition.[45,47] However, others have noted that if females are used to regular handling, they are less likely to cannibalize their young.[25,53] Some individual females are simply more tolerant of disturbance than others. Female hedgehogs with young can be surprisingly aggressive. One of the few times when a female hedgehog is likely to bite is when she has a litter of babies. She may hiss and snort and come out of the nest to attack if disturbed.[25] This behavior may be seen to a lesser degree in females who are habituated to human handling and regular disturbance.

The gestation period of most hedgehog species ranges from 28 to 40 days (average 35 days in *E. europaeus* and *A. albiventris*).[9,45] If the exact date of mating is uncertain, it can be very difficult to determine, merely by visual inspection, if a female is pregnant. Mammary gland development may be subtle and thorough palpation requires anesthesia. In general, if weekly weight checks reveal that a female has gained more than 50 g (1.7 oz) within 3 weeks of having access to a male, then she is probably pregnant.[53]

When parturition is pending, the female hedgehog will gather available material in her mouth and use it to make a nest for herself and her offspring.[21] Many females will not feed the night prior to parturition.[47] Once young are born, females will continue to feed at night and spend the days in their nest caring for their young.[3,52] Young of *E. europaeus* have been reportedly born most often during the night.[47] Whereas, reports of *A. albiventris* claim the young are usually born during the day.[9]

Hedgehog births are rarely witnessed since in the wild they usually occur underground or hidden from view in a nest. However, on the few occasions where captive births have been witnessed, the female hedgehog lays on her side or belly with her legs extended. She may shift position frequently and lick her genitalia periodically. She strains with each contraction that may last several seconds. After each birth, she severs the umbilical cord, consumes the placenta and birth fluids and in the process, licks the neonate clean (*pers. obs.*).[9,13,54] In captivity, she may move around the enclosure between births (*pers. obs.*) and the birth of the litter may take several minutes to hours. Fortunately, difficult births, requiring assistance, are uncommon.

If a litter of hedgehogs is removed from the dam or they die soon after birth she will return to a postpartum estrus rapidly and usually will become pregnant again on that cycle.[45]

The average litter size of *A. albiventris* is three.[9,24,45] Litter sizes of the European hedgehogs are somewhat larger with 4–5 being common.[37,45,49] Average birth weights of *E. europaeus* in captivity range from 8 to 22 g (0.28–0.77 oz) with an average of 15 g (0.52 oz).[47] Weights of newborn *A. albiventris* ranging from 5 to 11 g (0.17–0.38 oz) have been recorded with an average of 10 g (0.35 oz).[9,53] Baby African hedgehogs should gain an average of 2–3 g (0.07–0.1 oz) per day during the first few weeks of life. Increases of 4–5 g (0.14–0.17 oz) per day should then continue from the third or fourth week up until weaning.[53]

Hedgehogs are altricial animals. They are born pink and naked with eyes closed and pinnae sealed tightly.[3,9,54] Their skin is edematous and covered with small bumps like the warts of a toad. Within a few hours of birth, the skin appears to "deflate" and flexible, soft white spines begin to emerge from the bumps. Within 24 hours, the full length of these first spines should be apparent (about 7 mm (0.27 in.) long in *Erinaceus* and 4.9–5.5 mm (0.19–0.21 in.) in *Atelerix*).[3,9]

Fur development is more varied among species but most hedgehogs have a covering of short fur by the time they are 2 weeks old. However, *A. albiventris* babies have been noted to have some hair on their abdomen as early as a day of age.[9]

Newly born hedgehogs can vocalize loudly at birth. They can crawl, pull themselves around using their front limbs, and flip themselves over from their dorsum to their ventrum.[9]

They typically nurse while lying on their backs and begin nursing soon after birth.[53] Within 12–24 hours,[9,54] the baby hedgehogs can walk and mothers will return a straying, vocalizing baby to the nest by carrying it in her mouth until it is about 4 weeks of age.[3]

Within 24 hours, startled baby hedgehogs can partially curl up their bodies to protect their faces by pulling down their forehead spines, chirp in alarm, and "box."[9,21,24] By 2–3 weeks of age, the baby hedgehog can roll up completely when alarmed.[24]

By about 15 days of age, hedgehog's eyes and ears open and by about 21–25 days of age, they are eating solid food.[9,47] In the wild, young hedgehogs typically suckle for 3–4 weeks, then begin leaving the nest regularly to forage with their mother.[47] In one population of captive hedgehogs, the oldest young ever observed still suckling was 44 days of age.[47] Typically, in captive-bred hedgehogs weaning will begin at 4–6 weeks of age[53] and most young hedgehogs are fully weaned by 40–44 days.[47] However, some may be weaned as late as 10 weeks.[49]

Cross-fostering of abandoned or orphaned hedgehogs is usually successful as long as the mother's young are of a similar size to the baby being fostered.[47,53] In fact, when female hedgehogs are housed in groups, they have been observed to feed and care for each other's offspring.[53]

Weight amongst young hedgehogs of different species varies considerably. Weaning weights of young *E. europaeus* at 40 days range from 125 to 345 g (4.4–12.2 oz).[47] Weaning weights of 170–195 g (5.9–6.9 oz) have been recorded in young *A. albiventris*.[55]

Common behavior problems

"Unfriendliness" or "Aggression"

Few behavior problems have been reported in pet hedgehogs to date. The most common complaint by owners, in the author's experience, is a lack of tameness, often referred to by pet owners as aggression. In these situations, owners often complain that their hedgehog puffs and snorts, rolls into a ball, and pokes them with its quills when they attempt to handle it. This is normal defensive behavior and these hedgehogs have either never been habituated to human handling or are simply not handled often enough in a rewarding manner for them to remain habituated. If they are taken out rarely and these events are fear inducing, then while the owner may think they are taming their hedgehogs, they may in fact be sensitizing them to handling (see Chapter 18 for more information on these processes).

Dimelow noted that within a few days of capture, wild hedgehogs (*E. europaeus*) would stop rolling into a ball when handled.[21] In the author's experience, "tameability" or "friendliness" of hedgehogs varies greatly between individuals. It is possible that this may reflect a difference in

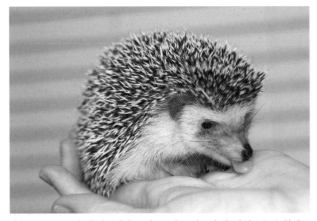

Figure 16.7   A hedgehog licking the author's hand. This behavior is likely to be followed by a bite so when this hedgehog began licking, it was simply placed back onto the ground.

the amount of handling that a hedgehog received when very young, or may even have a genetic component (i.e., "friendly" parents have "friendly" offspring and "unfriendly" parents have "unfriendly" offspring?). However, until further research is performed on development and temperament in hedgehogs, we must simply assume that a hedgehog resistant to handling may be made more tolerant through desensitization and/or counterconditioning procedures as described in Chapter 18. The author's pet hedgehogs took insects quite voraciously when offered, so mealworms were a treat that could be used effectively to teach the hedgehogs that good things happened when they were approached and handled by humans. Every hedgehog may have different preferred foods, so caretakers may have to try several different food items to determine which the hedgehog seems most fond of. Once that item has been identified, it can be used in very small amounts for desensitization and counter conditioning.

Hedgehogs rarely bite in an attempt to stop handling or escape. However, the author has noted that hedgehogs will often lick fingers several times and then if the hand is not withdrawn, they often bite (see Figure 16.7). While this never drew blood and rarely, left a mark, it could be startling and clearly, many pet owners will not want this experience! It is likely that this behavior is purely investigatory and it may be more likely to occur if fingers smell remotely of food. However, if using food items to tame or train the hedgehog, they will likely learn to approach fingers expecting food. Therefore, it is not recommended that you present fingers to the hedgehog when not offering food and once the food is offered, the hand should be withdrawn. In this manner, hedgehogs can often be lured onto one hand while holding a treat in the other. Once they accept the treat, the hand they are standing on can be carefully withdrawn from the cage while the hedgehog consumes the treat. While in the process of desensitizing and counterconditioning, it will be important to decrease

the amount of food fed during regular feeding, in direct proportion to the amount used as rewards so that training does not lead to obesity.

While hedgehogs can be tamed to accept regular handling, it is not known if they appreciate stroking or scratching, as other pets might, so they are probably a pet best enjoyed by simply observing them in their provided habitat. Nevertheless, desensitizing them to a certain amount of human handling will result in an animal that is less stressed when being removed for trips to the veterinarian, cage cleanings, etc. and may be important to ensuring that the animal experiences good welfare.

Nocturnal behavior

After acquiring a nocturnal species as a pet, many people discover that the nocturnal behavior can be disturbing and some people are disappointed to find that the pet will not be awake and interactive during daylight hours when most pet owners wish to interact with their pet. Fortunately, it has been noted that hedgehogs in captivity seem to display a more varied routine. One study noted that shifts in body position, location within the cage, and even awakening to eat and eliminate during the day were common in captive hedgehogs.[9] By feeding and handling hedgehogs during the daylight hours, we may be able to increase the flexibility of their schedule without undue stress. Hedgehogs that do continue to be active during the night should simply have their habitat removed to an area of the house where they will not disturb people.

Handling

Even the tamest hedgehog may resist handling when the time comes for a physical examination, toenail trim, or other veterinary procedure. Heavy leather gloves can be used to carefully pick up the hedgehog. A plastic slotted spoon has also proved useful for gently scooping a rolled-up hedgehog from a cage. If the hedgehog is used to being handled, it is often possible to use one hand to stroke it gently and then slowly grasp the quills and skin on the sides and back over the shoulder, scruffing it, similarly to what one might do with a cat (see Figure 16.8). Once scruffed, the hedgehog can be given a brief exam and some will tolerate nail trimming while in this position. The author has found this technique to be most effective in hedgehogs that have been well habituated to handling.

Some hedgehogs will roll into a ball when frightened, and remain that way, making it very difficult to examine them. Different authors have described a variety of methods for "unrolling" the frightened hedgehog.[3,25,56] Placing the rolled-up hedgehog into a shallow pan of warm water (3–5 cm so that the hedgehogs' nose and mouth will remain above water) will often entice it to unroll. Some hedgehogs will allow their hind limbs to be gently

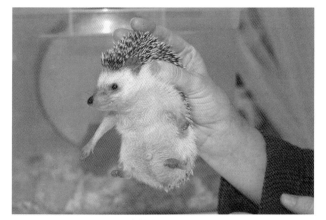

Figure 16.8   Scruffing a relatively tame hedgehog.

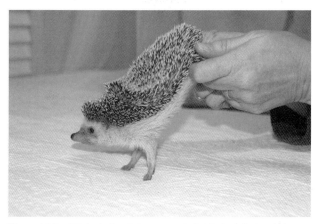

Figure 16.9   This hedgehog is tame enough that its back feet could be gently grasped and lifted. While attempting to maintain its hold on the ground with its front feet, it did not try to roll up.

grasped as they walk along the exam table. Once grasped, the hedgehog can be quickly lifted so that its front feet are forced to grasp for the table surface. Many hedgehogs, while attempting to gain a foothold, will remain unrolled (see Figure 16.9). However, some hedgehogs will still manage to roll up into a ball. When using this technique, it is important to not dangle the hedgehog for more than a few seconds without some degree of support for its front feet, as this seems very distressing to some individuals. In most cases, complete anesthesia is the most humane way of performing a thorough physical exam and most other procedures on the hedgehog.

Acknowledgments

Photos in this chapter courtesy of M. C. Tynes, copyright 2010.

References

1. Nowak RM. *Walker's Mammals of the World*. 5th ed. Baltimore and London: John Hopkins Press, 1991;114–122.

2. Morris PA. Nightly movements of hedgehogs (*Erinaceus europaeus*) in a forest edge habitat. *Mammalia* 1986;50:395–398.

3. Reeve NR. *Hedgehogs*. London: T&AD Poyser Natural History, 1994.

4. Easton ER. Observations on the distribution of the hedgehog (*Erinaceus albiventris*) in Tanzania. *Afr J Ecol* 1979;17:175–176.

5. Gregory M. Notes on the Central African hedgehog, *Erinaceus albiventris* in the Nairobi area. *E Afr Wildl J* 1976;14:177–179.

6. Corbett GB. The family Erinaceidae: A synthesis of its taxonomy, phylogeny, ecology and zoogeography. *Mamm Rev* 1988;18:117–172.

7. Herter K. The insectivores. In: Grzimek, ed. *Grzimek's Animal Life Encyclopedia*. New York: Van Nostrand Reinhold, 1968;176–257. (Cited in Reeve NR. *Hedgehogs*. London: T&AD Poyser Natural History, 1994.)

8. Fons R. Insectivores. In: Parker S, ed. *Grzimek's Encyclopedia of Mammals*. Vol. 1. New York: McGraw-Hill Publishing, 1990;425–472.

9. Merrit DA. Husbandry, reproduction and behavior of the West African hedgehog (*Erinaceus albiventris*) at Lincoln Park Zoo. *Int Zoo Ybk* 1981;21:128–131.

10. Carpenter JW. Hedgehogs. In: Carpenter JW, ed. *Exotic Animal Formulary*. 3rd ed. Missouri: Elsevier Saunders, 2005;369.

11. Heatley JJ, Mauldin GE, Cho, DY. A review of neoplasia in the captive African hedgehog (*Atelerix albiventris*). *Semin Avian Exotic Pet Med* 2005;14:182–192.

12. Bridges CDB, Quilliam TA. Visual pigments of men, moles and hedgehogs. *Vision Res* 1973;13:2417–2421.

13. Herter K. *Hedgehogs: A Comprehensive Study*. Phoenix House, 1965. (Cited in Reeve NR. *Hedgehogs*. London: T&AD Poyser Natural History, 1994.)

14. Bretting H. Die Bestimmung der Riechschwellen bei Igeln (*Erinaceus europaeus L.*) für einige Fettsäuren. *Z Säugetierk* 1972;37:286–311. (Cited in Reeve NR. *Hedgehogs*. London: T&AD Poyser Natural History, 1994.)

15. Lindeman W. Zur Psychologie des Igels. *Z Tierpsychol* 1951;8:224–251. (Cited in Reeve NR. *Hedgehogs*. London: T&AD Poyser Natural History, 1994.)

16. Wysocki CJ, Beauchamp GK, Reidinger RR et al. Access of large and nonvolatile molecules to the vomeronasal organ of mammals during social and feeding behaviors. *J Chem Ecol* 1985;11:1147–1159.

17. Chang Hsiang-Tung. An auditory reflex of the hedgehog. *Chinese J Physiol* 1936;10:119–124.

18. Attié C. Emission sonores chez le Hérisson européen *Erinaceus europaeus*, et signification comportmentale. *Mammalia* 1990;54:3–12. (Cited in Reeve NR. *Hedgehogs*. London: T&AD Poyser Natural History, 1994.)

19. Gregory M. Observations on vocalizations in the Central African hedgehog (*Erinaceus albiventris*) including a courtship call. *Mammalia* 1975;39:1–7.

20. Burton M. *The Hedgehog*. London: Andre Deutsch, 1969. (Cited in Reeve NR. *Hedgehogs*. London: T&AD Poyser Natural History, 1994.)

21. Dimelow EJ. The behavior of the hedgehog (*Erinaceus europaeus L.*) in the routine of life in captivity. *Proc Zool Soc Lond* 1963;141:281–289.

22. Ganchrow JR. Consummatory responses to taste stimuli in the hedgehog (*Erinaceus europaeus*). *Physiol and Behav* 1977;18:447–453.

23. Brockie RE. Observations on the food of the hedgehog (*Erinaceus europaeus*) in New Zealand. *N Z J Sci* 1959;2:121–136.

24. Brodie ED III, Brodie ED Jr., Johnson JA. Breeding the African hedgehog *Atelerix pruneri* in captivity. *Int Zoo Ybk* 1982;22:195–197.

25. Smith AJ. Husbandry and medicine of African hedgehogs (*Atelerix albiventris*). *J Sm Ex Anim Med* 1992;2:21–28.

26. Graffam WS, Fitzpatrick MP, Dierenfeld DS. Fiber digestion in the African white-bellied hedgehog (*Atelerix albiventris*): A preliminary evaluation. *J Nutr* 1998;128:2671S–2673S.

27. Morris PA. A study of home range and movements in the hedgehog. *J Zool Lond* 1988;214:433–449.

28. Campbell PA. Feeding rhythms of caged hedgehogs (*Erinaceus europaeus*). *Proc N Z Ecol Soc* 1975;22:14–18.

29. Harrison Matthews L. *British Mammals*. London: Collins, 1952. (Cited in Reeve NR. *Hedgehogs*. London: T&AD Poyser Natural History, 1994.)

30. Herter K. Das Verhalten der Insektivoren. *Handb Zool* 1956;8:Chapter 10. (Cited in Reeve NR. *Hedgehogs*. London: T&AD Poyser Natural History, 1994.)

31. Burton M. Hedgehog self-anointing. *Proc Zool Soc Lond* 1957; 129:452–453.

32. Brockie R. Self-anointing by wild hedgehog (*Erinaceus europaeus*) in New Zealand. *Anim Behav* 1976;24:68–71.

33. Brodie ED. Hedgehogs use toad venom in their own defense. *Nature* 1977;268:627–628.

34. Schoenfeld M, Yom-Tov Y. The biology of two species of hedgehog, *Erinaceus europaeus concolor* and *Hemiechinus auritus aegyptius*, in Israel. *Mammalia* 1985;49:339–355.

35. Reeve NJ, Morris PA. Construction and use of summer nests by the hedgehog (*Erinaceus europaeus*). *Mammalia* 1985;49:187–194.

36. Morris P. Winter nests of the hedgehog (*Erinaceus europaeus L*). *Oecologia* (Berlin) 1973;11:299–313.

37. Parkes J. Some aspects of the biology of the hedgehog (*Erinaceus europaeus L*) in the Manawatu, New Zealand. *N Z J Zool* 1975; 2:463–472.

38. Fowler PA. Thermoregulation in the female hedgehog, *Erinaceous europaeus*, during the breeding season. *J Reprod Fert* 1988; 82:285–292.

39. Wroot, A. Hedgehogs. In: MacDonald D, ed. *The Encyclopedia of Mammals*. New York: Facts on File Publications, 1984;750–757.

40. Gupta BB. Investigations of the rolling mechanism in the Indian hedgehog. *J Mammal* 1961;42:365–371.

41. Reeve NJ. The home range of the hedgehog as revealed by a radio tracking study. *Symp Zool Soc Lond* 1982;49;207–230.

42. Reeve NJ, Morris PA. Mating strategy in the hedgehog (*Erinaceus europaeus*). *J Zool Lond* 1986;210:613–614.

43. Riber, AB. Habitat use and behaviour of European hedgehog *Erinaceus europaeus* in a Danish rural area. *Acta Theriol* 2006; 51:363–371.

44. Dmi'el R, Shwarz M. Hibernation patterns and energy expenditure in hedgehogs from semi-arid and temperate habitats. *J Comp Physiol B* 1984;155:117–123.

45. Morris B. Some observations on the breeding season of the hedgehog and the rearing and handling of the young. *Proc Zool Soc Lond* 1961; 136:201–206.

46. Sainsbury AW, Cunningham AA, Morris PA et al. Health and welfare of rehabilitated juvenile hedgehogs (*Erinaceus europaeus*) before and after release into the wild. *Vet Rec* 1996;138:61–65.

47. Morris B. Breeding the European hedgehog *Erinaceus europaeus* in captivity. *Int Zoo Ybk* 1966;6:141–146.

48. Bedford JM, Mock OB, Nagdas SK et al. Reproductive characteristics of the African pygmy hedgehog, *Atelerix albiventris*. *J Reprod Fert* 2000;120:143–150.

49. Jackson DB. The breeding biology of introduced hedgehogs (*Erinaceus europaeus*) on a Scottish Island: Lessons for population control and bird conservation. *J Zool* 2006;268:303–314.

50. Ranson RM. New laboratory animals from wild species. Breeding a laboratory stock of hedgehogs (*Erinaceus europaeus L*.) *J Hyg Camb* 1941;41:131–138.

51. Prakash I. Cannibalism in hedgehogs. *J Bombay Nat Hist Soc* 1955; 52:922–923.

52. Morris PA. Pre-weaning mortality in the hedgehog (*Erinaceus europaeus*). *J Zool* 1977;182:162–167.

53. Smith AJ. Neonatology of the hedgehog, (*Atelerix albiventris*). *J Sm Ex Anim Med* 1995;3:15–18.

54. Gupta BB, Sharma HL. Birth and early development of Indian hedgehogs. *J Mammal* 1961;42:398–399.

55. Lienhardt G. Beobachtungen zur Morphologie, Judentwicklung und zum Verhalten von Weibauchigeln Erinaceus albiventris (*Atelerix pruneri* [Wagner 1841]) in Gefangenschaft. *Säugetier Mitt* 1982;30:251–259. (Cited in Reeve NR. *Hedgehogs*. London: T&AD Poyser Natural History, 1994.)

56. Johnson-Delaney CA. Other small mammals. In: Meredtih A, Redrode S, eds. *BSAVA Manual of Exotic Pets*. Gloucester: BSAVA, 2002;102–112.

17
Sugar gliders

Jennifer L. Sobie

The sugar glider (*Petaurus breviceps*) is a small, nocturnal, social marsupial endemic to the open woodland forests of the eastern and northern coasts of Australia and north to New Guinea.[1] The common name "sugar glider" is fittingly descriptive of two of *Petaurus breviceps*' unique and defining features: a sugar glider's primary means of distance locomotion is gliding—they possess gliding patagium membranes that extend between their fore and hind limbs and are able to soar from treetop or branch to a lower target sometimes hundreds of feet distant—and, although they're omnivorous, their preferred food is sweet sap and nectar of eucalyptus, acacia, and gum trees.[2]

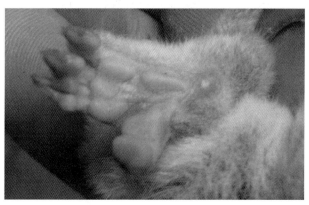

Figure 17.1 The plantar side of the syndactylous second and third digit of the sugar glider.

The sugar glider

A member of the family Petauridae and the genus *Petaurus*, the sugar glider is one of eleven petaurid possum species[3] and shares certain distinctive physical attributes with other family members, including dark-striped facial and dorsal markings and unique hind foot structure. The hind feet have five digits, the first of which is large, clawless and opposable, and similar to many other marsupials, including those in the *Phalanger* genus, the second and third digits are syndactylous (Figures 17.1 and 17.2). The syndactylous digits each retain a nail, and the resulting structure is used as a grooming tool. Their fourth digit is somewhat elongated and used in part to extract insects from bark.[4] The forefeet also have five digits each, the first of which is opposable, but none are syndactylous and all five terminate in a sharp, curved claw.[5] In addition, like many other marsupials, petuarids have distinctive dentition. They have diprotodont incisors, two developed incisor teeth at the front of their lower jaw and no lower canines, and brachyodont, bunodont molars, which are low, rounded cusps for grinding. The incisors are large and project slightly forward, and sugar gliders use

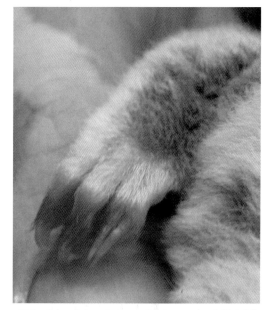

Figure 17.2 A dorsal view of a sugar glider's second and third digit.

them to gnaw into bark in search of exudates and insects. They then rely on their rounded molars to crush the arthropods and extract the nutrients.[6]

Also unique to petuarid marsupials is their gliding patagia. They look superficially very similar to flying squirrels, but the similarity is a stunning case of convergent evolution because the two species are not related. In fact, the physical structuring of their patagia is completely different. The sugar glider has a well-developed tibiocarpalis muscle in the most lateral portion of each patagium rather than styliform cartilage like the flying squirrel.[7] Glider patagia in sugar gliders stretch from the fifth finger of their forelimbs back to the first toe of their hind feet—wrist to ankle—earning them the nickname "wrist-gliders" or "wrist-winged gliders."

The pelage of a healthy sugar glider living in captivity is soft and gray. Those in the wild have a brownish tinge from life in their native eucalypt forests. As mentioned, sugar gliders have a black dorsal body stripe that runs from between their eyes to the base of their tail. Their tail—accounting for about half of their total length of 320–420 mm (12.5–16.5 in.)[5]—is furred similarly to their body and the last couple of inches is black. They are a pale cream ventrally, and their facial pelage is cream or silver. Their features—eyes, pinnae, and muzzle—are outlined in black or in the gray of their body coat, giving them a striking appearance.

Sugar gliders have a paedomorphic appeal. This is partly because they are small. Wild males generally weigh 115–160 g (4–5.6 oz) and females slightly less (95–135 g or 3.4–4.8 oz),[8] and their head and body combined are approximately 12–15 cm in length (4.7–5.9 in.). But their appeal is also likely due to facial features that are large in comparison to their head. As nocturnal omnivores, they have large, dark protruding eyes that are set relatively widely apart, facing forward and centered between the base of their nose and the base of their equally large, directional pinnae. These adaptations help them avoid nighttime predators and make the best use of the protective forest canopy of their habitat. For example, the position of their eyes on their head gives them a high degree of orbital convergence and the resulting binocularity improves visual acuity in foliage.[9] Nevertheless, their eyes also give sugar gliders an undeniably charming appearance.

Sugar gliders have an average lifespan of between 4 and 7 years in the wild,[10] and when kept in good health can be expected to live 10 and 12 years,[5,8] and possibly even up to 15 years in captivity.[10]

Table 17.1 shows reference physiological data and environmental data for healthy sugar gliders.

Out of Australia

Sugar gliders have a relatively extensive history as a captive species in their native Australia, not as pets but rather as

Table 17.1 Reference data for sugar gliders

Reference physiological data for healthy sugar gliders[2,5,8,10]	Values
Adult Size	
Body length	16–21 cm
Tail length	16.5–21 cm
Male weight	115–160 g
Female weight	95–135 g
Lifespan (years)	
Average captive lifespan	9–12
Reported maximum captive lifespan	15
Average wild male lifespan	4–5
Average wild female lifespan	5–7
Reported maximum wild lifespan	9
Body temperature	36.3°C (97.3°F)
Cloacal temperature	32–36°C (97.3°F)
Heart rate	200–300 beats/min
Basal metabolic rate	2.54 (weight in kg)$^{0.75}$

Reference environmental data for sugar glider captivity[5,8,10]	Values
Temperature zone	24–31°C (75–88° F)
Food consumption	15–20% body weight/day
Animals per enclosure	Minimum 2
Enclosure	200–300 beats/min
Suggested size	2 × 2 × 2 m
Material	Wire mesh
Mesh spacing	2.5 × 1.3 cm

residents in zoological and wildlife rehabilitation facilities.[6] In other countries, however, their popularity is not simply as zoological residents but also as exotic companion animals and has been growing steadily; they are relatively popular as pets in North America, Europe, and Japan.[11] They weren't introduced to the United States until 1994,[2] but they have become popular enough in the United States to be referred to as "pocket pets" in some United States Department of Agriculture (USDA) publications.[12] However, it should be kept in mind that they are still considered exotic animals and are not domesticated. Ownership is legal by national standards, but breeding is regulated by the USDA Animal and Plant Health Inspection Service, and four or more breeding females may qualify an owner as a breeder.[2] In addition, ownership itself may be regulated at the state level, or it may be legal at the state or country level but prohibited at the city level. Potential owners should check with the USDA (www.usda.gov) and with their state, county, and city web sites for up-to-date information on designations, regulations, and requirements regarding sugar gliders.[13,14]

Social behavior

Sugar gliders are a highly social species that naturally form strong and cohesive groups, commonly referred to as colonies. Colonies are populated by up to twelve adults,[8] including one to three males.[1] Colonies live together in the hollows of trees and form enduring social dependencies,[15] harmonizing wake–sleep behavior patterns, grooming, and general activity.[16] The social structure is hierarchal; both males and females establish strong hierarchies within colonies. However one male, conventionally identified as the dominant male, is responsible for most of the territorial patrolling, scent-marking, and aggression.[17] This male is likely the perpetrator of over 75% of all conceptions annually in the wild,[15] although his sons may play a supporting role in the hierarchal structure, cooperating with their sire to provide care of young and maintenance of social status. Dominant males weigh more than subordinate males and yet are quicker and more active, and they also manage to spend more time in the colony nest. They have extremely high levels of testosterone[15] and concomitantly lower cortisol concentrations than other colony males.[18]

Communication

Individual and community-specific information is conveyed through scent. It is possible that saliva has informational value,[17] but the primary means of socially cohesive communication is scent-marking. Sugar gliders mark themselves, their mates, and other members of their colony, and they can instantly distinguish the scent of individuals and groups.[19,20] Scent-marking in marsupials has been found to be sensitive to plasma testosterone concentrations in that it terminates with castration and renews with exogenous testosterone treatment.[21] However, studies indicate that social status also plays an integral part in scent-marking behavior in sugar gliders, both directly and indirectly. It is likely that only the dominant male scent-marks, irrespective of the plasma concentrations of testosterone in intermediate-ranking males[22]—including in those that have been recently translocated from a separate colony where they were the dominant, and therefore, the high testosterone male. However, social stimuli markedly suppress testosterone concentration in sugar gliders, and for the most part, subordinate males have significantly lower plasma concentrations of testosterone than dominant males.[18]

Adult male sugar gliders impart scent from four glands: two cutaneous glands, a frontal gland, and a sternal-throat gland;[23] and two paracloacal glands that open into the cloaca,[24] the proctodeal and paraproctal glands. All glands are testosterone dependent and follow an annual cycle of development and decline.[23] Peaks in the plasma concentration of testosterone have been found to coincide with the July–September breeding season in the Southern Hemisphere.[25] Adult females do not have frontal or sternal glands, which makes it simple to sex animals: the male's frontal gland is hairless, appearing as a pale patch within the dark facial striping on the forehead (see Figure 17.3). Females also have scent glands in their pouches, which are active from shortly before parturition until the young

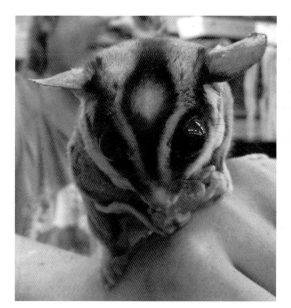

Figure 17.3   The frontal gland of the male sugar glider.

leaves the pouch.[17] The scent is attractive to a newborn sugar glider, and the young are able to distinguish their own mother from other mothers at about day 74, the time they normally begin to leave the pouch. By day 94, the young are able to discriminate between the odors associated with two different communities.[17]

Scent is transmitted by purposeful contact.[17] One animal clasps the neck of another and forces the head upward, and then rubs its forehead on the chest of the animal. If the initiator is male, secretions from his frontal gland are transferred to the chest area of the other animal; if the initiator is female and the other animal male, the secretions from the male's sternal gland are transferred to the female's forehead.[20]

Because sugar gliders are highly social, they are likely to experience behavioral and physiological distress if kept singly in captivity. They are very sensitive to environmental change, particularly when the change includes changes in colony members—so much so that sugar glider hierarchal-colony manipulation and the resulting loss of social status has been considered a model for the study of the sociobiological etiology of human depression.[26] Studies evaluating social behavior found that environmental context and the individuals with which animals associate have a dramatic impact on social positioning and resultant behavior. Specifically, when even a large and robust dominant animal from one colony is introduced into another colony with an existing hierarchy, the transferred formerly dominant individual often loses his social position regardless of size, and this social change significantly reduces the animal's access to resources such as food, water, communal grooming, and general social and sexual access.[26] He also loses size and weight, and as mentioned, his plasma testosterone levels drop.[18] In addition, intraspecific aggressive behavior is seen between colonies[20] and may also occur when an animal is removed from a colony and then returned after several days. A reintroduced animal will, at minimum be scrutinized immediately and marked when returned; if the animal was introduced into a new colony and marked there, it will be attacked upon its return.[19] Removing the dominant male also triggers marking in inter-mediate-ranking males,[20] and results in increased patrol activity, mating, and aggression by other males.

Introductions

Because sugar gliders are highly social and form territorial group dependencies recognizable by scent, both in the wild and in captivity, and because they aggressively ostracize any animal that has not been accepted into the colony, introduction of new animals must be done carefully. Resident members will readily bite nonmembers,[20] and attacks—particularly by residents of the same sex as the new animal—can quickly culminate in the death of the intro-duced animal.[8] Temporary removal of the dominant male may facilitate acceptance of a new colony member through disruption of the colony, but it will concomitantly increase aggression in resident members,[17] cause significant stress in the dominant male,[18] and may induce self-mutilation and other stress-related behaviors such as coprophagy, hyperphagia, polydipsia, and pacing[5,27] in the displaced animal. It could also create a problem upon reintroduction of the original male.[19] For these reasons, it is not recom-mended. One possible option is to use gliders' own scenting behavior to facilitate the introduction of a new animal. Rather than simply introducing the animals to each other face-to-face, scent should be mingled beforehand, particularly if there is more than one resident glider and if cage space is limited.

MacPherson[11] suggests that this be done using the nesting bags of the resident and new gliders. New ani-mals should always be quarantined for 3 weeks before being introduced to resident animals, and this time period can be used to begin the scenting process. Each evening when the gliders leave their nesting sacks, the residents' sack should be moved to the new animal's enclosure and a clean sack placed in the residents' enclosure. After the quarantine period is up, if the new animal is healthy, its enclosure can be moved beside the residents' enclosure, and the nest bags switched each evening between the two enclosures. Periodic wash-ing of the nest bags will be necessary, but, in general, switching nest bags allows transfer of scent without hos-tility. After 10 days or so, the new glider can be introduced to the resident colony during the day, when the resident animals are sleeping. If fighting that involves bloodshed takes place or if the new animal is rejected and found sleeping alone, the animals should be separated and scent

mingling reinstated for at least a week before reintroduction is attempted again.[11]

Activity patterns

Sugar gliders are largely nocturnal, emerging from their communal nests within 30 minutes of sunset.[28] They are active most all night, and as pets they can be described as playful, energetic, and even hyperactive.[5] Much of their active phase involves foraging for food, but they also spend a great deal of time engaged in social behavior, including grooming, marking colony members and territory, and copulating. They tend to synchronize some of their behav-ior with others in their colony, not necessarily expressing the same behavior at the same time—although grooming bouts are often shared—but rather coordinating their com-ings and goings to and from the nest.[16] Scent-marking takes place mainly inside the nest, and it is thought that this coor-dination facilitates intra-colony olfactory recognition and communication by maximizing the probability that colony members will be together a sufficient amount of time to mingle scent.[16,20]

Communal living also offers other advantages, such as energy conservation in low ambient temperatures. Colony members huddle together in their nests,[29] and shivering together helps them generate heat.[30] Sugar gliders' abilities to adapt to seasonal climate changes are intriguing, because climate changes can present problems for some marsupials due to their lack of brown adipose tissue and relative ina-bility to store energy.[31] Sugar gliders don't often experience temperature changes greater than 10°C (20°F) in their natural habitat, but they still must cope with longer and cooler nights and reduced food availability in winter. They apparently cope through changes in both their behavior and their thermal physiology that allow them to maintain their daily winter energy expenditure at levels similar to those in summer.[32] Physiologically, they adapt to seasonal changes in temperature by increasing or decreasing subcu-taneous fat, a strategy that can increase energy reserves and provide insulation.[33] They adapt behaviorally to tempera-ture changes by exposing or covering their body surface. In warm weather they often sprawl on their backs and splay their limbs in the air to expose their patagia, or they lick their paws and wave them slowly about, and it isn't unusual to see them salivating excessively in high heat. They conserve heat in cold weather by curling into a ball, first tucking their head, legs, and patagia under their body and then covering their head with their tail. The colder their sur-roundings are, the tighter the ball they make.[33] In addition, although their resting metabolism doesn't change, their relative activity patterns do change to decrease energy expenditure in winter[33], including the employment of torpor in response to low ambient temperature and food shortage.[31]

Torpor

Torpor is characterized by a controlled reduction of body temperature, metabolic rate, and other physiological processes involving energy expenditure.[28] There appears to be a correlation between thermoregulatory pattern and predictability of food supply,[34] and torpor is employed by many small mammals and birds to overcome energy shortages during adverse environmental conditions or limited food supply.[28,35] Animals in captivity or laboratory conditions use torpor in response to acute environmental stressors such as cold or food limitation.[31,36–38] Studies indicate that when captive sugar gliders use torpor, they usually do so early in the morning,[30] soon after entering their inactivity phase. Sugar gliders generally use torpor in an opportunistic manner, but captive sugar gliders do not follow the thermoregulatory patterns of gliders in the wild. Wild sugar gliders regularly employ torpor in winter, frequently experiencing torpor during their resting phases while continuing to forage during their active phases[30] but falling temperatures rarely trigger torpor of any duration in captive sugar gliders. It is hypothesized that this difference is due to two factors: first, captivity stress may inhibit torpor[39] and second, increases in body mass are correlated with decreases in daily torpor use[39] and most captive animals are fed *ad libitum*. Captive animals that do not experience torpor under temperature stress often respond if food is suddenly limited,[28] and studies evaluating torpor in sugar gliders often rely on 24 hours or more of food restriction.[28,29] Thus, torpor that is not intentionally induced in an indoor-housed captive sugar glider should be considered an indication of serious physiological stress of some sort, particularly stress relating to diet.

Controlled studies[28] indicate that captivity even in outdoor aviary colonies can also effect differential torpor patterns. Geiser, Holloway, and Körtner[28] found the average duration of torpor bouts in the wild to be about twice as long as those in captivity, that is, 13 hours compared to 7. They also found a difference between captive and wild populations in the maximum duration of torpor bouts, with the longest individual bouts just over 13 hours in captivity and 23 hours in the wild. Again, this difference might be due to differences in body mass since wild gliders are often more lean than captive ones[28] but activity patterns also differ. Wild sugar gliders reduce their activity to the point of inactivity on cold or wet nights, whereas captive gliders continue to be active throughout the night and are more active in general than wild gliders. They begin their nightly activity period almost immediately after sunset and continue to be active up to just minutes before sunrise, whereas wild sugar gliders may wait up to 20 minutes before becoming active after sunset, and they generally retire 1–2 hours before sunrise. In addition, sugar gliders in captivity are rarely seen leaving the nest during the day, whereas wild individuals occasionally forage in the late afternoon. It is likely that predictable food supplies and relative safety from predators affects activity patterns.

Locomotion

Sugar gliders are arboreal and uniquely adapted to forest living. *Petaurus* translates roughly to "rope-dancer," and aptly describes the animals' agility among the treetops.[11] Their limb structure allows them exceptional dexterity within the forest canopy, and they are active climbers, racing along branches and boughs and ascending and descending tree trunks rapidly headfirst in a manner similar to sciurid rodents such as tree, ground, and flying squirrels. In captivity they often scurry head first down the mesh of their enclosure, or hang head-down on the mesh to eat.

Their primary means of distance locomotion, however, is gliding. They have been reported to glide up to 50 m (150 ft).[5] Sugar gliders control their trajectory by limb and trunk movements that vary the curvature of the left or right patagia and through use of the tail as a rudder and stabilizer. The gliding membrane structure is unique to marsupials and distinct from that of gliding eutherians.[40]

To glide, a sugar glider points itself at its target and springs forward with a powerful thrust of its hind limbs, spreading its forelimbs wide to open the patagia (see Figure 17.4). In the instant just prior to landing—within 10 ft of the target—it straightens its legs beneath it and throws its head back, bringing it parallel to the target to meet the surface with its four feet and their securing claws. The sugar glider's eye set likely helps it navigate its gliding environment by allowing it optimal depth perception.

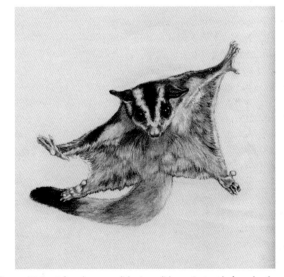

Figure 17.4 A female sugar glider in a glide, an instant before she throws her four legs forward to contact the landing target with her feet and securing claws.

Nevertheless, whether from injury, age, or other factors, sugar gliders occasionally underestimate the distance or angle of their target and have been found injured or dead at the base of trees.

Reproduction, development, and care of young

Sugar gliders are marsupials, and their reproduction is considerably different than that of placental mammals.[27] Gestation is very short, and the young then migrate out of the uterus and up into an external pouch, within which are mammae that provide the fetus its nourishment through the remainder of its development. Most female marsupials have epipubic bones (marsupial bones, ossa marsupialia or eupubic bones), which are small bones thought to function in support of the pouch. However, these bones are absent in gliders, possibly as an adaptive reduction in skeletal weight that aids gliding.[2,5] In other areas, the reproductive tract of the sugar glider is similar to all other marsupials.[27] The tract has paired uterine bodies with two lateral vaginal canals, as well as a median vaginal canal through which the glider gives birth. The lateral and median canals merge and join with the urethra to form the urogenital sinus before entering the cloaca.

The anatomy and physiology of the male sugar glider reproductive system is also similar to other marsupials. Males have a bifid penis that lies in the ventrum of the cloacal floor.[27] The scrotal pouch is pendulous and furred, and attached to the body wall proximal to the cloacal opening and penis.

Sugar gliders are seasonally polyestrus on a 29-day cycle[5] in their natural habitat, with a breeding season between June and November, when food is plentiful. However, they will breed throughout the year in captivity.[10,27] The female's pouch contains two mammae, each with two teats, and most often (81% of the time) two young, known as joeys, are produced.[2,5] Two litters in a single breeding season are not uncommon; the second litter is sometimes facilitated by the reproductive strategy of fetal diapause, whereby blastocysts that had been fertilized during postpartum estrus stop development until the suckling joeys mature and leave the pouch.[27]

Development

Undisturbed gestation in sugar gliders is 15–17 days. At that time, the fetal joeys emerge from the urogenital opening encased in an amniotic sac, having front claws but no visible ears or eyes and weighing only 0.2 g (0.007 oz). The joey must break the sac with its claws and migrate its way to the pouch entrance;[5] its enlarged cartilaginous shoulder girdle, later assimilated in development of the sternum and scapula,[27] aids in the migration. Migration is not marked by a change in behavior in the dam other than an increased interest in cleaning her pouch and licking her coat between the cloacal orifice and her pouch opening, and joeys dislodged during migration are not retrieved. Once within the pouch, the joey locates a teat and takes it into its mouth. The teat swells in the joey's mouth and secures the fetus.[27] At this point, the joeys are not detectable by external visual inspection of the pouch, but they may be visible as slight bulges within 2 weeks and as peanut-sized lumps in approximately 1 month.[10] Joeys will remain in the pouch for 70–74 days, attached to the teat for up to half their pouch life. Toward the end of pouch life the joeys will extend the pouch greatly, and appendages can be seen protruding at various times. They emerge tail first, with full but short pelage, and when the head does emerge the eyes may not be fully open.

After emergence the joeys will suckle periodically and will remain in the family nest even after weaning at 110–120 days of age. Joeys are considered independent and can locate and procure their own food at approximately 17 weeks.[27] They are forced to leave the colony at 7–10 months of age,[5] just before reaching puberty. In recognition of this behavioral pattern, some authors have recommended that female young in captivity should be removed after weaning to avoid attack.[2] However, since weaning occurs several months before the age at which the young leave the colony, this could result in the young failing to learn some important aspects of their normal adult behavior so caution should be used. Further study is warranted to determine if young removed from a colony prior to 7 months of age demonstrate any abnormal behavior later in life. Sexual maturity is reached at 8–12 months of age in females, and at 12–15 months in males.[27]

Mating and care of young

The dominant male breeds the adult females of the colony repeatedly during periods of abundant food. Although there is little published on mating rituals, it has been observed that the female will lower her body and the male will mount a posteriori but, rather than clasping her with his forelegs, he will grasp her coat in his fore paws and begin copulation. Males participate in the care of the emerged joeys and, like the female, will carry the young on their backs or stomachs. Observations indicate that the males are attentive to and tolerant of the young.[10]

Immature gliders, whether the offspring of wild or hand-reared adults, are not easily frightened by novel stimuli and will seek warmth and close spaces to help regulate their temperature. For this reason, they are relatively easy to handle and will even seek out a gentle human grasp. Older joeys, those that have been out of the pouch for a few weeks, are more discriminating and may avoid humans.[10] Offering small bits of sweet foods such as fruit can facilitate acceptance of human touch.

Husbandry and care

Dietary needs

Evaluation of several feeding ecology studies of sugar gliders in their natural habitat indicates that their diet is highly correlated with resource availability and that they are remarkably adaptable opportunistic feeders.[4] In captivity they are attracted to a diverse array of available foods, from fruit and insects to prepared pet and bird feeds. However, their readiness to accept a variety of foods belies the fact that their captive diet must be carefully considered to ensure their optimum health. Improper diet is a leading contributor to clinical problems in companion gliders, and pet gliders too often present for veterinary care with diet-related conditions such as malnutrition (including hypoproteinemia, hypocalcemia, and anemia), obesity, osteodystrophy, vitamin and mineral imbalances, and dental disease.[4-6]

Ingestive behavior of wild sugar gliders

Wild sugar gliders feed on plant exudates such as sap and gum, on nectar and pollen, on honeydew and lerp secretions from insects, and on nutrients within hemolymph and soft tissues of arthropods they access by crushing.[4,6,41] A number of studies[4,6,41–43] have evaluated the contents and nutritional value of the diets of both wild and captive sugar gliders, and it has been found that, in general, sugar glider diet is dependent on seasonal availability and physiological demands. Saps and gums are the staple of the wild sugar glider diet,[8] but throughout spring and summer (from September to February in the Southern Hemisphere), evaluation of feces indicates that pollen consumption for protein correlates with flowering seasons. Spring and summer diet have also been found to contain many arthropods, including moths, spiders, and scarabaeid beetles, even when saps are plentiful, perhaps because the high protein content of the arthropods better meets the reproductive needs of gliders.[4] During autumn and winter, from March to August, gliders spend the majority of their time consuming gum, sap, honeydew, and manna.[4,42]

Feeding captive gliders

Although it is impractical to attempt to provide captive, pet gliders their natural diet of plant and insect exudates,[6] a number of diets for captive sugar gliders have been formulated. *In vitro* evaluation of the basic nutritional parameters of three diet suggestions commonly found on the Internet, including fecal and physiological parameter analysis and thorough veterinary health checks, indicated that none of the diets evaluated were optimal; there was evidence of mineral and vitamin imbalances, especially vitamin D and iron, and of calcium/phosphorous imbalances.[6] It was found, however, that total protein was apparently sufficient and overall the diets evaluated were highly digestible. It was also noted that young, healthy male

Table 17.2 Sugar glider diet providing 159 kJ energy, 17% crude protein (1550 mg), 0.61% calcium, 0.44% phosphorus, and 0.9 IU/kg vitamin D

Diet 1[4]
12 g chopped, mixed fruit (any type, <10% citrus)
2.5 g cooked, chopped vegetables (50/50 starchy/non-starchy, steamed, or microwaved)
10 g peach or apricot nectar
5.5 g ground, dry, low-iron bird diet
1 g mealworm (or other invertebrates, e.g., grasshoppers, moths, fly pupae, crickets)

Table 17.3 Sugar glider diet providing 126 kJ energy, 21% crude protein (1750 mg), 0.77% calcium, 0.64% phosphorus, and 1.1 IU/g vitamin D

Diet 2[4,10]
12 g chopped, mixed fruit (any type, <10% citrus)
2.5 g cooked, chopped vegetables (50/50 starchy/nonstarchy, steamed, or microwaved)
10 g peach or apricot nectar
5.5 g ground, dry, low-iron bird diet
insects for dental hygiene

gliders don't require a lot of calories. Based in part on these findings and in part on evaluation of others' findings, Dierenfeld[4] suggests two sample daily diets. One provides 126 kJ energy, 21% crude protein (1750 mg), 0.77% calcium, 0.64% phosphorus, and 1.1 IU/g vitamin D (see Table 17.2). The other diet, designed by Pye[10] and blended into a slurry, provides 159 kJ energy, 17% crude protein (1550 mg), 0.61% calcium, 0.44% phosphorus, and 0.9 IU/kg vitamin D (see Table 17. 3).

Food should be limited to 15–20% of body weight to reduce the risk of obesity, and treat foods (including apple, nectarine, melons, grapes, figs, sweet corn, sweet potato, beans, pumpkin, sprouts, lettuce, broccoli, and parsley) shouldn't exceed 15% of the diet.[8,10]

Fresh water should be available continuously in multiple locations throughout the enclosure.

Diet and enrichment

Gliders use their incisors in their natural habitat to extract gum that has accumulated in crevices created by insects, as well as to strip bark to locate and extricate arthropods and gouge into sap columns; these behaviors may be important for maintaining tooth and gum health.[4] Wild sugar gliders also invest a lot of time scenting, licking, and prying leaves and branches aside searching for manna and nectar. These natural behaviors should be considered when setting up the environment of captive gliders. Providing natural materials that simulate foraging conditions, such as nontoxic tree branch materials drilled with holes and filled as food stuff receptacles, can afford captive animals the opportunity to express their natural feeding behaviors and thereby provide them important environmental enrichment.[4,8] Several feeding stations placed in various locations will help ensure sufficient food and enrichment opportunities in multiple-member colonies.

Housing

Because of the social nature of sugar gliders, they should be kept in groups of at least two in captivity. The species is energetic and highly active, with colonies in the wild occupying a territory of up to 1 ha (2.5 ac);[5] although a cage size of $1 \times \frac{3}{4} \times 1$ m (approximately $36 \times 24 \times 36$ in.)[5] has been suggested as the absolute minimum, a more appropriate $2 \times 2 \times 2$ m ($6 \times 6 \times 6$ ft)[8] better addresses the welfare needs of the species. Tall is better than squat, and commercial bird cages often are good choices for glider enclosures.[10] Enclosures should be wire mesh for good ventilation, with mesh spacing approximately 2.5×1.3 cm (1.0×0.5 in.).[5,8] Aviaries of sufficient size have been used successfully as enclosures for pet or companion gliders as well as for gliders in research laboratories.[8,28,33]

Nest boxes

Enclosures must include a nest box, bag, or pouch. Wild sugar gliders sleep huddled together in their nests in tree hollows, and continuous access to a similar sleep and hiding area is necessary to avoid stress in captive environments. Suggestions for appropriate nest boxes include wooden cylinders or hollow logs equipped with hinged openings for caregiver access and removable bases for cleaning,[5,8] as well as birdhouses or boxes made of wood, plastic, or rubber storage containers.[10] Nest boxes should be at least 13×13 cm (6×6 in.).[5] Entry openings should be no smaller than 3.75 cm (1½ in.) in diameter.[10] Nesting material is optional, but can include such things as hardwood shavings, shredded recycled paper products or dried leaves, coconut fibers, and sea grass.[5] Newspaper or magazine pages should be avoided because of the dyes, as well as most cloth strips and other materials that could snag the animals' fragile limbs and phalanges.

Accessories

Enclosures should include a number of branches and rods running both vertically and horizontally, similar to branches in the wild, to help meet the activity needs of sugar gliders and accommodate their natural inclinations to scurry, jump, climb, and glide. Perches, shelves, bird swings, and ladders can be situated at various levels around the cage. Bird toys and solid cat toys that cannot be shredded also make suitable enrichment objects. Exercise wheels other than those made of solid plastic or metal should be avoided, because the wire type can be hazardous to limbs.[5,10] Feeding stations and watering stations, preferably in forms that simulate natural foraging situations such as mentioned earlier, should be situated in various locations throughout the upper half of the cage. Shallow hanging dishes and sipper bottles are appropriate water

dispensers,[4] and water and food receptacles should be sanitized daily.

Cage location

Ideal ambient temperature for sugar gliders is 24–27°C (75–80°F), but gliders tolerate temperatures between 18°C and 32°C (65°F and 90°F).[5] Enclosures should be situated to avoid direct sunlight, although a room with windows is best. In addition, care should be taken to avoid daytime disturbances. Wild sugar gliders spend the majority of their time scampering along branches in the forest canopy, and this predisposition should be kept in mind when creating a suitable environment. They will feel safest if they can spend the majority of their time in the treetops, or at least in the top third or half of their enclosure, so nest boxes and accessories should be positioned accordingly. Cats should be kept out of the room that houses the enclosure as much as possible, particularly at night, and objects resembling winged or other predators, including stuffed animals and piles of clothing, should never be accidentally set on top of the cage.

Handling

Hand-reared sugar gliders adapt well to captivity and develop strong bonds with their human companions if given sufficient interaction with their owners.[5] Particularly when handled quietly, calmly, and frequently from an early age, they develop into gentle and entertaining pets.[8] Because scent is an important component of social recognition in gliders, newly acquired animals—even those hand-reared in captivity—require time to recognize their handlers' scents, and they may urinate frequently when held or perching on their handlers' head or shoulders. Ness and Booth[5] recommend socialization periods of at least 2 hours each day. They also suggest that handling for socialization and companionship be done at night, during the glider's activity period. Although many of these animals are now bred domestically and are fairly docile when hand-raised, they may react with ferocity when handled by individuals other than their owners.

Acknowledgments

Photos and original artwork, courtesy of the author.

References

1. Suckling GC. Population ecology of the sugar glider, *Petaurus breviceps*, in a system of fragmented habitats. *Aust Wildl Res*, 1984;11:49–75.

2. Booth RJ, Sugar gliders. In: Kahn CM, Line S, eds. *The Merck/Merial Manual for Pet Health*. Whitehouse Station, NJ: Merck & Co, 2007;1039–1043.

3. Groves C. Superfamily Petauroidea. In: Wilson DE, Reeder DM, eds. *Mammal Species of the World*. 3rd ed. Baltimore, Maryland: Johns Hopkins University Press, 2005;50–56.

4. Dierenfeld ES. Feeding behavior and nutrition of the sugar glider (*Petaurus breviceps*). *Vet Clin North Am Exot Anim Pract* 2009;12(2):209–215.

5. Ness RD, Booth R. Sugar gliders. In: Quesenberrry KE, Carpenter JW, eds. *Ferrets, Rabbits, and Rodents Clinical Medicine and Surgery.* 2nd ed. St. Louis: Elsevier Inc, 2004;330–338.

6. Dierenfeld ES, Thomas D, Ives R. Comparison of commonly used diets on intake, digestion, growth, and health in captive sugar gliders (*Petaurus breviceps*). *J Exot Pet Med* 2006;15(3):218–224.

7. Endo H, Yokokawa K, Kurohmaru M, Hayashi Y. Functional anatomy of gliding membrane muscles in the sugar glider (*Petaurus breviceps*). *Ann Anat* 1998;180:93–96.

8. Booth R. Sugar gliders. *Semin Avian Exotic Pet Med* 2003;12(4): 228–231.

9. Changizi MA, Shimojo S. "X-ray vision" and the evolution of forward-facing eyes. *J Theor Biol* 2008;254:756–767.

10. Pye G. Sugar gliders. In: Carpenter JW, ed. *Exotic Animal Formulary.* St. Loius, MO: Elsevier Saunders, 2005;347–357.

11. MacPherson C. *Sugar Gliders: A Complete Pet Owner's Manual.* New York: Barron's Educational Series Inc, 1997.

12. USDA Animal Care Resource Guide: Glossary. Available at: http://www.aphis.usda.gov/animal_welfare/downloads/manuals/eig/2.1_eig.pdf. Accessed Sep 17, 2009.

13. Johnson-Delaney CA. Common procedures in hedgehogs, prairie dogs, exotic rodents, and companion marsupials. *Vet Clin North Am Exot Anim Pract* 2006;9(2):415–435.

14. Maas AK. Legal implications of the exotic pet practice. *Vet Clin North Am Exot Anim Pract* 2005;8(3):497–514.

15. Stoddart DM, Bradley AJ. Plasma testosterone concentration, body weight, social dominance and scent-marking in marsupial sugar gliders (*Petaurus breviceps*; Marsupialia: Petauridae) *J Zool (London)* 1994;232:595–601.

16. Kleinknecht, S. Lack of social entrainment of free-running circadian activity rhythms in the Australian sugar glider (*Petaurus breviceps*: Marsupialia). *Behav Ecol Sociobiol* 1985;16(2):189–193.

17. Thiessen, D, Rice M. Mammalian scent gland marking and social behavior. *Psychol Bull* 1976;83:505–539.

18. Mallick J, Stoddart DM, Jones IH et al. Behavioural and endocrinological correlates of social status in the male sugar glider (*Petaurus breviceps*; Marsupialia: Petauridae). *Physiol Behav* 1994;55(6):1131–1134.

19. Ewer RF. *Ethology of Mammals.* New York: Plenum Press, 1968.

20. Schultze-Westrum T. Social communication by chemical signals. In: Pfaffman C, ed. *Olfaction and Taste.* New York: Rockefeller University Press, 1969.

21. Fadem BH, Erianne GS, Karen LM. The hormonal control of scent marking and precopulatory behavior in male gray shorttailed opossums (*Monodelphis domestica*). *Horm Behav* 1989;23:381–392.

22. Stoddart DM, Bradley AJ, Hynes K. Olfactory biology of the marsupial sugar glider—A preliminary study. In: Doty RL, Müller-Schwarze D, eds. *Chemical Signals in Vertebrates VI.* New York: Plenum Press, 1992; 532–528.

23. Stoddart DM, Bradley AJ. The frontal and gular dermal scent organs of the marsupial sugar glider (*Petaurus breviceps*). *J Zool (London)* 1991;225:1–12.

24. Bradley AJ, Stoddart DM. The dorsal paracloacal gland and its relationship with seasonal changes in cutaneous scent gland morphology and plasma androgen in the marsupial sugar glider (*Petaurus breviceps*; Marsupialia: Petauridae). *J Zool (London)* 1993;229:331–346.

25. Bradley AJ, Stoddart DM. Seasonal changes in plasma androgens, glucocorticoids and glucocorticoid-binding proteins in the marsupial sugar glider *Petaurus breviceps. J Endocrinol* 1992;132(1):21–31.

26. Jones IH, Stoddart DM, Mallick J. Towards a sociobiological model of depression: A marsupial model (*Petaurus breviceps*). *Br J Psychiat* 1995;166(4):475–479.

27. Johnson-Delaney CA. Reproductive medicine of companion marsupials. *Vet Clin North Am Exot Anim Pract* 2002;5(3):537–553.

28. Geiser F, Holloway JC, Körtner G. Thermal biology, torpor and behaviour in sugar gliders: A laboratory-field comparison. *J Comp Physiol B* 2007;177:495–501.

29. Fleming MR. Thermoregulation and torpor in the sugar glider, *Petaurus breviceps* (Marsupialia, Petauridae). *Aust J Zool* 1980;28:521–534.

30. Geiser F. Metabolic rate and body temperature reduction during hibernation and daily torpor. *Annu Rev Physiol* 2004;66:239–274.

31. Körtner G, Geiser F. Torpor and activity patterns in free-ranging sugar gliders *Petaurus breviceps* (Marsupialia). *Oecologia* 2001; 123:350–357.

32. Geiser F, Drury RL, McAllan BM et al. Effects of temperature acclimation on maximum heat production, thermal tolerance, and torpor in a marsupial. *J Comp Physiol B* 2003;173:437–442.

33. Holloway JC, Geiser F. Seasonal changes in the thermoenergetics of the marsupial sugar glider, *Petaurus breviceps. J Comp Physiol [B]* 2001;171(8):643–650.

34. Schleucher E. Torpor in birds: Taxonomy, energetics, and ecology. *Physiol Biochem Zool* 2004;77(6):942–929.

35. Wang LCH. Ecological, physiological, and biochemical aspects of torpor in mammals and birds. In: Wang LCH, ed. *Advances in Comparative and Environmental Physiology.* Berlin: Springer Verlag, 1989;361–491.

36. Geiser F, Brigham RMJ. Torpor, thermal biology, and energetics in Australian long-eared bats (*Nyctophilus*). *J Comp Physiol [B]* 2000;170(2):153–162.

37. Kelm DH, von Helversen O. How to budget metabolic energy: Torpor in a small Neotropical mammal. *J Comp Physiol [B]* 2007 Aug;177(6):667–677.

38. Lovegrove BG, Raman J. Torpor patterns in the pouched mouse (*Saccostomus campestris*; Rodentia): A model animal for unpredictable environments. *J Comp Physiol [B]* 1998 May;168(4):303–312.

39. Holloway JC, Geiser F. Reproductive status and torpor of the marsupial *Sminthopsis crassicaudata*: Effects of photoperiod. *J Therm Biol* 1996;21:375–380.

40. Johnson-Murray JL. The comparative mycology of the gliding membranes of *Acrobates*, *Petauroides* and *Petaurus* contrasted with the cutaneous mycology of *Hemibelideus* and *Pseudocheirus* (Marsupialia: Phalangeridae) and with selected gliding rodentia (Sciuridae and Anamoluridae). *Aust J Zool* 1987;53:101–113.

41. Smith AP. Diet and feeding strategies of the marsupial sugar glider in temperate Australia. *J Anim Ecol* 1982;51:149–166.

42. Howard J. Diet of *Petaurus breviceps* (*Marsupialia: Petauridae*) in a mosaic of coastal woodland and heath. *Aust Mammal* 1989; 12:15–21.

43. Smith AP, Green SW. Nitrogen requirements of the sugar glider (*Petaurus breviceps*), an omnivorous marsupial, on a honey-pollen diet. *Physiol Zool* 1987;60:82–92.

18

From parrots to pigs to pythons: Universal principles and procedures of learning

Susan G. Friedman and Lore I. Haug

Ms. Jones calls your clinic asking for help with her 7-year-old daughter's rabbit, Peaches. Peaches kicks and scratches when the daughter goes to put Peaches back into the cage after being let out to play. Ms. Jones is not sure what to do. The local pet store told her Peaches was too dominant and she should find another rabbit. Ms. Jones is distraught because her daughter is very attached to Peaches despite Peaches aggressive behavior. (See Case Study 1 at the end of the chapter for resolution of Peaches' problem.)

Introduction

Behavior is at the top of the list of problems that people have with their pets. As the number of exotic pets grows, so does the need for veterinarians who can help clients prevent and solve behavior problems effectively and humanely. As medical practitioners, veterinarians are trained to solve behavior problems that are symptoms of underlying physiological dysfunction associated with aging, injury, or disease. The medical model is used to categorically diagnosis, treat, and cure these problems. However, a substantial number of behavior problems are independent of physical health. These problems are due to the process of learning and the behavioral model is needed to help clients understand, predict, and solve them.

From a behavioral perspective, learning is defined as a change in behavior due to experience – i.e., certain types of interactions between an individual and the environment. Given the age-old debate regarding nature versus nurture, it is easy to overlook the fact that it is the nature of all animals to change what they do based on the experience of doing it. Chance explains, "Learning does not give the species the tendency to behave a certain way in a particular situation; rather it gives the individual the tendency to modify its behavior to suit a situation. It is an evolved modifiability."[1]

Unfortunately, much of what clients know about learning and behavior is based on conventional wisdom that persists mainly because it is repeated so often (e.g., dropping a parrot reduces biting because the parrot concedes the dominant alpha role to its human owner). However, conventional wisdom lacks the reliability that results from systematic observation and experimentation. Without scientifically validated information, caregivers inadvertently create persistent behavior problems that lead to needless suffering for themselves and their pet.

Learning has been studied with the scientific method for well over 100 years, and the general principles that describe how specific types of interaction with the environment affect behavior are well documented. Over the last 50 years, these principles have been honed into a technology to solve practical behavior problems in real-world settings. This is the foundation of contemporary applied behavior analysis (ABA), the technology of behavior change.

The goal of this chapter is to disseminate to veterinarians the basic principles and select procedures of ABA. However, this is an introductory chapter and many fascinating and essential topics have been treated cursorily or not at all. It is our hope that this relatively brief discussion serves to inspire veterinarians to seek more in-depth information and deepen their expertise with the science and technology of behavior change. With that in mind, the objectives of this chapter are to (1) review the fundamental, universal principles of animal learning, (2) describe the essential procedures needed for your behavior-change toolbox, and (3) demonstrate, with two case studies, how clients can use these principles and procedures to solve behavior problems with their exotic pets.

How animals learn

Behavior: What is it?

Most clients never consider how their descriptions of behavior are really just value labels of what they think an animal *is* rather than what it *does*. They wish for a ferret that is friendly, a degu that is docile, and a toad that is tame. Veterinarians can explain that no one can teach animals what to *be*; rather, we teach them what to *do* and when to do it. For example, we can train a ferret to approach people, relax while being touched, and take food from hands. When a ferret is observed to do these behaviors, we then call it friendly.

Among professionals, there is a tendency to describe behavior in terms of diagnostic labels that are often hypothetical, psychological constructs. Ostensibly, these constructs tell us what an animal *has* or *lacks*, such as anxiety, dominance, or motivation. A construct is a concept that is inferred from commonalities among observed phenomena and used to explain those phenomena. However, constructs are abstractions by definition, and abstractions cannot cause behavior. Although constructs can have a place in theory building, and conveniently summarize behaviors with a single word, they lack the specific information we need for the objective analysis of behavior.

The key to solving problem behaviors is to describe what an animal actually does and to place that behavior in a context, not inside the animal. Behavior does not occur in a vacuum or spray out of animals haphazardly. There are always conditions on which behavior depends. Therefore, changing conditions necessarily changes behavior. This is good news because, although clients do not have direct control over their pets' neural processes, they do have direct control over the conditions in which their pets behave.

For our purposes then, behavior is what an animal does in certain conditions, which can be measured. Behavior can be overt, i.e., public (chewing, scratching, running), or covert, i.e., private (thought and emotions). Likewise, the conditions that affect behavior can be inside and outside the skin. However, the focus in this chapter is the behavioral level of analysis, the level at which observable behavior and observable conditions act upon one another. It is one piece of the behavior puzzle without which no accounting of behavior is complete.

Two types of behavior: Two learning processes

Traditionally, behavior is classified in one of two ways—respondent and operant, which roughly corresponds to involuntary and voluntary behavior, respectively. Briefly, respondent behaviors include simple reflexes (jumping at a loud sound) and certain inherited, species-typical behavior sequences (nest building onset by seasonal changes). Respondent behaviors depend on particular events that occur immediately before the behavior to automatically elicit them. Thus, respondent behaviors are characterized as stimulus–response (S–R) relations. In contrast, operant behaviors depend on consequences, that is particular events that follow the behavior. Operant behaviors occur in some form, at some frequency, and increase or decrease depending on the outcomes they produce. Thus, operant behaviors are characterized as response–stimulus (R–S) relations, whereby the stimulus that follows the response influences (increases or decreases) future responses. For example, a hamster will continue to shimmy (response) down a tube that leads to food (consequent stimulus). Operant antecedent stimuli do not automatically trigger operant behavior in the same sense that a reflexive response is elicited by an antecedent stimulus. Between an operant antecedent and an operant behavior is choice, discussed further below.

Learning occurs with both respondent and operant behavior but what is learned is different. With respondent learning (also known as classical conditioning), new eliciting stimuli, not new behaviors, are learned. This occurs through the process of repeated, contiguous pairing of a neutral stimulus with an existing eliciting stimulus. This is stimulus–stimulus (S–S) learning and it is this process that accounts for such responses as the elicitation of the salivation at the sound of a can opener, and milk letdown in dairy cows at the sight of milking parlors. It is also the process by which emotional behaviors are triggered, such as blushing and increased heart rate exhibited by some parrots in the presence of a mate. Similarly, anxiety and fear (e.g., increased respiration, muscle tension, piloerection) can be elicited by seemingly benign conditioned stimuli, such as a white lab coat that has been repeatedly paired with painful injections or restraint. These emotional behaviors are of particular interest when they affect an animal's ability to learn and, therefore, its quality of life.

With operant learning, new behaviors are acquired and existing behaviors modified based on the past results of doing them. Operant behavior is a purposive tool to control one's environment, and consequences are feedback about how to behave in the future. Behaviors that produce valued results are repeated; behaviors that produce aversive results are modified or suppressed. This is contingency learning (in ABA nomenclature, if behavior B, then consequence C: B–C). With operant learning, antecedents are learned signals for the particular behavior–consequence contingency ahead (when A, if B, then C). For example, with experience, a potbellied pig will quickly learn that when the gate is open (A), if it walks through the gate (B), then the result will be novel foraging opportunities (C). However, a tired or satiated pig may choose to disregard the antecedent signal. As can be seen, operant learning (ABC) is quite different than respondent learning (S–S–R), a distinction that eludes professionals too often.

Respondent and operant behaviors are inextricably intertwined. For example, when a bird's flight response is elicited by a sudden, loud noise (respondent), the experience (consequences) of flying away may affect the bird's future flight speed, patterns, and destinations (operant), the next time it is startled. In general, problem behaviors and solutions are best viewed through an operant porthole. Operant behavior tends to be the larger repertoire and is more observable, requiring less inference than respondent interpretations. Where operant behavior leads, respondent behavior often follows. However, some respondent behaviors can interfere with operant learning, such as extreme anxiety and fear. When this is the case, the best course of action may be to deal with the respondent behavior problem first, clearing the way for operant learning.

Basic procedures for changing respondent fear

It is not uncommon for animals to learn new triggers for reflexive fear responses through the process of respondent learning. These elicited fear responses are often associated with operant escape or aggressive behaviors, as well. For example, when a ferret is handled at the clinic, restraint can often trigger the physiologic responses of fear such as muscular tension, tachycardia, tachypnea, elevated blood pressure, and cortisol release. This may result in biting to escape. There are three well-established procedures to reduce respondent fear to clear the way for animals to be more attentive to operant learning. These include systematic desensitization, counterconditioning, and response blocking (flooding).

Systematic desensitization

Systematic desensitization is a procedure by which a conditioned emotional response (e.g., fear of a harmless stimulus) is extinguished by gradually exposing the animal to the fear-eliciting stimulus. The first step in systematic desensitization is to arrange a stimulus hierarchy from no response eliciting to extreme response eliciting. Next, the animal is exposed to the first step on the hierarchy after which the next step is presented. This process of gradual exposure continues until the animal shows no fear responses at the last step on the hierarchy. Care must be taken to not elicit the fear response at any level of exposure. There can be several stimulus features to manage when conducting a systematic desensitization program. For example, a pig described as fearful of people may respond fearfully to intensity (e.g., volume of the person's voice or the rapidity of their behavior), proximity (how close the person is), duration (how long the person is in view), and number (one person versus several). Each stimulus feature should be arranged on the hierarchy and presented in turn to allow the animal to desensitize gradually to each trigger. The efficacy of systematic desensitization can often be improved by combining it with reinforcement[2] or counterconditioning.

Counterconditioning

With counterconditioning, the animal's conditioned emotional response to a stimulus is replaced with an opposite response. For example, if a parrot is afraid of the sound of the vacuum (the conditioned stimulus), this sound can be paired with food to elicit an opposite emotional ("pleasure") or physiologic (heart rate reduction) reaction. Counterconditioning will only occur if the new eliciting stimulus triggers a response powerful enough to supplant the problem response. Since this is difficult to accomplish with some stimuli, it is often advantageous to pair the counterconditioning procedure with systematic desensitization, particularly for extreme fear reactions.

Response blocking

Response blocking (flooding) is another exposure procedure but unlike systematic desensitization, it is not gradual and the animal has no power to move away. With response blocking, the animal is presented with the fear-eliciting stimulus at full strength without possibility of escape, until the fear responses are no longer observed. Flooding requires long duration sessions; if the session is aborted before reaching the goal of fear cessation, the process may actually exacerbate the animal's fearful response.[3]

While flooding can be effective, the procedure is a cause of grave concern as it can be traumatic for both the client and the patient. Flooding removes animals' power to choose, which can result in impaired behavior, a condition termed learned helplessness. The animal learns that its behavior has no effect on the environment resulting in decreased responding even when power to escape is restored. Learned helplessness can generalize to situations other than the one in which it was induced[4] and has been associated with detrimental physiologic side effects.[5]

Fundamental principles of operant behavior

The most fundamental law of operant behavior is the law of effect, which states: Behavior is a function of it consequences. Consequences that function to increase the frequency of a behavior are called reinforcers, and the process by which the behavior increases is called reinforcement. Consequences that function to decrease the frequency of a behavior are called punishers, and the process by which the behavior decreases is called punishment.

The operation used to deliver consequences describes another important dimension to consider. When a behavior results in the addition or presentation of a stimulus, the consequence is called positive ($+$) and when a behavior results in the subtraction or removal of a stimulus, the consequence is called negative ($-$). These terms are used like mathematical operations without value judgments about the pleasantness or unpleasantness of the consequence *per se*. Thus, every consequence can be described along two different dimensions: function (increasing

	FUNCTION	
	Increase	**Decrease**
OPERATION **Addition** +	Positive reinforcement (rewards)	Positive punishment (discipline)
Subtraction −	Negative reinforcement (escape)	Negative punishment (penalties/fines)

Figure 18.1 Consequences: Function by operation and common terms.

or decreasing) and operation (positive or negative), as described in Figure 18.1.

As each individual is unique, this makes ABA a study of one. True to form, consequences can affect different animals, even those from the same species, in very different ways. The characteristic of being a reinforcer or punisher is demonstrated solely by the future strength (e.g., frequency, duration, or intensity) of each individual animal's behavior. New reinforcers can be conditioned with the respondent process of repeated, contiguous pairing of a neutral stimulus with an existing reinforcer. The more reinforcers an animal behaves to get, the more successfully it can learn and clients can teach. New punishers are similarly learned. To influence behavior effectively with consequences, reinforcers and punishers should be delivered immediately and consistently, – i.e., consequences are most effective when they are certain, swift, and strong.

Examples to pick the principle

Although a certain amount of terminology tumult results from the fact that these terms have specific scientific meaning that can be different than common usage, the procedural differences are clear when viewed systematically. Four key questions will help clarify each process when answered in the following order:

1. What is the target behavior being assessed?
2. What is the immediate consequence the behavior produces?
3. Do you predict this consequence will maintain/increase (reinforce) the behavior or suppress/decrease (punish) the behavior?
4. Is the consequence something the animal gets (positive) or is something escaped/removed (negative), as a result of the behavior?

The following examples illustrate the effects of the four consequences with a single behavior and pet—a biting parrot. Of course any individual may respond very differently.

- *Positive reinforcement*—When client is on the phone (Antecedent, A), if the parrot bites (Behavior, B), then the client pets the bird (Consequence, C). Biting will likely increase.
- *Negative reinforcement*—When client offers hand (A), if the parrot bites (B), then the client removes his/her hand (C). Biting will likely increase.
- *Positive punishment*—As client passes doorway with bird on hand (A), if the parrot bites (B), then the client shakes hand sharply (C). Biting will likely decrease.
- *Negative punishment*—As client installs seed cup (A), if parrot bites cage bars (B), then the client briefly removes seed cup (C). Biting cage bars will likely decrease.

Operant behavior-change procedures

Considerations for designing a behavior-change plan

Reducing problem behaviors is not the only goal when planning an intervention. A good plan is one in which the physical and social context of the environment are redesigned to provide the animal with an opportunity to replace the function served by the problem behavior with an acceptable alternative behavior, and allows the animal to learn new skills that make the problem behavior less likely to occur. One key to respecting behaving organisms is understanding that the problem behavior has function, i.e., it serves a purpose for the animal. Therefore, focus on replacing the problem behavior with an appropriate alternative behavior that can serve the same function.

O'Neill et al.[6] describe four considerations to increase the effectiveness and efficiency of behavior-change plans: First, behavior support plans should describe how the client plans to change the environment to promote and maintain appropriate behavior. This is accomplished by changing a wide range of conditions such as medications, diet, physical settings, schedules, exercise, training procedures, and the use of rewards and punishers. It is also important to describe in detail exactly who in the family will do what and when.

Second, there should be a clear link between the functional assessment of the problem behavior (i.e., the related antecedents and consequences that maintain the problem behavior, discussed later) and the intervention plan. For example, a functional assessment may reveal that a sugar glider repeatedly bites offered hands to remove the hands from its immediate cage area. Therefore, the intervention plan to reduce this behavior should identify what alternative behavior the animal can use to accomplish this goal in a more acceptable way (e.g., the sugar glider can lean away from the hand rather than bite it). The intervention should also identify new behaviors to teach the animal (e.g., stepping onto a hand by choice and without hesitation). The main focus of an intervention plan should be on what an animal *should do* instead of the problem behavior, not on what it *should not do*. This is why it is important to ask the client, "What do you want the animal to do instead?" With in this in mind, behavior interventions should target one problem behavior at a time. It is not uncommon for a successful intervention to result in generalized improvements to other problem behaviors and to improve the relationship between caregiver and pet. Although caregivers will often choose to change the behavior most problematic to them, it is often a better strategy to start with the behavior that is easiest to change. In this way, caregivers will be reinforced for their efforts.

Third, behavior-change plans should be technically sound. A technically sound plan is one that adheres to the scientific principles of learning in order to make the problem behavior irrelevant, inefficient, and ineffective. A problem behavior becomes irrelevant when an alternative behavior provides the same, or more, reinforcement to the animal. A problem behavior becomes inefficient when, compared to the wrong behavior, the right behavior can be performed with less effort, fewer responses, and results in quicker reinforcement. A problem behavior becomes ineffective when the maintaining reinforcer is reduced or withheld each time the behavior is exhibited.

Fourth, the behavior-change program should fit the client's setting and skills. The best strategy is the one that can be implemented effectively by the people responsible for the plan. Interventions should fit the client's routines, values, resources, and skills. A good plan is effective in helping the animal and also results in reinforcing outcomes for the client, in both the short and long run (see Figure 18.2).

One mystery that often surrounds problem behavior is its very persistence. Clients may have a litany of failed behavior-change programs by the time they turn to you for help. As they wade through the personal recipes of one Internet charlatan after another, clients don't realize that with each failed attempt at behavior change, the window of opportunity to change the behavior closes a little bit because the problem behavior has been intermittently reinforced. Intermittent schedules of reinforcement build the highly persistent behavior of gamblers, animals willing to behave again and again and again, without reinforcement, for that one jackpot that inevitably arrives. Thus, there should be nothing casual about intervening on an animal's functional

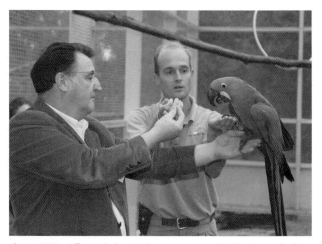

Figure 18.2   Effective behavior-change programs should empower both the animal and the caregiver. Caregivers should be taught skills that allow them to be an integral part of the animal's current and future learning. (Photo courtesy of Steve Martin.)

problem behavior. Each intervention should start with a careful functional assessment and the intervention should be designed to meet the needs of the animal using the most positive, least intrusive methods.

Functional assessment

Functional assessment is the first step in developing any behavior-change program. It is the process of developing hypotheses about the functional relations among antecedents, behaviors, and consequences—the ABCs, as demonstrated in the examples in the previous section. The hypothesis generated from a sound functional assessment improves our understanding of behavior and our ability to predict it. Functional assessment also improves the interventions we design in order to decrease problem behaviors, increase appropriate alternative behaviors, and teach new skills.

Functional assessment requires observation skills that clients can quickly develop. The following key questions can help focus their observations on the ABCs:

- What does the problem look like in terms of actual behavior, that is what do you see?
- Under what conditions does your animal do this behavior, that is what events predict it?
- What does your animal get, or get away from, by emitting this behavior?
- Under what conditions does your animal not do this behavior, that is when is the animal successful?
- What do you want the animal to do instead?

The answers to these questions will improve clients understanding of relationships between the problem behavior and the environment they provide. Examining the ABCs reveals that there are no problem *behaviors*; there are problem *situations*. The problem behavior is only one element of problem situations. The other two elements, occasion setting antecedents and functionally related consequences, are environmental elements that can be changed.

The functional assessment and intervention design worksheet

The functional assessment and intervention design (FAID) worksheet[7] was created to teach clients how to systematically solve behavior problems through the process of answering guiding questions. The worksheet can be filled out at home and reviewed during an appointment with the veterinarian or veterinary technician. Often, when one behavior is changed, it affects other behaviors. As a result, every problem behavior should be assessed separately, following the goal of changing one behavior at a time (see Figure 18.3 for the complete worksheet). Two case studies using an abbreviated form of the worksheet follow the chapter (Case Studies 1 and 2).

Changing behavior with antecedent strategies

A stimulus becomes an antecedent for a particular behavior if the stimulus is repeatedly present when the behavior is reinforced. A ringing doorbell can become a signal for loud vocalizations if the vocalizations result in social reinforcers when the bell rings. Opening the animal's cage door can become a signal for aggression if the aggression results in the animal being left outside the cage. The strength of a stimulus to signal, or cue, a particular behavior is related to the strength of the reinforcer that follows the behavior. To build strong cues, deliver strong reinforcers in the presence of the cues.

Add or remove the cue

One way to reduce the problem behavior is to remove the stimulus that cues the behavior. For example, buttons and jewelry often cue chewing because chewing results in social and sensory reinforcers in the presence of the buttons and

---

1. Observe and operationally define the target behavior.
   a. What does the animal do that can be observed and measured?
2. Identify the distant and immediate physical and environmental antecedents that predict the behavior.
   a. What general conditions or events affect whether the problem behavior occurs?
      i. Medical or physical problems?
      ii. Sleep cycles?
      iii. Eating routines and diet?
      iv. Daily schedule?
      v. Enclosure and activity space?
   b. What are the immediate antecedents (predictors) for the problem behavior?
      i. When, where, and with whom is the behavior problem most likely to occur?
      ii. Does the behavior immediately follow a caregiver's demand or request, or a person entering or leaving the environment?
   c. When is the animal most successful, that is, when doesn't the problem occur?
3. Identify the consequences that maintain the problem behavior, that is the immediate purpose the behavior serves.
   a. What does the animal gain by behaving in this way, such as attention, an item or activity, or sensory feedback?
   b. What does the animal avoid by behaving in this way, such as particular people, a demand or requests, items or activities, or sensory stimulation?
   c. To what extent does the animal's natural environment support the behavior (i.e., what function might it serve)?
4. Develop a summary statement describing the relationships among the antecedent predictors, the behavior, and consequence for each situation in which the behavior occurs.

> **Functional Assessment Summary Statement**
>
> Distant Antecedents: This parrot was re-homed after spending its first 6 months loose in a dark basement with 9 others parrots. It was malnourished and undersocialised.
>
> | | |
> |---|---|
> | Antecedent: | When I offer my hand |
> | Behavior: | Parrot bites |
> | Consequence: | To remove my hand |
> | Prediction: | Biting will continue/increase |

After the functional assessment summary statements have been developed, the primary caregiver can respond to the following questions to design the behavior-change program.

1. Replacement behavior: What existing alternative behavior would meet the same purpose for the animal?
   a. Rather than _____
                (Identify the problem behavior)
   b. This animal can _____
                (Identify the replacement behavior)
   Example: Rather than biting my hand, this parrot can lean away.

Figure 18.3   The functional assessment and intervention design (FAID) worksheet.

2. Desired behavior: What behavior do you ultimately want the animal to exhibit?
   a. When _____
      (Summarize antecedents)
   b. This animal _____
      (Identify desired behavior)
   c. In order to _____
      (Summarize "payoffs")

   Example: When I offer my hand, this parrot can step up, in order to get a ride to the play tree.

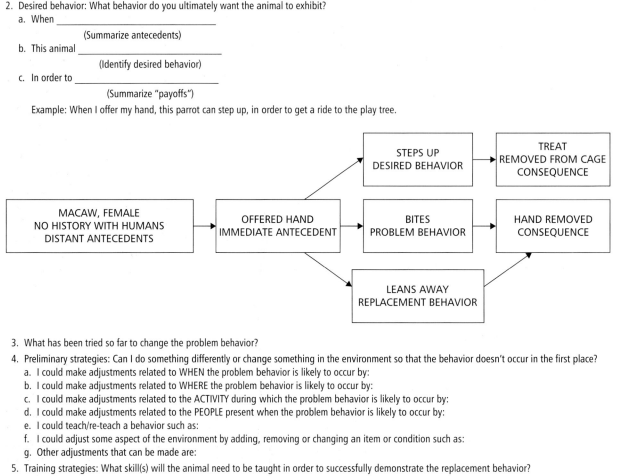

3. What has been tried so far to change the problem behavior?
4. Preliminary strategies: Can I do something differently or change something in the environment so that the behavior doesn't occur in the first place?
   a. I could make adjustments related to WHEN the problem behavior is likely to occur by:
   b. I could make adjustments related to WHERE the problem behavior is likely to occur by:
   c. I could make adjustments related to the ACTIVITY during which the problem behavior is likely to occur by:
   d. I could make adjustments related to the PEOPLE present when the problem behavior is likely to occur by:
   e. I could teach/re-teach a behavior such as:
   f. I could adjust some aspect of the environment by adding, removing or changing an item or condition such as:
   g. Other adjustments that can be made are:
5. Training strategies: What skill(s) will the animal need to be taught in order to successfully demonstrate the replacement behavior?
   a. Who will provide the training?
   b. When will the training take place?
   c. Where will the training take place?
   d. How often will training take place?
   e. How and how often will opportunities for practice be provided?
6. Reinforcement procedures: What will I do to increase the occurrence of the replacement/desired behavior?
   a. Identify potential reinforcers: What preferred items, activities, or people might be used as incentives in an intervention for this animal?
   b. Establish specific behavior criteria: What exactly must the animal do to earn the above reinforcers?
   c. Determine the schedule of reinforcement: How frequently can the animal earn the above reinforcers. Typically, continuous reinforcement (a reinforcer for every correct behavior) is best.
7. Reduction procedures: What will I do to decrease the occurrence of the problem behavior?
   a. I will ignore all occurrences, immediately attending to something else by:
   b. I will stop and redirect each occurrence of the behavior by:
   c. I will implement time-out from positive reinforcement by:
   d. Other strategies:
8. Implementation details: What other details or explanations would help another person implement this plan accurately and consistently?
9. Tracking change: How can I monitor the animal's behavior so I have a reliable record of progress and can continue or modify the plan as needed?
   a. Describe exactly how data will be collected and recorded.
      i. Frequency count of the target behaviors across the day.
      ii. Frequency count from ___:___ am/pm to ___:___am/pm
      iii. Timing duration of target behaviors.
      iv. Other.
10. Evaluating outcomes: This program will be considered successful if what outcome is achieved by both the animal and the caregivers, under what conditions?

Figure 18.3   Continued

jewelry. By removing the cues (wearing T-shirts and removing jewelry) chewing necessarily decreases. Adding a cue for an alternative behavior is another way to reduce the frequency of a problem behavior. For example, opening the food door may cue lunging because lunging has been reinforced with the delivery of food. Teaching an animal to stand in a particular location when the food door is opened prevents lunging at the door.

Increase or decrease effort with setting events

Setting events are the context, conditions, or situational influences that affect behavior. For example, coming out of the cage can be made easier by selecting cages with large doors, which may ultimately reduce biting. We can make chewing the window frame harder by locating the play area in the middle of the room. The relation between setting events and problem behavior should be considered carefully as the setting is often one of the easiest things to change, to change behavior.

Strengthen or weaken motivation

Motivating operations (also known as establishing operations) are antecedent events that temporarily alter the effectiveness of consequences. For example, a few food treats may be a highly motivating consequence to a pet that rarely has access to them but not motivating at all to one that has unlimited access to treats every day. A ferret may be more motivated to go into its cage after a long play session when it is tired and ready to sleep. Chasing the family cat may be less reinforcing after an energetic training session, and stepping onto a hand may be more reinforcing to a bird when the bird is on the floor.

Antecedent behavior-change strategies are often preventative solutions rather than learning solutions. As a result, antecedent strategies are often the most positive, least intrusive, effective behavior-change procedures. Clients often feel they must change the behavior by fixing the animal. Teaching clients that simple changes in the antecedent environment can result in effective solutions to behavior problems is often a big relief.

Decreasing behavior with consequences

Extinction

Once the reinforcer for a problem behavior is identified, it can be permanently withheld or eliminated to reduce the behavior. When the contingency between a behavior and its consequence is eliminated, the behavior serves no function and eventually decreases or is suppressed. This process is called extinction. Extinction is most effective the very first time a problem behavior occurs, that is do not give the behavior a reinforcing function in the first place.

There are very few problem behaviors that are well suited to extinction. First, extinction can be a slow process. This is typically the case with behaviors with an intermittent reinforcement history. Second, there is often an intolerably sharp increase in the frequency and intensity of the problem behavior, called an extinction burst, before it eventually decreases. This escalation in behavior often results in clients reinforcing even more problematic behavior. If extinction is the selected process, clients must be forewarned of the possibility of an initial extinction burst so they don't give up and reinforce the animal at the peak of its behavioral response. Third, extinction can result in frustration-elicited aggression, which adds another problem to contend with. Fourth, the reinforcement for some behaviors is difficult or impossible to control. Physiologic changes associated with the cue or the behavior can also provide intrinsic (e.g., sensory, neuro-chemical) reinforcement. Last, the problem behavior may recover over time requiring the extinction procedure to be implemented again.

Punishment

Punishment is the process by which consequences decrease or suppress behavior. Behavior can be punished by contingently adding an aversive stimulus, called positive punishment (discipline), or by contingently removing positive reinforcers, called negative punishment (fines, penalties, and time-out). For example, when a client passes through a doorway with her bird on her hand (A), if the parrot bites (B), then the client shakes her hand sharply (C). In this scenario biting will likely decrease (punishment) given the addition (positive) of the sharp shake of the hand. Alternatively, when a client installs a seed cup through a cage door (A), if parrot bites cage bars (B), then the client temporarily removes seed cup (C). Biting cage bars will likely decrease (punishment), given the temporary, contingent removal (negative) of the filled seed cup.

As with all consequence procedures, punishers must be delivered consistently and immediately. Punishment should also be strong enough to suppress behavior but not result in fear or harm. Decades of scientific studies demonstrate the detrimental problems with positive punishment. As a result, positive punishment should only be used to solve behavior problems when more positive, less intrusive procedures have failed (an uncommon occurrence among experienced practitioners). Punishment is associated with four detrimental side effects: Increased aggression, generalized fear, apathy, and escape-avoidance behaviors.[8] Equally important to consider is that punishment doesn't teach the animal what *to do* in place of the problem behavior. Punishment also does not teach caregivers how to teach alternative behaviors. Caregivers become focused on the problem behavior rather than on productive solutions. Punishment is really two aversive events—the onset of a punishing stimulus and the forfeiture of the reinforcer that has maintained the problem behavior in the past. Additionally, punishment often requires an increase in aversive stimulation to maintain initial levels of behavior reduction. The potential arises for caregivers to deliver physically harmful interventions. Perhaps the most detrimental side effect of punishment is that when it is effective, punishment reinforces the punisher who is therefore more likely to punish again in the future, even when antecedent arrangements or positive reinforcement is the better choice. This can become a vicious cycle where the animal's relationship with the caregiver centers on the caregiver's attempts to punish rather than teach the animal what to do.

Time-out from positive reinforcement

Time-out from positive reinforcement is a negative punishment procedure that can effectively reduce problem behavior with fewer detriments than positive punishment. Time-out is the temporary removal, or reduction, of access to positive reinforcers contingent on a problem behavior. When a client reaches down to pet a ferret (A) and the ferret explores her hand by nipping it (B), the client moves away, withdrawing attention (C). Nipping when the client pets the ferret will likely decrease due to the process of negative punishment in which attention, a positive reinforcer, is removed. Time-out can be a relatively unintrusive behavior-change procedure if it is implemented correctly, that is consistently, with close contiguity (immediacy) to the problem behavior, and short duration of just a few seconds. The animal should be quickly brought back into the situation and given a chance to do the right behavior and earn positive reinforcement. The client should also let the procedure do the job and avoid injecting emotional responses into the process, which may be reinforcing to the pet.

Increasing behavior with consequences

Without question the two sharpest behavior-change tools are variations of differential reinforcement. Differential reinforcement is the process of reinforcing one class of behaviors while at the same time extinguishing another behavior. Differential reinforcement of alternative behavior (DRA) is used to replace problem behavior with a more appropriate behavior, and differential reinforcement of successive approximations (shaping) is used to teach new skills. Both procedures avoid the problems and side effects of positive punishment and result in high rates of positive reinforcement so vital to behavioral health. This is why both procedures are close to the top of the ethical hierarchy of behavior-change strategies (discussed later in the chapter) (Figures 18.4a–c).

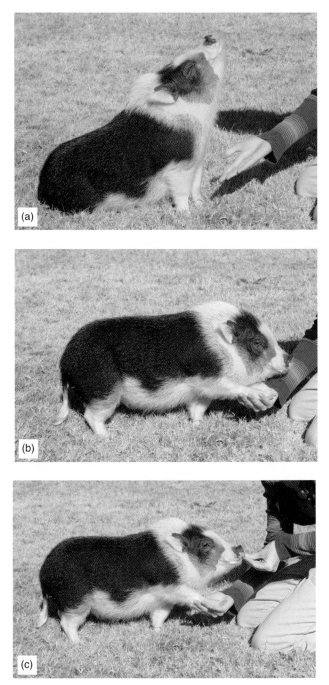

Figures 18.4 (a–c)   The most striking advantages to positive reinforcement training include empowerment and strengthening of the animal–caregiver bond. Here a pig is asked to perform a previously shaped behavior. The pig can choose to perform this behavior or offer some other response; however, the caregiver will only reinforce the desired response. (Photos courtesy of M. C. Tynes, copyright 2010.)

Differential reinforcement of alternative behavior

With DRA, a desirable replacement behavior is reinforced (increased) while the problem behavior is extinguished (i.e., suppressed or returned to baseline levels due to withdrawal of reinforcement). A functional assessment is necessary to identify the reinforcer that has been maintaining the problem behavior in the past, in order to withhold it.

There are three things to consider when selecting an alternative behavior. First, although the behavior targeted for reduction is a problem to people, it serves a legitimate function to the animal or it would not continue to exhibit the behavior. The function is either to gain something of value – for example screaming to gain attention (positive reinforcement), or the function is to remove something aversive – for example lunging to remove intruding hands (negative reinforcement). An alternative or incompatible behavior should be selected that replaces the function served by the problem behavior but in a more appropriate way. If the alternative behavior is incompatible with the problem behavior (i.e., if both behaviors can't physically be performed at the same time), the behavior-change program can proceed more quickly. For example, talking is incompatible with a bird screaming, and standing in the back corner is incompatible with lunging at the feed door.

Second, the alternative behavior should produce even more reinforcement than the problem behavior in order to successfully compete with and replace it. According to the principle called the matching law, the distribution of behavior between alternative sources of reinforcement is equal to the distribution of reinforcement for these alternatives.[3] Thus, given a choice between two alternative behaviors, animals preferentially exhibit the behavior that results in the greater reinforcement. The matching law is itself a powerful tool for managing behavior. For example, if stepping onto an offered hand produces twice the reinforcement as biting it, the animal will tend to choose to step on the hand.

Third, the alternative behavior should be one the animal already knows how to do. During the extinction component for the problem behavior, a well-established alternative behavior is more likely to be performed than one that is newly acquired. When alternative behaviors are strengthened and maintained, differential reinforcement can provide long-lasting results. As this method relies on positive reinforcement to teach animals what *to do*, it offers a positive, constructive, and practical approach to managing animals in captivity and meets a high ethical standard.

Shaping

Differential reinforcement of successive approximations is also known as shaping. Shaping is used to teach new behaviors by successively reinforcing subtle variations in responses, called approximations, along a continuum that leads to the final goal behavior.

Shaping starts by reinforcing the closest approximation, the related form or estimate of the target behavior, that the animal already exhibits. Next, an approximation slightly closer to the target behavior is reinforced, at which time reinforcement for the first approximation is withheld. Once the second approximation is performed without hesitation, an even closer approximation is reinforced while withholding reinforcement for all previous approximations. In this manner, the criterion for reinforcement is incrementally shifted closer and closer to the target behavior, until the animal eventually exhibits the final goal. At this stage, every instance of the completed target behavior is reinforced. For example, to teach a parrot to play with a toy, the following approximations can be reinforced in turn: looking at the toy, leaning toward the toy, moving a foot in the direction of the toy, taking one step toward the toy, taking several steps to arrive beside the toy, touching the toy with the beak, touching the toy with a foot, holding the toy with a foot while manipulating it in the beak, and finally reinforcing longer durations of toy-play. If the animal experiences difficulty at any criterion, the client can back up and repeat the previous successful step, or reinforce even smaller approximations. Ultimately, it is the learner who determines the pace, the number of repetitions, and the size of the approximations in a shaping procedure, but in general, smaller approximations tend to produce a more fluid progression and more stable learning.

Implementing a shaping procedure requires keen observation of the subtle, natural variation in the way behaviors are performed. For example, each time a parrot lifts its foot, it is naturally done differently than the last time (e.g., left or right; high or low; fast or slow, with toe movement or without, and so on). In daily life, these variations are unimportant and simply classified as one behavior, or operant class, called "lifting a foot." However, the subtle variations in foot lifting are exactly what allows us to shape new behaviors, such as offering a steady foot for nail trims.

With shaping we can theoretically teach any behavior within the biological constraints of the animal. Husbandry, medical, and enrichment behaviors can be shaped to reduce stress and increase physical and mental stimulation. Animals can learn behaviors such as going in and out of crates, staying calm wrapped in towels, moving to designated stations or perches, and playing games. Shaping can also be used to change different dimensions of existing behaviors such as their duration, rate, intensity, topography, and latency (response time).

A matter of ethics: Effectiveness is not enough

What makes behavior analysis unique according to Bailey and Burch[9] is also relevant to veterinarians and other animal professionals working with behavior: Both behavior analysts and veterinarians supervise others, such as paraprofessionals and clients, who carry out the behavior intervention plans. The interventions are usually implemented where the behavior problem actually occurs, rather than in an office. The participants are often very vulnerable and unable to protect themselves from harm.

These interdisciplinary commonalities suggest that the ethical standards established for behavior analysts may also have widespread relevance.

There is a 30-year-old standard that promotes the least restrictive, behavior interventions (LRBI) with human participants (also referred to as most positive, least intrusive, behavior intervention). This standard appears in public federal law protecting children (IDEA, 1997) and the Behavior Analyst Certification Board Guidelines for Responsible Conduct for Behavior Analysts (2004). According to Carter and Wheeler,[1] intrusiveness refers to the level of social acceptability of an intervention and the degree to which the participant maintains control. Although this definition leaves room for a great deal of judgment at the edges, it is clearer in the middle where most behavior consultations lie. Procedures with aversive stimuli are more intrusive and would be recommended only after less intrusive procedures have been tried.

Figure 18.5 shows a proposed hierarchy of intervention strategies working with animals that takes into account distant and immediate antecedent arrangements. The examples are with pet parrots but apply to all animals. The overwhelming majority of behavior problems can be prevented or resolved with one or more strategies represented in Levels 1–4 (i.e., arranging distant and immediate antecedents, positive reinforcement, and DRA). Level 5

Level 1:
Distant antecedents—address medical, nutritional, and physical environment variables.
Example: Resolve feather picking by removing the ingested earring, improving diet, adding soft wood and paper items to cage, and increasing exercise.

Level 2:
Immediate antecedents—redesign setting events, change motivations, and add or remove discriminative stimuli (cues) for the problem behavior.
Example: Move play gym away from window frame to redirect chewing; provide focused 1:1 time before leaving parrot on play gym to reduce wandering; remove earrings before holding bird to reduce snatching.

Level 3:
Positive reinforcement—contingently deliver a consequence to increase the probability that the right behavior will occur, which is more reinforcing than the problem behavior.
Example: When client is on the phone (A), if the parrot perches (B), then the client pets the bird (C). Perching will likely increase.

Level 4:
Differential reinforcement of alternative behavior—reinforce an acceptable replacement behavior and remove the maintaining reinforcer for the problem behavior.
Example: When client walks in the room (A) if the bird keeps 2 ft on perch (B) then the client praises and offers a treat. When the client walks in the room (A), if the bird frantically rocks back and forth (B), then the client ignores the bird. Keeping both feet on the perch will likely increase and rocking will likely decrease.

Level 5 (no sequential order of intrusiveness intended):
a. Negative punishment—contingently withdraw a positive reinforcer to reduce the probability that the problem behavior will occur.
Example: As client installs seed cup (A), if parrot bites cage bars (B), then the client removes seed cup for 5 seconds (C). Biting cage bars will likely decrease.
b. Negative reinforcement—contingently withdraw an aversive antecedent stimulus to increase the probability that the right behavior will occur.
Example: When client offers hand, holding a towel with other hand (A), if the parrot steps up (B), then the towel is removed (C). Stepping up will likely increase.
c. Extinction—permanently remove the maintaining reinforcer to suppress the behavior or reduce it to baseline levels.
Example: Enlist children's help to ignore the parrot's attention-maintained swear words.

Level 6:
Positive punishment—contingently deliver an aversive consequence to reduce the probability that the problem behavior will occur.
Example: As client passes through doorway with bird on hand (A), if the parrot bites (B), then the client shakes hand sharply dropping the bird on the floor (C). Biting will likely decrease.

Figure 18.5 Hierarchy of behavior-change procedures using the most positive, least intrusive, effective criteria (Level 1 most recommended—Level 6 least recommended).

(i.e., negative punishment, negative reinforcement, and extinction) may occasionally be the ethical choice under certain circumstances. Level 6, positive punishment (i.e., the application of aversive stimuli that reduces the probability of the behavior occurring again), is rarely necessary or suggested by standards of best practice when one has the requisite behavior knowledge and teaching skills. Clearly, the animals in our care would benefit from such an intervention hierarchy that is both ethical and feasible to implement.

Conclusion

In the medical field, practitioners are trained to focus on physiological problems. Veterinarians tend to use the same medical modality when presented with an animal displaying an undesirable behavior. Both clients and practitioners are typically focused on determining how to change the *animal* and eliminate the behavior. When you fixatedly stare at an obstacle in the road, your likelihood of a crash is greater than if you evaluate the entire scene for an easier and more successful path of travel. Similarly, an effective behavior-change plan should evaluate the animal's environment and behavior in a comprehensive and systematic way, permitting construction of a clear route to success. The science of behavior analysis provides the map and the vehicle with which to structure a humane, effective behavior-change plan.

Functional assessment delineates the essential dependency between environmental antecedents, the animal's behavior, and its consequences. This knowledge permits development of strategies for antecedent change (e.g., setting events) and manipulation of consequences (e.g., differential reinforcement, shaping) with the focus on teaching the animal what we want it to *do* rather than concentrating on what it should not do.

Perhaps, most importantly when changing behavior is that we recognize that animals are sentient, feeling beings, and as such, choice is not only a right but also a biological need for behavioral health. Behavior-change methodologies should not be things we do *to* an animal, but interactions we have *with* an animal—a conversation, not a monologue. Arrangements for behavior change should empower both the owner and the animal, ultimately resulting in an enhanced quality of life for both.

Case Study 1: Peaches

Now back to Ms. Jones and Peaches. After taking a thorough behavioral history, you discover some of the following points.

1. Peaches is a 2-year-old female mini-lop weighing approximately 6 lbs.
2. Peaches is kept in a wire cage measuring approximately 71 × 71 cm (28 × 28 in.) and 40 cm high (16 in. high) which is kept in the laundry room.
3. Peaches is fed commercial rabbit pellets, some alfalfa hay, and a few pieces of vegetables (mostly lettuce and carrots) daily. These are generally given to her in the evening around the time the owner eats dinner.
4. Peaches is let out of her cage for approximately 30–60 minutes per day, usually in the evening when Ms. Jones daughter has time to play with her.
5. Peaches only struggles and kicks when the person holding her approaches the laundry room door. Sometimes they can get her into the cage, but other times they must put her down in order to avoid being hurt.

Initial interpretation may conclude this is a complex issue because the owner and the practitioner may become bogged down in the belief that Peaches is "dominant" and therefore inherently defective. In actuality, this is a single and simple behavioral complaint: kicking and scratching, specifically when being returned to her cage, and makes the functional assessment straightforward.

Functional assessment

1. **Identify the behavior:** Peaches kicks and scratches.
2. **Identify the distant and immediate physical and environmental antecedents that predict the behavior.**
   a. **What general conditions or events affect whether the problem behavior occurs?**
      - Peaches is a moderately large rabbit.
      - Peaches is typically fed before her exercise outing.
      - Peaches is let out in the evening when rabbits tend to be most active.
      - Peaches is kept in a small cage in a closed room.
      - Peaches receives only 30–60 minutes of exercise per day.
      - Peaches has one wooden chew toy in her cage at all times. She is given alfalfa cubes once daily in the morning.
   b. **What are the immediate antecedents (predictors) for the problem behavior?**
      - The kicking and scratching occur when carried back to her cage and with all family members but more so with the daughter.
      - Onset of the behavior occurs as the owner, holding Peaches, approaches the laundry room door.

   c. When is the animal most successful, that is when doesn't the problem occur?
- When she goes into her cage on her own (which happens rarely).
- When she is held or carried away from her cage or in locations away from her cage.

3. Identify the consequences that maintain the problem behavior, that is the immediate purpose the behavior serves.
   a. Peaches intermittently avoids being placed in the cage. The daughter often sets her down which results in Peaches having more time outside the cage. This intermittent consequence (reinforcement) has probably built very persistent behavior.

After the functional assessment summary statements have been developed, the primary caregiver can respond to the following questions to design the behavior-change program

4. Replacement behavior: What existing alternative behavior would meet the same purpose for the animal?
   a. Teach the owners to set Peaches down as soon as they feel her tense on her body or at the immediate onset of any struggling, rather than waiting until she is actually kicking and scratching.

5. Desired behavior: What behavior do you ultimately want the animal to exhibit?
   a. When Peaches is carried, she remains calm in the owners' arms.
   b. Peaches goes willingly into her cage on her own when cued to do so.

6. Can I do something differently or change something in the environment so that the behavior doesn't occur in the first place?
   a. Obtain a larger cage and move it out of the laundry room. Because approach to the laundry door is a specific signal for kicking and scratching, moving the cage to a new location allows for the owner and Peaches to more successfully develop a new history with cage entry behavior.
   b. Be sure the cage is located low enough to the ground that Peaches can readily enter the cage on her own.
   c. Allow Peaches out of the cage more frequently so she obtains more exercise.
   d. Allow Peaches out of the cage during the training sessions in the *afternoon* when she is most likely to want to rest and therefore may be more willing to go back inside.
   e. Let Peaches out for exercise prior to feeding her meals so these meals can be used to reinforce cage return behavior.

7. Training strategies: What skill(s) will the animal need to be taught in order to successfully demonstrate the replacement behavior?
   a. Train Peaches to return to the cage on cue (e.g., hand signal, verbal cue, or a bell).
   b. Train Peaches to rest calmly on a large towel (which then can be used to pick her up safely and securely).
   c. Place enrichment items (toys, chewing objects) in the cage and, if necessary, encourage their use by using a shaping procedure to increase Peaches' interaction with them.

8. Reinforcement procedures: What will I do to increase the occurrence of the replacement/desired behavior?
   a. Returning to cage on cue:
   - Use a portion of her daily ration of pellets and all of her treats (e.g., vegetables) to reinforce returning to the cage.
   - The behavior is trained initially by placing her close to the cage and reinforcing cage entering. Over training sessions, she will be placed further from the case in small increments to shape cage returning in approximations.
   b. Sitting on the towel:
   - Peaches can be cued to sit on the towel just inside the cage or on the floor just outside the cage door in order to be taken outside to a safe enclosed area for exercise. (Towel stationing will be taught separately prior to using this strategy.)
   - Being let of out the cage reinforces calm towel-sitting behavior.
   - Food/treats can be used to reinforce calm behavior during shaping approximations for folding the towel around her and eventually lifting her off the ground.
   c. Behaviors will be reinforced on a continuous schedule of reinforcement.

9. Tracking change: How can I monitor the animal's behavior so I have a reliable record of progress and can continue or modify the plan as needed?
   a. The owner can keep a training log listing each session, number of trials (repetitions) of the behavior, and the number of trials on which Peaches is successful. (Too many unsuccessful trials mean that the criteria for reinforcement should be lowered so that Peaches is more successful.)

10. Evaluating outcomes: This program will be considered successful if what outcome is achieved by both the animal and the caregivers, under what conditions?
    a. The owner should specifically define the goal behavior, for example from how far away from the cage is Peaches expected to return on her own when cued to do so?
    b. How long/far is Peaches expected to remain calm in the towel when she is being carried?
    c. High levels of reinforcement while being held in a towel will allow for gradual fading of the towel over time so peaches can be carried calmly without the towel.

Case Study 2: Pepe

Pepe is a 20-year-old male Mexican red-headed parrot (*Amazona viridigenalis*). The owners' complaint is that Pepe screams, bites people when attempting to pick him up, and tries to attack their other bird, a Senegal parrot ("Jasper") of unknown sex and age.

Your behavioral history uncovers the following:

1. Pepe is housed in 61 × 56 × 76 cm (24 × 22 × 30 in.) parrot cage. Jasper is housed in a slightly smaller cage on the opposite side of the breakfast room approximately 20 ft from Pepe's cage. Both birds have playpens on top of their cages but they are not allowed out of the cages at the same time. Both birds also have a play stand in the living room on opposite sides of the room. Both cages have approximately 3–5 parrot toys that the owner changes out when the birds have destroyed them.
2. The birds are each let out onto the top of their cages or on their play stands for approximately 30 minutes in the morning and 1–1.5 hours in the evening. The owners directly play with the bird for approximately 30% of this time and sometimes carry the bird around the house with them on their hands or shoulders.
3. Pepe has always bitten when anyone has tried to pick him up. He bites both his owners and strangers. He is most likely to bite when on or in his cage, on his play stand, or on any piece of furniture. Pepe is less likely to try to bite if picked up off the floor. When Pepe bites, he generally leaves marks on the person's hand and has actually drawn blood approximately 20% of the time. Immediately after biting, Pepe screams and then "laughs." This makes the owners angry and they often yell at him or try to squirt him with water. They have attempted to pick him up with gloves, a perch, and towels. These interventions have not reduced Pepe's biting behavior. At this time, the owner generally coerces Pepe onto a perch to move him from one place to another. Pepe bites at the perch and backs away but eventually will step up onto it.
4. Pepe also sometimes bites unpredictably when sitting on the owner's shoulder. He will suddenly screech and then bite at the owner's ear or cheek. The owner has not identified an antecedent for this behavior.
5. Pepe frequently screams or makes loud piercing noises when the owners try to watch television, read, or cook. This occurs when Pepe is in his cage or on his play stand. The owners try to ignore this, but admit that sometimes they yell at him or squirt him with water to get him to stop. Squirting him with water does interrupt the behavior for a while but yelling does not.
6. When Pepe is on his cage or playpen, he periodically flies over to Jasper's cage and tries to bite Jasper through the bars. If both birds were out together, Pepe would fly over and try to attack Jasper. The owner immediately takes Pepe and puts him in his cage. The owners did try clipping Pepe's wings to discourage this behavior. While this did reduce the frequency of the problem, Pepe would sometimes climb down off his cage and walk over to Jasper's cage. Pepe's wings are no longer clipped as the owners do enjoy having Pepe flighted and also found that sometimes Pepe would try to fly and then fall to the floor.

This case demonstrates the multitude of complaints that many owners bring to practitioners. Wading through the information to determine what is relevant to the functional assessment and what is not can be daunting, but it is a crucial step in designing an effective strategy for behavior change. Learning to discard irrelevancies and focus on the behaviors directly related to the functional assessment is part of the educational process for practitioners and the owners.

The history above reveals four behavior issues:

- Biting when the owner tries to pick up the bird.
- Screaming and making loud noises when the owners are relaxing.
- Screaming and biting the owner's ear when on the owner's shoulder.
- Flying to Jasper's cage and trying to bite Jasper.

While all of these issues are of concern to the owner, tasking the owners with multiple behavior plans simultaneously lowers the likelihood of success for any one behavior. Additionally, the resolution of one behavior may improve or otherwise influence the others (thereby changing the functional assessment).

A sound approach is initially to focus on the behavior change that has the greatest likelihood of success. In this particular case, the biting behavior is a sensible place to start because the owner's ability to safely handle Pepe strengthens their bond and increases their enjoyment of his companionship. Additionally, the attention that Pepe receives during training sessions may eliminate the bird's attention-seeking screaming as well as reducing his attacks on Jasper (which also garner him attention). Although the biting behavior is the initial focus of the intervention program, antecedent management changes can be made immediately to try to reduce reinforcement for some of these undesirable behaviors. Antecedent change for these behaviors can include:

- Screaming when the owner is relaxing/cooking.
  - Provide enrichment and foraging items during this time to limit screaming as an attention-seeking behavior.
  - Give Pepe a training session just prior to the time the owner wants to relax so Pepe may be more inclined to rest quietly on his play stand.

- Screaming and biting the owner's ear/cheek.
  - Do not allow Pepe to sit on the owner's shoulder.
  - Limit interaction to times when Pepe is on his play stand or cage to prevent shoulder climbing behavior.

- Flying over and attacking Jasper through the cage.
  - Move Jasper's cage further away from Pepe.
  - Allow Pepe out of his cage only under direct owner supervision when the owner is able to keep him engaged in another activity (e.g., training, play, and so on) to prevent him from flying over to Jasper's cage.

Functional Assessment

1. **Observe and operationally define the target behavior.**
   a. Pepe bites the owner's hand
2. **Identify the distant and immediate physical and environmental antecedents that predict the behavior.**
   a. What general conditions or events affect whether the problem behavior occurs?
      - Pepe is more likely to bite when he has been out of his cage for less than 1 hour.
      - Pepe is more likely to bite when he is on his cage, on a piece of furniture, or on the owner's shoulder.
   b. What are the immediate antecedents (predictors) for the problem behavior?
      - Someone reaching toward Pepe with their hand.
   c. When is the animal most successful, that is when doesn't the problem occur?
      - Pepe is least likely to bite when he is picked up off the floor and from inside his cage.
3. **Identify the consequences that maintain the problem behavior, that is the immediate purpose the behavior serves.**
   a. Biting causes people to withdraw their hands.
   b. Pepe avoids being placed back in his cage or taken off his play stand.
   c. Pepe get to remain on the owner's shoulder

After the functional assessment summary statements have been developed, the primary caregiver can respond to the following questions to design the behavior-change program

4. **Replacement behavior: What existing alternative behavior would meet the same purpose for the animal?**
   a. Rather than biting, Pepe can lean or move away from the hand.
5. **Desired behavior: What behavior do you ultimately want the animal to exhibit?**
   a. Pepe steps up calmly, without hesitation, when a hand is offered.
6. **What has been tried so far to change the problem behavior?**
   a. Picking Pepe up with gloves, a towel, or a perch
7. **Preliminary strategies: Can I do something differently or change something in the environment so that the behavior doesn't occur in the first place?**
   a. Limit Pepe's handling during the initial training process. If the problem is severe enough, this may mean leaving Pepe in his cage and conducting initial training sessions with behaviors, such as targeting and waving, which can be taught in-cage with the door closed. This will build a positive relationship that can be leveraged for later training of the step-up behavior.
   b. Do not allow strangers to try to pick Pepe up.
   c. Withdraw the hand at the first indication that Pepe is leaning or moving away. (Withdrawing the hand will reinforce Pepe for leaning away rather than biting.) This gives the parrot control/empowerment, which tends to reduce behaviors typically associated with fear and anxiety. This response from the owner also teaches the owner to be observant of Pepe's communication efforts to allow for a more sophisticated interaction between the owner and bird.
8. **Training strategies: What skill(s) will the animal need to be taught in order to successfully demonstrate the replacement behavior?**
   a. Teach Pepe a "step-up" cue by using successive approximations for lifting his foot and then stepping up onto the offered hand.
   b. Each owner should participate in daily training. Each owner should engage Pepe in a separate training session.
   c. Training initially should take place in an area where the bird can be most successful, that is away from his cage or even on the floor. Training is repeated in more challenging areas as Pepe and the owner have success at each stage. (Removing Pepe from his cage for these sessions means finding a nonthreatening way to remove him from the cage.)
   d. If Pepe is more likely to step up onto a perch, then the owner can begin training with a perch. Successive approximations are used to shape perch-stepping behavior. Over sessions, the owner should continue to shape this behavior with his/her hand moving closer to the area where Pepe is stepping up with the goal being the successful fading of the perch altogether so that Pepe is reliably stepping up directly onto the owner's hand.

9. **Reinforcement procedures: What will I do to increase the occurrence of the replacement/desired behavior?**
   a. Reinforcement for stepping up can include: food treats, verbal/auditory interaction with owner, and the opportunity to come out of the cage.
   b. Reinforcement will be provided when Pepe meets the current criteria for stepping up. The behavior should be shaped in small increments using a differential reinforcement procedure to allow Pepe to be successful.
   c. Each correct trial will receive reinforcement (continuous reinforcement schedule).
10. **Tracking change: How can I monitor the animal's behavior so I have a reliable record of progress and can continue or modify the plan as needed?**
    a. The owner should keep at least a simple training log describing the number of training sessions and trials per day as well as Pepe's success rate for each session.
11. **Evaluating outcomes: This program will be considered successful if what outcome is achieved by both the animal and the caregivers, under what conditions?**
    a. Pepe steps up onto the owner's hand reliably and calmly when the hand is offered.

References

1. Chance P. *Learning and Behavior*. Belmont, CA: Thomson Wadsworth, 2006;24–26.
2. Friedman, SG. Pavlov's parrots. *Good Bird Mag* 2007;3(2):27–30.
3. Staub E. Duration of stimulus-exposure as determinant of the efficacy of flooding procedures in the elimination of fear. *Behav Res Ther* 1968;6:131–132.
4. Maier SF, Seligman, MEP. Learned helplessness: Theory and evidence. *J Expl Psychol: Gen* 1976;105:3–46.
5. Laudenslager ML, Ryan SM, Drugan RC et al. Coping and immunosuppression: Inescapable but not escapable shock suppresses lymphocyte proliferation. *Science* 1983;221:568–570.
6. O'Neill RE, Horner RH, Albin RW et al. *Functional Assessment and Program Development for Problem Behavior: A Practical Handbook*. 2nd ed. CA: Brooks/Cole, 1997.
7. Friedman SG. A framework for solving behavior problems: Functional assessment and intervention planning. *J Exotic Pet Med* 2007; 16(1):6–10.
8. Azrin NH, Holz WC. Punishment. In: Honeg WK, ed. *Operant Behavior: Areas of Research and Application*. New York: Appleton-Century-Crofts, 1966.
9. Bailey JS, Burch MR. *Ethics for Behavior Analysts*. New Jersey: LEA, 2005.

19

Behavioral pharmacology in exotic pets

Lynne M. Seibert

Exotic pets, particularly pet birds, may be presented to the veterinarian with a variety of behavioral complaints, including feather plucking or barbering, self-inflicted trauma, excessive vocalization, aggression, stereotypies, persistent reproductive behaviors, redirected sexual behaviors, anxiety- and fear-related responses.[1] Effective management of behavior problems of exotic pets requires that the veterinarian address a variety of factors affecting both mental and physical well-being.[2] In some situations, the behavior problem can result in potentially serious medical complications, such as dystocia resulting from chronic egg laying, cloacal prolapse from chronic masturbation, injuries resulting from intra- or inter-specific aggression, or infections secondary to self-trauma. A holistic treatment approach to behavioral health may need to include medical interventions, pain management, modifications to the environment, social enrichment, nutritional improvements, behavior modification exercises, and in some cases, psychoactive medications.

Psychoactive agents cause changes in mood or behavior through their actions in the central nervous system. Drugs are being used with increasing frequency in a variety of species presenting with behavioral abnormalities, particularly when nonmedical therapies alone have failed to resolve the problem. Use of these medications can be considered after obtaining complete medical, behavioral, and nutritional histories, completing appropriate diagnostic testing, and establishing a behavioral diagnosis and the need for pharmacotherapy. Due to the complicated nature of behavioral disorders, and the multitude of contributing factors, it is rare for a behavior medication alone to provide a cure.[3] In addition to medication for the patient, the caregiver should receive instructions for behavioral interventions that will facilitate more appropriate behavioral responses, and environmental modifications aimed at reducing stress and improving husbandry.[4] Treatment of concurrent primary or secondary medical conditions will often be necessary, and hormonal therapies may be indicated in some cases.

The use of behavioral medications in exotic species is not typically supported by dose-titration studies, pharmacokinetic studies, toxicity studies, or placebo-controlled trials documenting efficacy. Very few controlled studies have been completed in exotic species, requiring the practitioner to rely primarily on anecdotal case studies or uncontrolled trials, often involving a small number of subjects, and experiential or practical clinical impressions regarding dosing, safety, and efficacy. Data from studies targeting other species, including humans, can provide useful information. However, caution is imperative when extrapolating data from one species to another, as significant physiological differences between species can result in lack of efficacy or unexpected adverse reactions.

For most exotic species, optimal therapeutic doses and dosing intervals for behavioral medications have not been established, nor is the required duration of treatment for clinical response known. Antidepressants are used to treat a variety of conditions in dogs and cats and often require up to 8 weeks of therapy before significant improvement is reported. Due to the lack of data, it is recommended that therapy be initiated using low or conservative doses and the dose gradually titrated, or dosing interval adjusted, until clinical improvement is noted. Dose titration allows for reduction or discontinuation of the medication in the event of an adverse reaction.

Psychoactive medications are often used to treat chronic conditions in humans, and long-term therapy is expected. The long-term effects of these medications are unknown in veterinary patients, and it is advisable to determine the expected duration of treatment and a plan for the gradual discontinuation of drug therapy once the behavior problem is controlled. If the medication cannot be discontinued without recurrence of the behavior, then the patient should be maintained on the lowest dose that controls the problem behavior.

Pet owners should be advised of any potential risks associated with the use of psychoactive medications and should sign an informed consent statement regarding their

CLINIC NAME
CLINIC ADDRESS AND TELEPHONE NUMBER
INFORMED CONSENT STATEMENT

It has been recommended that your pet be treated with _____ (drug name), a medication that is not licensed for use in this species. This means that using it for your pet is considered "extra label." This does not mean that the drug is dangerous to your pet, just that this species was not the subject tested for approved use.

_____ (drug name), is a medication that has been used in humans and other species for the treatment of behavioral disorders. This medication has been chosen for your pet because it has been deemed to have the potential to be efficacious. This does not guarantee that the medication will be effective.

As with all medications, this drug may have potential side effects. While side effects are rare, and every effort is made to minimize them, the occasional pet may not be able to tolerate the medication.

Possible Discomforts and Risks

Potential adverse effects include regurgitation, sedation, diarrhea, loss of balance, anxiety, increased agitation, increased heart rate, loss of appetite, lowering of the seizure threshold, central nervous system toxicity, neurological symptoms, increased aggressiveness, and death.

Side effects are rare, and when experienced are usually transient. However, if your pet experiences any of these symptoms, it is important that you stop the medication and contact us immediately, so we can make informed decisions about your pet's care.

As with any medication, your pet may have unique and unforeseen side effects.

I, the undersigned, acknowledge that I am the owner of _____.
I consent to the use of this medication in my pet. Questions regarding the medication were answered to my satisfaction, and the possible benefits and risks of its use have been explained to me.

_____

(Patient, Species, Case Number)

_____   _____

(Signature of Owner)   (Date)

_____   _____

(Signature of Clinician)   (Date)

Telephone numbers to call if questions or problems:
Normal business hours   _____
After-hours emergencies   _____

Figure 19.1   Informed consent statement.

understanding of the extra-label nature of the use of the drug (Figure 19.1). Extra-label drug use requires that the use of a particular drug has a specific rationale, that a diagnosis and the need for treatment have been established, and that the drug's use is considered acceptable for the patient's condition.[3]

Neurotransmitters and behavior

Psychoactive drugs are thought to produce their behavioral effects through their actions on neurotransmitters in the central nervous system. Neurons communicate via chemical messengers called neurotransmitters. Neurotransmitters are involved in regulating a variety of behavioral systems relevant to an organism's survival, such as social interactions, aggression, sexual behavior, predator defense, sleep cycles, feeding behavior, and stress responses.[5] Neurotransmitters of primary importance in psychopharmacology include serotonin,

norepinephrine, dopamine, and gamma-amino-butyric acid (GABA). The biogenic amines (monoamines) are related by their chemical structure and include catecholamines (norepinephrine, epinephrine, dopamine), which are synthesized from dietary tyrosine, and indoleamines (serotonin, melatonin), which are synthesized from tryptophan.

Monoamine neurotransmitters are stored in granular vesicles within axons at nerve terminals and are released from the presynaptic neuron into the synaptic space. The release of neurotransmitter from the presynaptic neuron results in binding of neurotransmitter to specific target receptor sites on both presynaptic and postsynaptic neurons, which transmits the signal to the target cell and produces the cellular response.[6] A variety of cellular activities can be triggered by binding of the ligand (neurotransmitter or drug) to its receptors.

The principle means of inactivation of neurotransmitter are by reuptake at the synaptic cleft or by enzymatic breakdown. Drugs that block or inhibit the reuptake of neurotransmitter (reuptake inhibitors) increase neurotransmitter availability and activity at synaptic receptor sites. Drugs can also block the postsynaptic effects at receptors. One example is the antipsychotics, which block activity at postsynaptic dopamine receptors.

Major drug classes with relevance in veterinary behavior

Benzodiazepines

GABA, or gamma-amino-butyric acid, is generally an inhibitory neurotransmitter, synthesized from glutamate and widely distributed in the brain. Benzodiazepines and barbiturates are GABA agonists, potentiating the effects of GABA activity at the GABA-A receptor. The regulatory functions of GABA-A receptors in the central nervous system include vigilance, anxiety control, seizure control, muscle tension, and memory functions. Benzodiazepines increase the binding affinity of the GABA-A receptor for GABA. Benzodiazepines produce specific antianxiety (anxiolytic) effects that are distinct from the nonspecific consequences of central nervous system depression. Benzodiazepines in common use in veterinary medicine include diazepam, alprazolam, clonazepam, chlorazepate, oxazepam, and lorazepam.

Side effects associated with benzodiazepine use may include muscle relaxation, ataxia, sedation, hyperphagia, paradoxical reactions, decreased locomotor activity, disinhibition of aggression, memory deficits, and increased muscle spasticity. There are rare reports of hepatic failure within 3–5 days of starting oral diazepam treatment in cats.[7] Benzodiazepines should be used with caution with obese patients, or when renal or hepatic impairment is present. Long-term use in humans can result in jaundice, neutropenia, anemia, and can lead to tolerance or dependence. After chronic dosing (daily administration for more than 1 week), these medications should be withdrawn gradually to avoid discontinuation syndrome. Anxiety, tremors, and seizures are possible if benzodiazepine therapy is abruptly withdrawn.

Benzodiazepines are indicated for the treatment of acute fear responses or phobias, muscle relaxation, seizure control, mild sedation, and as appetite stimulants. Diazepam has been suggested as a treatment for feather picking in birds.[8] Johnson suggested that the sedative effects of diazepam could be detrimental, and it is most appropriately used to suppress an acute episode of self-mutilation and not appropriate for chronic treatment.[9] Benzodiazepines have also been used to help facilitate initial acceptance of restraint devices in the hospital setting (Table 19. 1).

Anticonvulsant agents

Antiepileptic medications have been used extensively to treat psychiatric conditions in humans, including panic disorder, post-traumatic stress disorder, obsessive-compulsive disorder, generalized anxiety disorder, mania, schizophrenia, and bipolar disorder, as well as a variety of neurological conditions, including neuropathic pain.[10] Anticonvulsants are being used with increasing frequency to treat behavioral conditions in veterinary patients, although no controlled studies exist at this time.

Gabapentin is an anticonvulsant structurally similar to GABA. It has been used to treat refractory epilepsy in canine patients at a dose of 10 mg/kg q8h, with minimal side effects.[11] It has also been used to manage pain in a variety of species, including dogs and cats.[12] In a case report involving a Little Corella cockatoo, gabapentin was used successfully to treat self-mutilation of the distal extremities resulting from presumed neuralgia. Self-mutilation resolved within days of starting therapy. Attempts to discontinue gabapentin therapy were unsuccessful, so the medication was continued without any adverse effects, but monitoring of uric acid was recommended.[13]

A review of available clinical data suggests that gabapentin is an effective treatment option for social anxiety in human patients.[14] Gabapentin has also been shown to shorten the time to onset of improvement in human patients with obsessive-compulsive disorder when combined with fluoxetine, compared to patients treated with fluoxetine alone.[15] Gabapentin has potential as a primary or adjunctive treatment option for anxiety conditions, including generalized anxiety, noise phobia, and obsessive-compulsive disorder in veterinary patients, but more clinical data is needed.

Carbamazepine is another anticonvulsant agent that has been used to treat behavioral disorders in veterinary patients.[16,17] It has been suggested for use in birds with feather-picking disorder and is reported to cause mild sedation and anticholinergic effects[18] (Table 19.1). Regular monitoring of complete blood counts is recommended due to the possibility of blood dyscrasias during treatment with carbamazepine.

Opioid antagonists

Endogenous opioid peptides are released during stress and induce analgesia. An increase in activity at opioid receptor sites has been associated with stereotypic and self-directed behaviors. The release of endogenous opioid peptides can have a reinforcing effect, resulting in persistence of the stereotypic behavior. Opioids also activate the dopaminergic system, and dopamine agonists have been shown to induce stereotypic behaviors under experimental conditions. Pure opioid antagonists reverse opioid-induced analgesia and potentially block the reinforcing effects of self-directed behaviors, such as feather picking or soft tissue mutilation. Pure antagonists, such as naloxone and naltrexone, have been used successfully to treat compulsive disorders and self-mutilation. Mixed agonists/antagonists have been used

Table 19.1 Dosages for psittacine birds

Drug generic (brand)	Dosage	Forms available	Drug class
Amitriptyline (Elavil)	1.0–5.0 mg/kg PO q12–24h[43]	10, 25, 50, 75, 100, 150 mg tablets 10 mg/ml injectable	Tricyclic antidepressant
Butorphanol (Torbugesic, Torbutrol)	0.5–2.0 mg/kg IM[18] 2.0–4.0 mg/kg PO q8h[6]	1, 5, 10 mg tablets Injectable forms 10 mg/ml nasal spray	Agonist at kappa-opioid receptors and a mixed agonist–antagonist at mu-opioid receptors
Carbamazepine (Tegretol)	3.0–10.0 mg/kg PO q24h[18] 20 mg/120 ml drinking water[18]	100, 200, 300, 400 mg tablets or capsules 100 mg/5 ml suspension Extended-release tablets are available in 100, 200, and 400 mg sizes	Anticonvulsant, may cause bone marrow suppression and hepatotoxicity[18]
Clomipramine (Anafranil)	0.5–1.0 mg/kg PO q12–24h[42] 3.0 mg/kg PO q12h[28] 4.5–9.0 mg/kg PO q12h[30]	25, 50, 75 mg capsules	Tricyclic antidepressant
Diazepam (Valium)	2.5–4.0 mg/kg PO prn or q6–8h[18] 0.6 mg/kg IM q8–12h[18] 1 mg/180 ml drinking water[18] 1.25–2.5 mg/120 ml water[18]	2, 5, 10 mg tablets 5 mg/ml solution	Benzodiazepine, anxiolytic agent for acute distress Sedation, appetite stimulation, anticonvulsant
Doxepin (Sinequan)	0.5–1.0 mg/kg PO q12h[18] 1.0–2.0 mg/kg q12h[41] 1.0–5.0 mg/kg q24h[9]	10, 25, 50, 75, 100, 150 mg capsules 10 mg/ml solution	Tricyclic antidepressant
Fluoxetine (Prozac)	1.0–5.0 mg/kg q24h[41] 2.0 mg/kg PO q12h[18] 2.0–3.0 mg/kg q12–24h[23]	10, 20, 40 mg capsules 10, 20 mg tablets 20 mg/5 ml solution	Selective serotonin reuptake inhibitor
Gabapentin (Neurontin)	10.0 mg/kg PO q12h[13]	100, 300, 400 mg capsules 600, 800 mg tablets 250 mg/5 ml solution (contains xylitol)	Anticonvulsant, analgesic
Haloperidol (Haldol)	0.2–0.4 mg/kg q12h[32] 0.15–0.9 mg/kg PO q24h[34] Begin at lowest dose and increase by 0.02 mg/kg increments q2d to effect	0.5, 1, 2, 5, 10 mg tablets 2 mg/ml oral solution 5 mg/ml short-acting injectable	High potency antipsychotic Lower dose to 0.05 mg/kg q24h for Quakers, grays, and cockatoos
Haloperidol decanoate	1.0–2.0 mg/kg IM q14–28d[18]	50 mg/ml, 100 mg/ml long-acting injectable	Lower dose for Quakers, grays, and cockatoos
Leuprolide acetate (Lupron depot)	400–800 mcg/kg IM q14–28d[35]	3.75, 7.5, 11.25 mg suspension for IM injection	GnRH analog
Melatonin	0.5–1.0 mg/kg PO q24h 0.25–2.5 mg/kg 1 hr before bed[38]	1, 2, 3, 5, 10, 20 mg tablets, capsules, liquid	Neurohormone
Naltrexone (Trexan)	1.5 mg/kg PO q8–12h[19]	50 mg tablets	Opioid antagonist
Paroxetine (Paxil)	1.0–2.0 mg/kg q12–24h[25]	10, 20, 30, 40 mg tablets 10 mg/5 ml solution	Selective serotonin reuptake inhibitor

as analgesics and for the treatment of compulsive behavior (Table 19.1).

Possible side effects of opioid antagonists include gastrointestinal problems (nausea, vomiting, constipation) and increased anxiety. Naltrexone is contraindicated with liver disease.

Treatment with naltrexone in an open trial of psittacine birds with behavioral feather picking resulted in positive responses in 34 out of 41 birds.[19] Some of the birds that experienced favorable responses to treatment were wearing restraint devices at the beginning of the trial (26 birds) and continued to wear collars for the first several months of treatment. However, many resolved with treatment, and the restraint collars could be removed. The duration of treatment required for responses was not reported in this study. Dosing intervals ranged from q12h to q6h (1.5 mg/kg). No side effects or laboratory changes were noted in the report.

Opioid agonists are useful for analgesia and may be indicated in cases of feather picking with soft tissue mutilation to help make the patient more comfortable. Pain-elicited fear responses may also benefit from treatment with analgesics. For a review of analgesia in birds, reptiles, and small mammals, see Hawkins.[20]

Selective serotonin reuptake inhibitors

Serotonin (5-hydroxytryptamine or 5-HT) receptors are found predominantly in the brain and gastrointestinal tract and act primarily in an inhibitory manner. Different serotonin receptor subtypes are responsible for modulating sleep–wake cycles, feeding behavior, mood, fear responses, pain perception, motor control, sexual behavior, impulsive behavior, and aggression. Central serotonergic dysfunction has been implicated in the pathogenesis of depression, anxiety, panic disorder, obsessive-compulsive disorder, and certain types of aggression.[21,22] The performance of feather pecking in laying hens has been shown to be triggered by low serotonin neurotransmission.[23]

Selective serotonin reuptake inhibitors, SSRIs, selectively block the reuptake of serotonin into presynaptic neurons, thus increasing the amount of active neurotransmitter in the synaptic space. Reuptake effects occur rapidly, but the effects on receptor sensitivity with chronic dosing may correlate more closely with the timing of clinical improvement. Specificity for serotonin reuptake transporter sites is believed to minimize the incidence of side effects when compared to the less selective tricyclic antidepressants (TCAs). SSRIs have minimal to no effect on norepinephrine, acetylcholine, and histaminic receptors.

Although SSRIs have a wide margin of safety in most species studied, adverse effects are possible and may include lethargy, nausea, loss of appetite, insomnia, agitation, and possible lowering of the seizure threshold. There are anecdotal reports of increased agitation in birds treated with paroxetine, and other SSRIs. SSRIs should not be used in combination with monoamine oxidase inhibitors, other serotonergic agents (TCAs), barbiturates, or antipsychotics (major tranquilizers). Overdose with serotonergic agents can result in a serious, potentially fatal condition known as serotonin syndrome. Substances that can contribute to serotonin syndrome include high doses of one or a combination of the following: foods or supplements high in tryptophan, medications that increase presynaptic release of serotonin (amphetamine), medications that inhibit the reuptake of serotonin (SSRIs, TCAs, tramadol, chlorpheniramine, trazodone), medications that inhibit enzymatic breakdown of serotonin (amitraz, selegiline), and other serotonin modulating substances (buspirone).[24] Clinical signs consistent with serotonin syndrome are variable, but may include diarrhea, tachycardia, myoclonus, tremors, seizures, and altered mental status. Treatment of serotonin syndrome involves discontinuation of serotonergic agents, supportive care, and administration of serotonin antagonists.

Selective serotonin reuptake inhibitors constitute some of the most useful and efficacious behavioral medications in veterinary practice and are indicated for the treatment of compulsive disorder, including some cases of feather picking and self-mutilation, panic disorder, impulse control, and anxiety. Chronic dosing is required, with effects noted within 2–6 weeks of treatment. There is very little published information about the use of SSRIs in exotic pets. Table 19.1 contains recommended dosages for commonly used SSRIs in pet birds.

An open clinical trial with fluoxetine for the treatment of feather picking resulted in early improvement in 12 of 14 birds, but relapses were common.[25] An initial dose of 2.3 mg/kg/day was used, which was increased up to 3.0 mg/kg q12h when the lower dose proved ineffective. Reported side effects included sneezing, ataxia, and lethargy.

A cockatiel with repetitive toe chewing behavior was successfully treated with a combination of behavior modification and fluoxetine administered orally at a daily dose of 1 mg/kg.[26] The bird began to improve after 3 weeks of treatment with fluoxetine, and the toe chewing behavior had completely resolved within 2 months of therapy. Gradual tapering of the dose was initiated after 3 months of treatment, and by 5 months, the medication had been completely discontinued with no recurrence of the problem behavior.

The author has used paroxetine as a first-line therapy in combination with appropriate environmental and behavioral interventions for the treatment of feather picking and self-mutilation in birds, with minimal to no adverse effects. A starting dose of 2 mg/kg PO q24h is used, and if well tolerated, doses have been safely increased from once daily dosing to twice daily dosing and up to 2–3 mg/kg PO q12h if needed. Martin also prefers paroxetine for treating feather picking and has used it successfully for the treatment of phobias.[6,27]

Tricyclic antidepressants

As a group, the TCAs affect serotonin, norepinephrine, acetylcholine, and histamine. They cause potentiation of central nervous system biogenic amines to varying degrees by blocking their reuptake presynaptically (reuptake inhibition).

Norepinephrine is formed by the hydroxylation of dopamine, which is derived from the dietary amino acid, tyrosine. Noradrenergic cell bodies are localized in the locus coeruleus area of the brain stem. Noradrenergic pathways in the brain control learning, vigilance, arousal, cardiovascular function, mood, and the stress response (post-ganglionic sympathetic neurons). Norepinephrine deficiency or dysfunction is associated with depression in human patients, and TCAs inhibit norepinephrine reuptake thereby enhancing noradrenergic activity. In general, TCA metabolites and secondary amines are more potent inhibitors of norepinephrine reuptake, while parent compounds and tertiary amines are more potent inhibitors of serotonin reuptake.

Cholinergic pathways are located throughout the central and peripheral nervous systems. Blockade of muscarinic cholinergic receptors is responsible for the atropine-like side effects of antipsychotics and TCAs.

The therapeutic effects of TCAs are believed to result from noradrenergic and serotonergic reuptake inhibition. Alpha-adrenergic blockade, antihistaminic, and anticholinergic effects account for the various side effects seen with these drugs.[28] Table 19.2 shows the relative biochemical activities for several TCAs, listed in order of decreasing serotonin selectivity. The first two columns, labeled 5-HT and NE, generally account for the anxiolytic properties of the TCAs. Serotonin selectivity is important for the effective management of compulsive disorder, making clomipramine the only anticompulsive agent in this category. The last three columns labeled alpha-1, H1, and MUS generally account for the side effects seen with TCAs. Side effects can appear acutely, but anxiolytic effects will require chronic dosing. Therefore, TCAs cannot be used intermittently to treat acute fears.

Table 19.2 Relative biochemical activities of tricyclic antidepressants

	5-HT (serotonin) reuptake	NE (norepinephrine) reuptake	Alpha-1 receptor antagonism	H1 antihistaminic activity	MUS anticholinergic effects
Clomipramine (Anafranil)	+++	+	++	+	++
Amitriptyline (Elavil)	++	±	+++	++++	++++
Imipramine (Tofranil)	+	+	++	+	++
Doxepin (Sinequan)	+	++	++	+++	++
Nortriptyline (Pamelor)	±	++	+	+	++
Desipramine (Norpramin)	0	+++	+	0	+

Side effects resulting from alpha-adrenergic blockade may include syncope, sedation, vasoconstriction, and smooth muscle contraction. Side effects resulting from antimuscarinic effects may include dry mouth, stomatitis, decreased tear production, and urinary retention. Cardiac arrhythmias, heart block, and stroke have been reported in human patients. Potential gastrointestinal side effects include constipation, change in appetite, diarrhea, vomiting, and nausea. Lowering of the seizure threshold, alterations in blood glucose levels, testicular hypoplasia, and bone marrow suppression have also been reported.[29]

Tricyclic antidepressants should not be used in breeding males, or patients with seizure disorders, hepatic disease, cardiovascular problems, glaucoma, diabetes mellitus, or adrenal tumors. TCAs should not be used in combination with monoamine oxidase inhibitors, antipsychotic agents (haloperidol, acepromazine), anticholinergic agents, antidepressants, antithyroid agents, barbiturates, or thyroid supplements. Table 19.1 contains recommended dosages for commonly used TCAs in birds.

TCAs are indicated as adjunctive therapy for anxiety, neuropathic pain, and pruritic skin conditions that may benefit from the antihistaminic effects.

Clomipramine is distinct among TCA drugs in its relative serotonin selectivity. It was studied in a placebo-controlled trial for cockatoos (genus *Cacatua*) with feather-picking disorder, with and without soft tissue mutilation.[30] Subjects were randomly assigned to either placebo or treatment groups in a double-blinded study. The treatment group received 3 mg/kg PO q12h of clomipramine compounded in a fruit-flavored suspension, and placebo subjects received a visually identical placebo formulation. During a 6-week trial period, treatment with clomipramine had no significant effects on body weight, Gram's stains, complete blood count values, or chemistry values, and no adverse events were recorded by owners during the trial.

According to caregiver assessments and physical assessments by an avian veterinarian, approximately 73% or 8 of 11 birds treated with clomipramine were considered to be improved after 6 weeks of treatment. Clomipramine-treated birds had significantly greater improvement over placebo-treated birds. Clinical signs resolved in one clomipramine-treated bird, three of the birds experienced substantial improvement, and four of the birds were judged to be somewhat improved. The presence of soft tissue mutilation did not affect responses compared to birds that damaged feathers only. There was also no significant effect of duration of feather picking on the response to treatment. Of the eight birds that were improved at 6 weeks, seven of them had begun to show improvement as early as 3 weeks.

In an open trial, 11 birds (various species) with feather-picking behaviors and soft tissue mutilation were treated with clomipramine at gradually increasing doses ranging from 0.5 mg/kg PO q24h up to 1.0 mg/kg PO q12h.[31] Reduction of feather picking and/or self-mutilation was reported for four birds within 4 weeks of treatment. Side effects included drowsiness, ataxia, and post-treatment regurgitation.

In a published case study involving a Congo African gray parrot with feather picking and self-injurious behavior, relatively higher doses of clomipramine were used.[32] The bird was initially started on 4 mg/kg PO q12h. At this dose, the caregiver noted increased wariness and increased appetite, with some improvement in feather condition after 4 weeks of treatment. The dosage was increased to 9.5 mg/kg PO q12h. Four months after starting clomipramine, the owner elected to increase the dose to 18.8 mg/kg PO q12h and reported that the bird appeared to be hallucinating. The dosage was decreased, and the bird was maintained on 9.5 mg/kg PO q12h (combined with buspirone to control anxiety). The bird was fully feathered 17 months after beginning therapy, and 3 months after the final dosage adjustment.

Amitriptyline has also been used as a treatment for feather picking in birds.[33] Eleven psittacine birds (various species) were treated with amitriptyline at a dose of 2 mg/kg PO q24h for 30 days. Eight birds showed improvement. Adverse events included worsening of feather picking, sedation, and agitation, particularly in the cockatoo species treated. Improvement tended to occur in the first 2 weeks of treatment.

Doxepin has been used in birds with feather-picking disorder at doses ranging from 1 to 5 mg/kg/day, and caregivers reported that their birds were less agitated, easier to handle, less aggressive, less anxious, had increased appetites, and decreased picking behavior.[9]

Amitriptyline, and other nonselective tricyclic agents, do not have proven efficacy for the treatment of compulsive disorder in any species. Antihistaminic effects, anticholinergic effects, and sedative effects may account for changes in behavior in some cases. Controlled studies are needed before concluding that nonselective TCAs are indicated for the treatment of feather-picking disorder.

While side effects in these case reports and clinical trials were rare, the author has had two patients with fatal reactions that were potentially a result of treatment with TCAs. A green-winged macaw developed neurological signs 2 days after starting clomipramine (3 mg/kg PO q12h) and expired before supportive care could be initiated. There were no abnormal necropsy findings to explain the cause of death. An apparently healthy Moluccan cockatoo that was being treated with imipramine (2 mg/kg PO q12h) also developed similar neurological symptoms and expired despite supportive care after several doses of the medication were given. This patient had previously taken clomipramine and became agitated on the medication, so it was discontinued. Medication should be discontinued for any bird that develops neurological symptoms or exhibits unusual changes in behavior. Sudden death has been reported in children, and some individuals are more sensitive to side effects than others (poor metabolizers). Overdose of TCAs can lead to potentially fatal cardiac conduction disturbances.

To address the possibility that there are individual birds that do not metabolize TCAs well, just as there is a subset of the human population who are "poor metabolizers," it is recommended that TCAs be used at lower doses initially and gradually increased if necessary, with close attention to behavioral changes and side effects.

Antipsychotic agents

Antipsychotic agents are used to treat psychotic symptoms in humans, such as those associated with schizophrenia, mania, and cognitive disorders. They act as dopamine antagonists, blocking dopamine receptors in the basal nuclei and limbic system, which produces behavioral quieting or a state of decreased emotional reactivity and relative indifference to stressful situations. Dopamine blockade depresses the reticular activating system and brain regions that control thermoregulation, basal metabolic rate, emesis, vasomotor tone, and hormonal balance. Antipsychotics also suppress spontaneous movements without affecting spinal and pain reflexes.[32] A large proportion of the brain's dopamine is located in the corpus striatum, which mediates the part of the extrapyramidal system concerned with coordinated motor activities. Motor side effects resulting from dopamine blockade in the extrapyramidal system are called extrapyramidal signs (EPSs). Like the structurally similar TCAs, many of the antipsychotics will also cause anticholinergic effects, antihistaminic effects, and alpha-adrenergic blockade.

Dopamine depletion, and the use of drugs that block dopamine, are associated with behavioral quieting, depression, and extrapyramidal motor symptoms, like those associated with Parkinson's disease. Excess dopamine, and drugs that release dopamine, have been associated with the development of stereotypies.[34]

With the exception of chemical immobilization, antipsychotics are rarely used in modern veterinary behavioral medicine. Psychosis is not diagnosed in companion animals, and antipsychotic agents have no notable anxiolytic effects. The side effects associated with antipsychotic use are generally unacceptable. A low potency antipsychotic in use in veterinary practice is acepromazine, used for chemical restraint or as a preanesthetic agent.

Side effects of antipsychotic agents may include hypotension, ataxia, anticholinergic effects, sedation, decreased seizure threshold, aggression, bradycardia, bone marrow suppression, cardiac arrhythmias, hepatitis, extrapyramidal motor signs, such as muscle tremors, stiffness, motor restlessness, difficulty initiating movements, and tardive dyskinesia, torticollis, and the inability to control movements, with chronic use. Effects on prolactin levels can result in infertility, galactorrhea, and weight gain.

Haloperidol (Haldol) is the least hypotensive, least sedating, and the least anticholinergic of the high potency antipsychotic agents, but is more likely to produce extrapyramidal (motor) signs. It is indicated as a last resort treatment option in some cases of self-mutilation, when the patient's physical well-being or survival is at risk, and the owner understands that potentially serious side effects are possible (Table 19.1).

Treatment of a Moluccan cockatoo with severe feather picking and mutilation of skin and muscle with haloperidol at an oral dose of 0.2 mg, resulted in increased agitation, inability to sit still, and other bizarre behaviors.[35] The dose was decreased to 0.15 mg, which was given q12h, and within 48 hours, the plucking and mutilating stopped. Additional avian patients were treated at doses ranging from 0.15 to 0.2 mg/kg q12h. Dosage adjustments were made in 0.02 mg increments. Reported side effects included decreased appetite, depression, agitation, and excitability. The best outcomes were reported for cockatoo species with soft tissue mutilation, but some caregivers were disturbed by the side effects and discontinued treatment.

In another case report, haloperidol was added to the drinking water of two gray parrots with feather-picking disorder (estimated dosage range of 0.2–0.9 mg/kg/day).[36] No improvement occurred until 10 weeks of treatment, and the birds were maintained on 0.4 mg/kg/day of haloperidol.

Hormone therapies

Seasonal behavioral changes in reproductively intact exotic pets are often observed by caregivers and can present some challenges for management. In pet birds, seasonal aggression, cage defense, chronic egg laying or nesting, recurrent masturbation, and some cases of feather-picking disorder may be induced by hormonal changes. Drugs that alter hormone secretion may be helpful in patients presented for undesirable reproductive behaviors.

Leuprolide acetate (Lupron) is a synthetic analog of gonadotropin releasing hormone (GnRH), which will inhibit gonadotropin secretion, luteinizing hormone, and follicle stimulating hormone via a negative feedback mechanism. With chronic administration, ovarian and testicular steroidogenesis is suppressed. In exotic animal practice, lupron has been used primarily for the treatment of adrenal disease in ferrets, to suppress egg laying in psittacine birds, and to reduce seasonal aggression. Mitchell reports using leuprolide acetate to treat aggression in an intact male iguana at a dose of 0.15 mg/kg q4weeks.[37]

Since serious medical consequences, such as egg binding, cloacal prolapse, or osteoporosis, are possible with untreated reproductive behavior in birds, hormonal therapy should be considered in addition to behavioral and environmental interventions. For the treatment of chronic egg laying, 37 birds were treated with depot lupron with an 89% improvement rate, compared with a 65% response rate with chorionic gonadotropin.[38] No significant side effects were noted.

Melatonin

Melatonin is a neurohormone secreted primarily by the pineal gland. Tryptophan is converted to serotonin, which is then converted to melatonin. Melatonin secretion is stimulated by the dark and inhibited by the light, and influences sleep–wake cycles and other circadian rhythms. Under short-day photoperiods, the duration of melatonin secretion generally increases.

Melatonin is also an important antioxidant, efficiently neutralizing hydroxyl radicals resulting from aerobic metabolism. Melatonin may function to protect the brain from oxidative damage. A survey of human medical literature reveals a variety of potential indications for melatonin supplementation, including sleep disturbances, cognitive decline, seasonal depression, neuroendocrine disorders, and cancer treatment.[39,40]

In birds, the role of melatonin as an indicator of day length for seasonal processes is not completely clear. Studying European starlings, Bentley found that melatonin influences seasonal changes in immune function and neural plasticity in the forebrain song-control system via a thyroid-dependent mechanism.[41] In ringdoves, melatonin administered at oral doses of 0.25 mg/kg and 2.5 mg/kg given 1 hour before bedtime (lights out) resulted in reduced nocturnal activity and improved rest, with higher doses effecting diurnal activity as well as nocturnal activity.[42]

Melatonin was found to act directly to induce release of gonadotropin inhibitory hormone (GnIH) in the paraventricular nucleus in the brains of Japanese quail, suggesting a potential mechanism for melatonin's role in seasonal reproductive behaviors.[43]

Melatonin has been used as adjunctive therapy in dogs with noise phobia because of its effect on psychomotor vigilance.[44] Further investigation is needed to determine the potential for melatonin in the treatment of behavioral disorders in exotic pets.

Conclusions

The variety of applications for psychoactive medication use in the treatment of various behavioral disorders in exotic pets has been reviewed.[6,9,27,45–47] However, very little data exists with regard to pharmacokinetics, safety, toxicity, therapeutic dosage ranges, and efficacy. Controlled studies are essential in order to enhance our ability to use psychoactive medications effectively in the treatment of behavioral disorders in exotic pets. Placebo controls will allow us to assess the efficacy of drug therapies, given that medications are often combined with environmental, behavioral, and nutritional modifications, and to determine the presence of adverse reactions associated with the active treatment. Without placebo controls, the cyclic nature of feather picking in particular creates uncertainty about the actual effectiveness of any treatment, particularly when drug therapies are combined with other interventions. The duration of a clinical trial is also relevant since many psychoactive medications require chronic dosing. Without the knowledge of required treatment duration, drug therapies may be abandoned before a fair trial is even completed.

Dose-titration trials will be important in establishing safe and effective doses of psychoactive medications for the variety of exotic pets treated in veterinary practices. Anecdotal reports of sudden death with TCAs and antipsychotics create concern about safety, even when relatively low doses are used. Determining safety and efficacy across a wide variety of exotic animal species will be challenging. Data from laboratory studies support that avian species show responses to psychoactive medications that are similar to those of mammals.[48,49] With more clinical data for exotic pet species, behavioral pharmacotherapy can be used more effectively, along with behavioral therapy, to prevent rehoming or euthanasia, reduce anxiety, protect the patient from self-injury, and improve overall quality of life.

References

1. van Hoek CS, ten Cate C. Abnormal behavior in caged birds kept as pets. *J Appl Anim Welf Sci* 1998;1(1):51–64.
2. Seibert LM, Landsberg GM. Diagnosis and management of patients presenting with behavior problems. *Vet Clin North Am Small Anim* 2008;38:937–950.
3. Crowell-Davis SL. Introduction. In: Crowell-Davis SL, Murray T, eds. *Veterinary Psychopharmacology*. Ames, IA: Blackwell Publishing, 2006:3–24.
4. Seibert LM. Mental health issues in captive birds. In: McMillan FD, ed. *Mental Health and Well-Being in Animals*. Ames, IA: Blackwell Publishing, 2005:285–294.
5. Riva J, Bondiolotti G, Michelazzi M et al. Anxiety related behavioural disorders and neurotransmitters in dogs. *Appl Anim Behav Sci* 2008;114:168–181.

6. Martin KM. Psittacine behavioral pharmacotherapy. In: Luescher UA, ed. *Manual of Parrot Behavior*. Ames, IA: Blackwell Publishing, 2006;267–279.

7. Center SA, Elston TH, Rowland PH et al. Fulminant hepatic failure associated with oral administration of diazepam in 11 cats. *J Vet Emerg Crit Care* 1996;6:618–625.

8. Galvin C. The feather picking bird. In: Kirk RW, ed. *Current Veterinary Therapy VIII Small Animal Practice*. Philadelphia, PA: WB Saunders Co, 1983;646–652.

9. Johnson CA. Chronic feather picking: A different approach to treatment. In: *Scientific Proceedings. Int Conf Zoo and Avian Med* 1987;125–142.

10. Johannessen LC. Antiepileptic drugs in non-epilepsy disorders: Relations between mechanisms of action and clinical efficacy. *CNS Drugs* 2008;22(1):27–47.

11. Platt SR, Adams V, Garosi LS et al. Treatment with gabapentin of 11 dogs with refractory idiopathic epilepsy. *Vet Rec* 2006;159(26):881–884.

12. Robertson SA. Managing pain in feline patients. *Vet Clin North Am Small Anim Pract* 2005;35(1):129–146.

13. Doneley B. Use of gabapentin to treat presumed neuralgia in a Little Corella (*Cacatua sanguinea*). In: *Proceedings. Assoc of Avian Vet Australasian Comm* 2007;169–172.

14. Mula M, Pini S, Cassano GB. The role of anticonvulsant drugs in anxiety disorders: A critical review of the evidence. *J Clin Psychopharmacol* 2007;27(3):263–272.

15. Onder E, Tural U, Gokgakan M. Does gabapentin lead to early symptom improvement in obsessive-compulsive disorder? *Eur Arch Psychiat Clin Neurosci* 2008;258(6):319–323.

16. Schwartz S. Carbamazepine in the control of aggressive behavior in cats. *J Am Anim Hosp Assoc* 1994;30:515–519.

17. Holland CT. Successful long-term treatment of a dog with psychomotor seizures with carbamazepine. *Aust Vet J* 1988;65:389–392.

18. Carpenter JW, Mashima TY, Rupiper DJ. *Exotic Animal Formulary*, 2nd ed. Philadelphia, PA: W.B. Saunders Company, 2001.

19. Turner R. Trexan (naltrexone hydrochloride) use in feather picking in avian species. In: *Scientific Proceedings. Annu Meet Assoc Avian Vet* 1993;116–118.

20. Hawkins MG. The use of analgesics in birds, reptiles, and small exotic mammals. *J Exotic Pet Med* 2006;15(3):177–192.

21. Reis HJ, Guatimosim C, Paquet M et al. Neuro-transmitters in the central nervous system and their implication in learning and memory processes. *Curr Med Chem* 2009;16(7):796–840.

22. Rapoport JL, Ryland DH, Kriete M. Drug treatment of canine acral lick. An animal model of obsessive-compulsive disorder. *Arch Gen Psychiat* 1992;49(7):517–521.

23. van Hierden YM, de Boer SF, Koolhaas JM et al. The control of feather pecking by serotonin. *Behav Neurosci* 2004;118(3):575–583.

24. Crowell-Davis SL, Poggiagliolmi S. Serotonin syndrome. *Compendium* 2008;Sept:490–493.

25. Mertens PA. Pharmacological treatment of feather picking in pet birds. In: *Scientific Proceedings. 1st Int Conf Vet Behav Med* 1997;209–211.

26. Seibert LM Animal behavior case of the month: Toe chewing in a cockatiel. *J Am Vet Med Assoc* 2004;224(9):1433–1435.

27. Martin KM. Behavioral approach to psittacine feather picking. In: *Scientific Proceedings. Annu Meet Assoc Avian Vet* 2004;307–312.

28. Crowell-Davis SL. Tricyclic antidepressants. In: Crowell-Davis SL, Murray T, eds. *Veterinary Psychopharmacology*. Ames, IA: Blackwell Publishing, 2006;179–206.

29. Sherman Simpson B, Papich MG. Pharmacologic management in veterinary behavioral medicine. *Vet Clin North Am Small Anim* 2003;33:365–404.

30. Seibert LM, Crowell-Davis SL, Wilson GH et al. Placebo-controlled clomipramine trial for the treatment of feather picking disorder in cockatoos. *J Am Anim Hosp Assoc* 2004;40:261–269.

31. Ramsey EC, Grindlinger H. Treatment of feather picking with clomipramine. In: *Scientific Proceedings. Annu Meet Assoc Avian Vet* 2003;379–382.

32. Juarbe-Diaz SJ. Animal behavior case of the month: Feather picking and self-injurious behavior in an African grey parrot. *J Am Vet Med Assoc* 2000;216(10):1562–1564.

33. Eugenio CT. Amitriptyline HCl: Clinical study for treatment of feather picking. In: *Scientific Proceedings. Annu Meet Assoc Avian Vet* 2003;133–135.

34. Seibert LM. Antipsychotics. In: Crowell-Davis SL, Murray T, eds. *Veterinary Psychopharmacology*. Ames, IA: Blackwell Publishing, 2006;148–165.

35. Lennox AM, VanDerHeyden N. Haloperidol for use in treatment of psittacine self-mutilation and feather plucking. In: *Scientific Proceedings. Annu Meet Assoc Avian Vet* 1993;119–120.

36. Iglauer F, Rasim R. Treatment of psychogenic feather picking in psittacine birds with a dopamine antagonist. *J Sm Anim Pract* 1993;34:564–566.

37. Mitchell MA. Leuprolide acetate. *Sem in Avian Exotic Pet Med* 2005;14(2):153–155.

38. Bowles HL, Zantop DW. Management of chronic egg laying using leuprolide acetate. In: *Scientific Proceedings. Annu Meet Assoc Avian Vet* 2000;105–108.

39. Witt-Enderby PA, Radio NM, Doctor JS et al. Therapeutic treatments potentially mediated by melatonin receptors: Potential clinical uses in the prevention of osteoporosis, cancer and as an adjuvant therapy. *J Pineal Res* 2006;41(4):297–305.

40. Lewy AJ, Emens J, Jackman A et al. Circadian uses of melatonin in humans. *Chronobiol Int* 2006;23(1–2):403–412.

41. Bentley GE. Unraveling the enigma: The role of melatonin in seasonal processes in birds. *Microsc Res Tech* 2001;53(1):63–71.

42. Paredes SD, Terron MP, Valero V et al. Orally administered melatonin improves nocturnal rest in young and old ringdoves (*Streptopelia risoria*). *Basic Clin Pharmacol Toxicol* 2007;100(4):258–268.

43. Ubuka T, Bentley GE, Ukena K et al. Melatonin induces the expression of gonadotropin-inhibitory hormone in the avian brain. *Proc of the Natl Acad Sci* 2005;102(8):3052–3057.

44. Graw P, Werth E, Krauchi K et al. Early morning melatonin administration impairs psychomotor vigilance. *Behav Brain Res* 2001;121:167–172.

45. Seibert LM. Psittacine feather picking. In: *Scientific Proceedings. West Vet Conf* 2003;1–6.

46. Welle KR. A review of psychotropic drug therapy. In: *Scientific Proceedings. Annu Meet Assoc Avian Vet* 1998;121–124.

47. Lawton MPC. Behavioural problems. In: Beynon PH, Forbes NA, Lawton MPC eds. *BSAVA Manual of Psittacine Birds*. Ames, IA: Iowa State University Press, 1996;106–114.

48. Feltenstein MW, Sufka KJ. Screening antidepressants in the chick separation-stress paradigm. *Psychopharmacology* 2005;181:153–159.

49. Wolff MC, Leander JD. Selective serotonin reuptake inhibitors decrease impulsive behavior as measured by an adjusting delay procedure in the pigeon. *Neuropsychopharmacology* 2002;27(3):421–429.

20

Welfare of exotic animals in captivity

Paul E. Honess and Sarah E. Wolfensohn

Introduction

Humans have a long history of associations with animals dating back to prehistoric hunting and the earliest attempts to domesticate animals either as hunting tools, pest controllers or secure food resources. Refinement of domestication has involved selective breeding and the development of training practices. However, initial animal keeping was predominantly utilitarian; only later did humans begin to keep animals for curiosity and later still, following the travels of the early explorers, did people begin to keep animals classed as exotic (i.e., "Belonging to another country, foreign, alien" or more narrowly: "Introduced from abroad, not indigenous").[1]

As technology has evolved it has become possible to keep exotic species, particularly the more challenging ones, more successfully. In some cases, captive breeding programmes have been managed in a way that controls costs and increases productivity such that it brings ownership of exotic species within the financial range of more people. There is, however, a clear responsibility to plan for the animal's optimum welfare *before* obtaining the animal and this may entail a considerable amount of research and potential expense. The understanding and acceptance of roles and responsibilities is one of the five themes of the UK's Animal Health and Welfare Strategy[2] and is also reflected in the scope of the European Union Animal Health Strategy.[3] Unfortunately, the expertise for providing the minimum acceptable conditions in which animals thrive may only rarely be passed on at point of sale.[4] This may mean that, without extensive research, those committed to keeping exotic species may experience a number of failures, which will likely be accompanied by varying degrees of suffering for the animals concerned, before any degree of success is experienced. Indeed, any owner seeking veterinary care for an exotic animal may need to seek specialist advice as their local clinic may lack the required expertise or specialized equipment for optimum treatment.[5-7] Mayer and Martin[8] highlight that although exotic animal medicine is an area of growth within veterinary medicine, there is nevertheless a general lack of training opportunities and pharmacological data concerning exotics, and that a general absence of context-specific literature can be problematic.

While technology has made the maintenance of exotic species in captivity easier—the Internet as a first port of call on husbandry and welfare of these species provides a mixed quality of advice.[9] This ranges from specialist sites established by experienced, often professional, keepers supplying good quality evidence-based advice, through to amateur/hobbyist sites that may recommend practices based essentially on folklore, which may at best be harmless or at worst give the wrong advice. Similar problems arise in the use of lay literature misused as if it had a scientific basis.[8]

Many taxon-centred professional societies of biologists and veterinarians (e.g., International Primatological Society: www.internationalprimatologicalsociety.org; Association of Avian Veterinarians: www.aav.org; American Society of Ichthyologists and Herpetologists: www.asih.org) contain expertise on welfare provision for the animal group in question. Many counsel against keeping exotic species as pets due to the very demanding conditions (e.g., dietary, social, activity) they require for even the minimum acceptable level of welfare, but nevertheless provide guidance on the care of the animals for those already legally owning them or determined to do so.[10]

Good welfare is not the same as simply maintaining an animal's physiological function to keep it alive and reproducing. In this chapter, we will set out the basic principles of welfare for exotic species and how taking a biologically systematic approach can enable a keeper of exotic species to plan and refine welfare conditions for the animals in their care. A combination of improving knowledge, increasing species' availability, and a continual pursuit for the ultimate exotic pet has meant that the range of species being kept as pets increasingly approaches that which is kept in zoos. As a result of this, much of the literature based on traditionally zoo-kept species becomes increasingly relevant in the context of exotic pets and therefore a number of examples cited in this chapter come from that literature.

Welfare: What should we be achieving for animals held in captivity?

While there is much discussion in society about the issue of attributing rights to animals along the lines of existing human rights, this remains contentious and many prefer less extreme frameworks for the protection of animals and their quality of life. One such framework is that promoted through the UK Farm Animal Welfare Council and which focuses on The Five Freedoms, specifically:

- freedom from thirst, hunger, or malnutrition;
- freedom from discomfort;
- freedom from pain, injury, and disease;
- freedom to express normal behavior;
- freedom from fear and distress.

At the most basic level these Five Freedoms ensure the survival of the animal but when implemented fully and diligently should optimize their welfare.

While traditional approaches to animal welfare have focused on the removal of negative states (e.g., thirst, thermoregulatory stress, social deprivation, boredom, fear, and so on), new approaches have been proposed that place greater emphasis on the provision of positive welfare states for animals, such as happiness, comfort, security, satiation, and so on.[11] The measurement of negative welfare states has always presented a number of methodological challenges (e.g., the measurement of autonomic responses and stress hormone levels) especially since many of the measurable responses to negative stimuli/stressors are convergent in preparing the body for a flight-or-fight response.[12] Indeed, the sampling/recording process itself can be stressful and may produce a response that swamps any measurable response to the presentation of a negative stimulus.[13] However, the assessment of positive welfare states is not immune to these problems and may suffer interpretative problems and accusations of anthropomorphism. New techniques (e.g., Ref. [14]) aim to probe the emotional state of animals as an indicator of their welfare status.

Even in their natural environment in the wild, most animals are unlikely to exist in positive welfare states at all times, and for much of the time, avoiding/escaping from negative welfare states may be the motivation for many of the essential functions of life in a wild animal (traveling to find food, surveillance behavior and predator avoidance, grooming to

remove ectoparasites, etc.). For this very reason, it may not be desirable to attempt to recreate all natural conditions in captivity; imposing the stress of presenting the animals with a predator may elicit natural behavior but is unlikely to be viewed as constituting good welfare or ethical treatment of the animals. Conversely, presenting live prey to animals in captivity will elicit natural predatory behavior but may again be considered ethically unacceptable due to the stress imposed on the prey;[15] indeed, in some countries feeding live vertebrate prey may be illegal.[16] Of course views on this are tainted with speciesism such that it might be seen as acceptable or even desirable to feed live invertebrates such as *Daphnia* or brine shrimp to aquarium fish but presenting a live rabbit to a python or a cow to lions would be considered unacceptable.

There is a consistent theme of meeting the "ethological needs" of animals running through the literature on the provision of welfare in captivity.[17–19] While not all natural behaviors are considered desirable in captivity,[20] there is a general belief that if animals are given the opportunity to express a natural range and balance of behaviors in their activity budget they will be more psychologically healthy than if these opportunities are stifled by inadequate environmental (physical, physiological, and social) provision. The application of consumer theory in order to infer the "needs" or "necessities" of captive animals[17,19] provides a valuable framework for advancing animal welfare. It assists welfare scientists in their efforts to define what animals want or do not want in their environment through the examination of their motivation for access to, or avoidance of, the aspect under investigation.[12] This has been demonstrated elegantly by a number of studies examining how hard animals will work for desirable opportunities, for example mink for access to water[21] and primates for social stimuli.[22] This approach provides a valuable framework for determining environmental and husbandry parameters for species for which these aspects remain poorly defined.

Implications of context

The context in which exotic species are kept in captivity vary widely and include: personal pets; mascots; zoos, safari parks, aquaria, aviaries, and menageries; laboratories and breeding facilities; production (agriculture and other animal products, e.g., fur); and helpers (including: military dolphins, mine-detecting rats, monkeys for the disabled, monkeys for tea-picking, coconut harvesting, etc.). Of course the degree to which keepers try to mimic natural conditions either in functional or aesthetic aspects will depend largely on both the species in question and the purpose for keeping them in captivity. If the purpose is educational, for example in zoos, then there will be some imperative to exhibit the animal in an environment that resembles the natural setting and replicates the animals' biology (social, ecological, behavioral). In terms of the behavior, whether a given species is kept in a laboratory or in a zoo, the goal is to allow it to exhibit as natural a repertoire of behavior (range and time) as possible. Visitors will learn more about wild counterparts under such conditions and laboratory researchers will have a more natural, unstressed model for their research producing more valid results. However, a climbing apparatus for arboreal primates in a zoo, for example, may need to resemble a tree in color, texture, and form whereas in a laboratory, the form is the most important aspect, allowing the animals to make good use of the vertical component of their caging and, where group-housed, to space themselves in a socially appropriate way.[23] While the aesthetics of environmental provision may vary between captive contexts, so do other aspects of welfare monitoring and provision including health care provision and decisions. In areas of animal production, laboratories, or domestic pets, the balance of financial, biosecurity, suffering/regulation, personal attachment considerations will change and result in inconsistent treatment for the animal even from the same person working across context.[24]

It may be simplistic to try to create a dichotomy between "wild" and "domesticated" species in respect to their welfare requirements, in particular because of the various feral and commensal states that exist between these extremes. It is, however, valuable to distinguish between those animals that have been domesticated and those that have not, as centuries and even millennia of selective breeding and shaping has modified the biology of a range of domesticated species such that they may now only faintly resemble their wild analogues.[25] We have been aware for a long time about the results and consequences of domestication across a wide range of animal and plant species, indeed Charles Darwin produced a detailed two-volume study on the subject in 1868.[26] In addition to producing variation in a range of "hard" characteristics such as pelage, body size and growth, fertility, and brain size[27] in a range of domesticated animals from chickens to cattle, there have also been changes in the behavior or habit of most domesticated species; a good example being the difference between wolves and the various breeds of dog selected for hunting, being eaten, herding, racing, or petting.[25] Price[28] points out that it is possible to generalize about the behavioral effects of domestication, whereas it is not possible to do so for genetic and phenotypic characteristics. He accounts for this through a simple habituation process, a raised threshold to trigger behavior (e.g., agonism), and the role of humans that have formed a buffer between the animal and the natural ecological pressures (e.g., foraging and predation) allowing the development of a more compliant temperament and the retention of juvenile characteristics. In summary, wild and captive animals (particularly domesticated ones) are capable of exhibiting approximately the same range of behaviors but the substantial difference in their behavior lies in the extent to which these behaviors are expressed. In essence the behavioral differences are quantitative rather than qualitative.[28,29]

Despite the notable successes that there have been in domestication, it remains the case that relatively few animals have been successfully domesticated with the unsuccessful ones failing at least one of Diamond's six tests of domestication: A diet suppliable by humans, fast enough growth rate and short enough interbirth interval, amenable disposition, readiness to breed in captivity, presence of a "follow-the-leader" hierarchy, and relative calmness when held in captive enclosures or faced with a predator.[25] Of course not all of these tests necessarily apply to whether an exotic species might make a suitable pet and it is easy to see how more of these tests might be satisfied by small-bodied animals, or their failure at least has less significant consequences.

While not necessarily being domesticated, it has been demonstrated that many exotic species may survive well and breed in captivity. However, the challenge is to make sufficient welfare provision for them to prevent the development of significant behavioral and clinical problems.[30,31] Certain species, or groups of species, seem to be particularly prone to developing behavioral problems in captivity; for example, among large, wide-ranging carnivores[32–34] and ungulates (e.g., giraffes[35]) as well as in parrots[36] and elephants.[37] Despite the belief that in the absence of predators and with continuous veterinary attention longevity is improved in captivity, there is evidence that this is not always the case, in particular for elephants.[38,39]

Sourcing and transportation

The origin of an animal will have an impact on its welfare in captivity. While individual temperament should always be taken into account, it is nevertheless the case that captivity and its attendant manipulations will present a more significant challenge to a wild-caught animal than to one bred in captivity.[13,40] The immobilization and capture, in some species (e.g., deer, horses, and birds), can lead to stress responses (capture myopathy) that can be so severe as to cause death.[41–43] Where cyanide is used in the harvest of marine fish for the aquarium trade, initial levels of mortality can be as high as 50%[44] and transport-related losses may be as high as 80%.[45]

International treaties and regulations govern cross-border trade in threatened animals and plants and their products (e.g., CITES: http://www.cites.org/eng/disc/what.shtml). However, these do not cover national trade or trade within some political/economic blocks (e.g., the European Union). It is therefore important to consider that sourcing an exotic animal may be part of a significant, and sometimes illicit, trade and therefore all appropriate paperwork should be secured in advance. The species may exist at low density with a limited distribution, as determined by ecological parameters and its current threat status (see IUCN Red List[46]). However many rare, beautiful, interesting, and exotic species are poorly known, both in terms of their conservation status as well as general aspects of their biology that may be fundamental to good welfare provision. The removal of even a few individuals from the wild may have a dramatic and even catastrophic effect on the viability of their source population. While not specifically an aspect of welfare, this is an important consideration in terms of general ethics.

For some exotic species, the process of transport (international, national, or local) can be extremely stressful and results in significant loss of stock (birds,[47] tortoises,[48] fish[45]). National and international regulations govern transport and define minimum conditions for live animals, for example air transportation is subject to IATA Live Animal Regulations[49] which define the responsibilities of shippers and carriers and container requirements, and are updated annually. Within the EC, the transport of animals is also regulated by EC Council Directive 91/628/EEC on the Protection of Animals During Transport,[50] whereas in the United States regulations vary between States (via each State Veterinarian, see www.aphis.usda.gov/vs/sregs/). The import or export of animals must comply with the relevant international legislation and transport regulations. The needs for individual species are listed, including those covered by CITES. These regulations have been adopted as standard by many countries. Arrangements for the transport of animals should ensure that their well-being is not jeopardized, and that they arrive at their destination in good health. Particular attention should be paid to the health and welfare prior to shipment in order to ensure that there are no subclinical infections that could cause clinical disease during or shortly after transport. Animals should be examined by a competent person as soon as they arrive, and the transport should be arranged in advance so that animals can be unboxed and placed in fresh ready-prepared housing immediately on arrival.

It is important that appropriate measures are taken to control and monitor animal health. Full consideration should be given to appropriate quarantine procedures and health screening, in particular against emerging zoonotic diseases (e.g., avian influenza, psitticosis, salmonella (reptiles), simian herpes B virus, and monkey pox).[8,51] Some animals may have predisposing factors such as a genetic variant which contribute to the development of disease. The susceptibility of some animals may be difficult to predict. Nutritional status of the animal will also be a factor in susceptibility to disease. The single most important predisposing factor in the animal is stress, which can lead to physiological disruption, immunosuppression, and the subsequent development of disease.[13,29] It is therefore very important to do everything possible to reduce the stress caused to animals.

Occasionally, exotic animals escape as a result of lack of diligence or not being contained properly, or are deliberately released due to unanticipated keeping costs, growth beyond expected parameters, changes in circumstances of the owner, or criminal behavior. The escapee is unlikely to be able to survive in the face of the challenges of feeding and protecting (predators, thermoregulation, disease) itself in a new environment to which it is not adapted. It may therefore suffer significantly before dying. However, where exotic escapees are able to survive, they may present predation, habitat alteration/degradation,[52] or disease threats to native wildlife, pets, livestock,[51,53] and humans,[8] or even thrive to plague proportions (e.g., lagomorphs and rodents in Australia)[53] in the absence of their usual diseases or predators that contain their number where they are native.

Planning a welfare strategy

When planning a welfare strategy of an exotic species, it is important that the full range of their biological requirements and needs are considered. Anything known about an animal's natural history is an important resource for understanding its requirements and the environmental parameters in which it should be kept in captivity. Therefore published research articles on the species' biology may assist in the construction of a welfare strategy in the absence of specific welfare provision guidance. The range of exotic species being kept in captivity is considerable and this taxonomic range is reflected in differences in their biology. It is therefore not possible to define a "one size fits all" welfare strategy in this chapter. Instead, we promote an approach designed to make the reader aware of the range of biological aspects that may need consideration when planning the provision of welfare for an exotic animal in captivity. By necessity we will therefore only highlight a limited selection of biological parameters that the animal care provider should consider; further research will be required on a case-by-case basis if even adequate welfare provision is to be made.

Evolutionary considerations

Typically, those species that are more phylogenetically closely related will have a more similar biology. This is due to their greater compliment of shared characteristics, some of which are primitive (e.g., general mammalian characteristics) and others, which help distinguish them from other more distantly related forms, are "derived"; being inherited from a more recent ancestor.[54] Therefore, in the absence of species-specific experience or guidance, literature on the welfare provision for a phylogenetically closely related species provides a valuable starting point for determining the welfare requirements of a novel species. Many texts exist that present taxonomic classifications of animals; however, only those that explicitly state they are based on phylogenetic principles should be used for finding the nearest appropriate relative to the species under consideration. This process is not only useful for behavioral, ecological, and reproductive parameters but has clinical as well as general welfare applications. Mayer and Martin[8] present a useful decision-making algorithm for choosing drugs for treatment that incorporates the same comparative principle.

It is important to consider the adaptations and specializations of the species. Evolutionary history has shaped species through natural selection; the suite of adaptations they possess enables them to survive and reproduce under the particular ecological conditions and selective pressures of their natural environment. Providing an environment that accommodates these adaptations and specializations is a key element of ensuring good welfare;[55] for example providing access to water for farmed ducks[56] and mink,[21] and appropriate housing temperature for rodents.[57] Understanding the life-history strategy of the species is important: it includes parameters such as lifespan, maturation, reproductive rate and investment, and senescence. It provides vital information not just on the overall suitability of the species for captivity but also on particular provisions that may need to be made for its welfare. For example, if the species is long-lived then, over an extended period, a suboptimal environment and restricted conditions may result in institutionalization with psychological (e.g., stereotypies[58]) and physical health problems (e.g., skeletal problems[59]). If being kept for breeding or in mixed sex pairs/groups, what is known of their reproductive parameters? Do they produce multiple offspring? What is the interval between offspring? Are facilities available to accommodate and manage a potential population explosion? Are young altricial or precocial? Are special conditions required for infants? If so, what are they, and can they be provided? What are the risks of infanticide associated with disturbance or adult presence? Are there temperature or humidity factors that may affect the sex ratio of offspring (e.g., some reptiles[60])?

Physiology

The correct functioning of an animal's physiology is essential to its survival. One of the most fundamental aspects of this is to understand how it regulates its body temperature. Is the species an endotherm (able to maintain body temperature by internal metabolic heat production) or an ectotherm (depending on external heat sources such as solar radiation?)[61] The answer to this question, combined with information about the ambient temperature of the environment where the animal is to be kept and the typical body temperature of the species or a phylogenetically close species will inform the keeper about either the need to maintain the animal's calorific intake or whether to provide an artificial heat source (e.g., heat lamp), or a combination of the two. Conversely, where the animal may become overheated, the provision of shade and bathing water will allow the animal to display natural behavioral thermoregulation. Ectothermic reptiles may gain their heat from radiant

(e.g., solar) or conductive sources (e.g., rocks, sand) and the provision of these should be appropriate depending on the habits of the species. Clearly, if they are nocturnal, an overhead heat lamp is less appropriate than heat from background or under-the-floor heaters.[62] It is also important to know whether there is a need to provide a specific humidity and lighting regime. Where artificial light is used, consideration should be given to the appropriate wavelengths of light required as some species require specific light regimes for the production of important vitamins (e.g., reptiles and amphibians,[63] marmosets[64]). Bulbs designed to produce specific light qualities, for example in the ultraviolet spectrum, may cease to produce the required wavelengths long before they appear, to the human eye, to malfunction and should be replaced before this point and in accordance with manufacturers' instructions.

The provision of readily available clean drinking water will be essential to most species, others may derive sufficient hydration from their food. For those that are aquatic or amphibious, the quality of their water habitat is likely to be critical. Keepers of exotics should be aware whether the additives and other chemical levels in tap water (e.g., chlorine and chloramines) will prove toxic or physiologically challenging to the animal. Commercially available products are available for testing the water quality and for the removal of chemicals. In addition to maintaining appropriate oxygenation, it is also necessary to avoid the buildup of toxic excreted metabolic products (e.g., ammonia and nitrites) and suspended solids in the water through regular water changes and appropriate filtration[65,66] (regular cleaning of the environment of terrestrial animals is also needed to prevent the buildup of toxic levels of ammonia). Maintaining clean water (drinking and bathing) also helps discourage potential pathogens.[66]

Diet tends to be one of the first areas of provision that concerns a keeper of a new, exotic species. However, providing for the animal's dietary needs is not as simple as supplying it with the necessary nutrition; other factors such as the frequency of feeding, method of presentation of the food as well as distribution of the food in time and space may be as important. For example, feeding a nocturnal species during the day may well affect its feeding success and therefore its nutritional well-being.[62] It is common for nocturnal exotics that are being kept as pets or for exhibition in zoos to be kept under reverse lighting conditions (light at night and simulated moonlight during the day)[31] to coincide their activity patterns with those of humans. Some species, particularly some carnivores, crocodilians, and large constricting snakes, are adapted to consuming a very large amount of food in a short period of time and then perhaps not feeding again for an extended period. Clearly, these species should be fed in accordance with their natural behavior. Other species, however, feed constantly on poor quality food (e.g., grazing ungulates) and there are also those that feed often on relatively small amounts of food that may be irregularly or sparsely distributed in their natural environment.[67,68] Behind these behavioral feeding adaptations frequently lie physiological and anatomical adaptations. Inappropriate feeding regimens can result in obesity, nutrient imbalance, anorexia, and developmental problems (e.g., shell deformities in tortoises[62]). Where animals are pair- or group-housed, social factors including aggressive competition and monopoly of food by dominant animals can limit the feeding of some individuals. Scattering food can reduce aggression in socially housed animals[69,70] and ensure that subordinate animals have an opportunity to feed.[71] Training animals to feed cooperatively can also be used to reduce within group aggression.[72] Gathering information about a species' natural foraging ecology will provide vital information for their nutritional maintenance. Mimicking natural distribution of food by feeding little and often for species that feed that way will also help maintain a cleaner environment (e.g., water quality in aquaria) and potentially reduce wastage.

Attention should also be paid to the animal's sensory interaction with its environment: where possible environmental structures should be constructed out of thermoneutral natural materials (e.g., wood).[64,73] Over-engineering by using metals will result in a noisy environment with surfaces that are cold to the touch. Consideration should also be given to smells and sounds in the environment. Prey species are likely to be stressed if they can see or smell a predator and therefore should be housed in a way that avoids this. There are some views, however, that antipredator behavior may be a desirable part of a natural behavioral repertoire,[74] particularly in zoos, and essential for those animals that may be released into the wild, and therefore controlled stimulation of this behavior may be appropriate in some instances. Equally, housing prey species in the sensory range of a predator may result in frustration in the predator.[73] Animals may also be very sensitive to noise in their environment. Understanding of the potential consequences of noise, including ultrasound, is viewed as increasingly important and was the subject of a focused issue of the *Journal of the American Association for Laboratory Animal Science*.[75] At its extreme, the ultrasound from a television in standby mode was reported to have killed a chipmunk in 2 days.[76]

Sociality

When discussing a species' sociality, it is perhaps more useful to distinguish between those that are gregarious and those that are solitary foragers living in dispersed social systems, rather than between social and solitary (e.g., Ref. [77]). It is nevertheless the case that species should be kept in a social environment that, wherever possible, reflects that of the species in its natural environment. If a species occurs gregariously in the wild, accommodating this may present challenges in also achieving an appropriate stocking density that allows each individual sufficient "personal space" and

enables them to retreat from undesirable social interactions. Crowding can result in undesirably high levels of aggression and can even result in cannibalism.[78] Animals that manage crowding by reducing levels of contact aggression and increasing appeasement behavior can nevertheless display behavior that indicates they find these conditions stressful.[79] There is a considerable body of literature on the impact on welfare of social isolation for species that are naturally gregarious. While it may be somewhat of a truism to conclude from this literature that the best enrichment for an individual of an intensely social species (e.g., many primates) is an appropriate conspecific, nevertheless there is also plenty of literature detailing how problematic it can be to produce stable pairs or groups. This is despite the existence of published protocols designed to improve the chances of success.[20] Conversely it can also be dangerous, and is unlikely to benefit the animals' welfare, to group-house a species that is not gregarious or is highly territorial.

It is very rare, with the exception of some domesticated pets, that human company provides a suitable alternative to that of a conspecific. On the other hand, in instances where people have to work closely with animals (e.g., in a laboratory environment with regular blood sampling or weighing), it is important that regular human contact or disturbance is neither stressful for the animal (altering its physiology and potentially making it a less valid experimental model) nor elicits behavior which is either dangerous or simply makes the animal difficult to manage. Both compromise the animal's welfare and therefore it is important that the animal is appropriately habituated to its human caretakers. Positive reinforcement training can also be used to train the animal to cooperate in a less stressful and also safer manner with a range of procedures.[80]

Good animal handling techniques will reduce the risk of injury from bites and scratches and will increase the confidence of both the owner and the animal. All animals will respond in some way to the presence of a human and most species can recognize individuals and will be nervous of strangers and those with whom they associate unpleasant procedures. It is therefore important to establish a friendly relationship with the animal to reduce nervousness on both sides. An animal that is confident and relaxed with its owner or caretaker will be more co-operative and less stressed with better welfare.

Behavior

The importance of accommodating a full behavioral repertoire when planning a welfare strategy has already been touched on earlier. This is not only a factor of the housing provided for the animal that will enable it to locomote, rest, nest, forage, hide, play, etc. in a way that reflects the natural tendencies appropriate for that species and age–sex class, but also derives from many of the factors discussed earlier relating to environmental factors such as lighting, humidity, temperature, and sensory stimuli. Our understanding of the welfare benefits of facilitating animals to exhibit a full, balanced species-typical behavioral repertoire has coincided with a changing view, in some circles, of environmental enrichment as an essential part of the holistic provision of welfare for captive animals rather than solely a responsive treatment for behavior abnormalities.[74] Even in the absence of behavioral abnormalities, enrichment of the structural, social, feeding, and manipulable environment provides a useful way of balancing the animal's behavioral repertoire, improving its display of natural behavior, and preventing boredom, aggression, and frustration all of which can lead to the development of unwanted abnormal behavior.[20] In reality there are as many environmental enrichment strategies as there are different species and many of the key elements of these are covered elsewhere. In particular the reader is referred to Rob Young's excellent text[73] on the subject which covers historical, functional, and practical aspects of environmental enrichment including techniques for assessing its effectiveness. It is not only important to assess the effectiveness of enrichment but for it to be successful it must be targeted.[20,73,74,81] That means it is focused on a specific behavior, age–sex class, species, etc. such as the ingenious enrichment devices targeted at species-typical feeding behaviors, for example artificial termite mounds for chimpanzee termite-fishing behavior,[82] gum feeder for marmosets,[83] or prey manipulation opportunities for carnivores.[84]

Assessment of welfare

We have given some pointers in some of the key aspects of designing a welfare strategy for exotic animals and it is appropriate to add a note about the assessment of welfare. Having researched the basic biology and welfare requirements of an exotic animal and formulated a welfare strategy, how can you tell whether it is working, or more importantly whether it is failing? Initial concerns are likely to focus on the need to ensure the best possible general clinical health of the animal. Standard veterinary health screening, differential diagnoses and, where necessary, referral to a specialist on the species or taxonomic group will resolve most clinical issues and key aspects of this are covered elsewhere (e.g., Ref. [85]). There is less formal guidance available on the assessment of psychological/behavioral welfare despite the increasing pressure for this.[86] As discussed previously, the use of techniques to examine the affective state of animals is becoming a particularly important aspect of laboratory-based psychological studies of welfare and quality of life, but as yet these techniques have little practical application outside the laboratory. Frequently, perceptions of an animal's welfare state are based on subjective (and inevitably anthropomorphic) judgements: "he is happy" or "he is sad." To counter this, there are those that promote the use of demonstrably objective welfare scoring systems that assess a phenomenon

used as an index of stress (e.g., Ref. [87]) or purists who may advocate the direct measurement of physiological parameters associated with the stress response. In reality we are still some way off from finding a fool-proof way to objectively assess absolute welfare that is practical for use across all captive contexts. Having said that, if an animal is struggling to adapt to its captive environment, then the stress placed on it by housing and husbandry is likely to be apparent in its behavior. If the animal begins to exhibit a restricted behavioral repertoire, spends a disproportionate amount of its time budget in one or a few behaviors, or develops new nonfunctional behaviors, then it is clear that its welfare is being challenged and measures to rectify this should be taken. Even small changes in the balance and diversity of an animal's repertoire are worthy of note; they may act as "iceberg" indicators of greater problems ahead, and they and further changes in response to new or increased enrichment, should be monitored closely over time. Finally, we should not totally discount the value of apparently subjective assessments of an animal's state; our ability to empathize provides an important barometer of concern that can usefully trigger more objective assessment. A good example of this was the observation that a slumped, depressive posture in monkeys was found to be associated with serotonin levels in the brain consistent with humans with a major depressive disorder.[88]

Conclusion

Many exotic species may not be appropriate for captivity as pets[89] or in any context because of their very specific environmental, nutritional, or social requirements. Others are only adaptable to captive conditions in specific contexts where the expertise and resources enable them to be maintained in a physically and psychologically/behaviorally healthy condition. It should also be noted that some exotic species may present a significant risk to their owners/caretakers. Maintaining dangerous animals in captivity necessitates a secure environment for housing the animal so as to minimize the escape risk and the risk of injury/death to those who care for these species, for example venomous snakes[90] and large, dangerous animals (tigers[91]). While there are certain species such as these that automatically would suggest additional care is needed, it is less immediately apparent in others. For example, an otherwise innocuous, slow-moving primate, the slow loris, *Nycticebus coucang*, proved to be an unusual, poisonous mammal capable of presenting a fatal risk to other animals it is housed with and even humans.[92] Taking the necessary precautions to safely house a dangerous animal (e.g., barrier caging, segregation of the animal for common husbandry procedures) may undermine the purpose of maintaining the animal in captivity (e.g., open exhibition), have prohibitively high cost implications and a negative impact on the ability to provide optimally for the animal's welfare.

When considering taking on an exotic species considerable caution should be exercised. This relates as much to the safety and security of both animal and caretaker as well as to the consequences of escape (e.g., from trauma, predation, envenomation, and disease) for people and other animals in the captive or wild environment. Painstakingly, careful planning needs to be in place to ensure that the best possible welfare conditions are in place for the animal and there is no substitute for extensive research from reliable sources in providing the vital information about physiological, clinical, and ethological parameters for the species in question or its nearest relative for which such information is available.

References

1. OED. *Oxford English Dictionary.* Simpson S, Weiner E, eds. Oxford: Oxford University Press, 1989.
2. DEFRA. *Animal Health and Welfare Strategy for Great Britain.* London: Department for Environment, Food and Rural Affairs, 2004;1–40.
3. EC. *A New Animal Health Strategy for the European Union (2007–2013) Where "Prevention is Better Than Cure".* Luxembourg: European Commission, Office for Official Publications of the European Communities, 2007;1–26.
4. RSPCA. *Measuring Animal Welfare in the UK 2007.* Horsham, UK: RSPCA, 2008;1–107.
5. Fisher PG. Equipping the exotic mammal practice. *Vet Clin North Am Exot Anim Pract* 2005;8(3):405–426.
6. Humphreys P. Care of wild and non-domestic species. *Vet Rec* 1992;130(20):454.
7. Harris DJ. Promoting the exotic pet practice. *Vet Clin North Am Exot Anim Pract* 2005;8(3):469–474.
8. Mayer J, Martin J. Barriers to exotic animal medicine. *Vet Clin North Am Exot Anim Pract* 2005;8(3):487–496.
9. Keeble E. Addressing the welfare needs of exotic pets. *J Small Anim Prac* 2003;44(11):517–518.
10. International Primatological Society Web Site. IPS international guidelines for the acquisition, care and breeding of nonhuman primates. Available at: http://www.internationalprimatologicalsociety. org/docs/IPS_International_Guidelines_for_the_Acquisition_Care_ and_Breeding_of_Nonhuman_Primates_Second_Edition_2007.pdf. Accessed Feb 22, 2010.
11. Yeates JW, Main DCJ. Assessment of positive welfare: A review. *Vet J* 2008;175:293–300.
12. Dawkins MS. The science of animal suffering. *Ethology* 2008; 114(10):937–945.
13. Honess PE, Marin CM. Behavioural and physiological aspects of stress and aggression in nonhuman primates. *Neurosci Biobehav Rev* 2006;30(3):390–412.
14. Harding EJ, Paul ES, Mendl M. Animal behavior: Cognitive bias and affective state. *Nature* 2004;427(6972):312.
15. Young RJ. The importance of food presentation for animal welfare and conservation. *Proc Nutr Soc* 1997;56(3):1095–1104.
16. Ings R, Waran NK, Young RJ. Attitude of zoo visitors to the idea of feeding live prey to zoo animals. *Zoo Biol* 1997;16(4):343–347.
17. Hughes BO, Duncan IJH. The notion of ethological need, models of motivation and animal welfare. *Anim Behav* 1988; 36(6):1696–1707.
18. Newberry RC. Environmental enrichment: Increasing the biological relevance of captive environments. *Appl Anim Behav Sci* 1995; 44(2–4):229–243.
19. Dawkins MS. Battery hens name their price: Consumer demand theory and the measurement of ethological "needs". *Anim Behav* 1983; 31:1195–1205.
20. Honess PE, Marin CM. Enrichment and aggression in primates. *Neurosci Biobehav Rev* 2006;30(3):413–436.
21. Mason GJ, Cooper J, Clarebrough C. Frustrations of fur-farmed mink. *Nature* 2001;410(6824):35–36.
22. Deaner RO, Khera AV, Platt ML. Monkeys pay per view: Adaptive valuation of social images by rhesus macaques. *Curr Biol* 2005; 15(6):543–548.
23. Waitt C, Honess P, Bushmitz M. Creating housing to meet the behavioural needs of long-tailed macaques. *Laboratory Primate Newsletter* 2008;47(4):1–5.
24. Wolfensohn SE, Honess PE. Laboratory animal, pet animal, farm animal, wild animal: Which gets the best deal? *Anim Welf* 2007; 16(S):117–123.
25. Diamond J. Evolution, consequences and future of plant and animal domestication. *Nature* 2002;418:700–707.
26. Darwin C. *The Variation of Animals and Plants Under Domestication.* Vol. 2. London: John Murray, 1868;488.
27. Clutton-Brock J. *A Natural History of Domesticated Mammals.* 2nd ed. Cambridge: Cambridge University Press, 1999.
28. Price EO. Behavioural aspects of animal domestication. *Q Rev Biol* 1984;59(1):1–32.
29. Carlstead K. Effects of captivity on the behavior of wild mammals. In: Kleiman DG, Allen ME, Thompson KV et al., eds. *Wild Mammals in Captivity: Principles and Techniques.* Chicago, USA: University of Chicago Press, 1996;xvi+639 p.
30. Kleiman DG, Allen ME, Thompson KV et al., eds. *Wild Mammals in Captivity: Principles and Techniques.* Chicago: University of Chicago Press, 1996;639+xvi.
31. Hosey G, Melfi V, Pankhurst S. *Zoo Animals: Behaviour, Management, and Welfare.* Oxford: Oxford University Press, 2009;661+xxii.
32. Wechsler B. Stereotypies in polar bears. *Zoo Biol* 1991;10:177–188.
33. Clubb R, Mason G. Captivity effects on wide-ranging carnivores. *Nature* 2003;425:473.
34. Mallapur A, Cheelam R. Environmental influences on stereotypy and the activity budget of Indian leopards (*Panthera pardus*) in four zoos in southern India. *Zoo Biol* 2002;21:585–595.
35. Bashaw MJ, Tarou LR, Maki TS et al. A survey assessment of variables related to stereotypy in captive giraffe and okapi. *Appl Anim Behav Sci* 2001;73(3):235–247.
36. Meehan CL, Garner JP, Mench JA. Isosexual pair housing improves the welfare of young Amazon parrots. *Appl Anim Behav Sci* 2003; 81:73–88.
37. Sherwin CM, Harris MJ, Harris S. "The elephant in the room"—The welfare of elephants in UK zoos. In: *UFAW Animal Welfare Conference: Recent Advances in Animal Welfare Science.* Birmingham, UK: Universities Federation for Animal Welfare, 2008.
38. Clubb R, Rowcliffe M, Lee PC et al. Compromised survivorship in zoo elephants. *Science* 2008;322(5908):1649.
39. Clubb R, Mason G. *A Review of the Welfare of Zoo Elephants in Europe: A Report Commissioned by the RSPCA.* Oxford: Animal Behaviour Research Group, Department of Zoology, University of Oxford, 2002;280, xi.
40. Crockett CM, Shimoji M, Bowden DM. Behavior, appetite, and urinary cortisol responses by adult female pigtailed macaques to cage size, cage level, room change, and ketamine sedation. *Am. J. Primatol* 2000;52(2):63–80.
41. Beringer J, Hansen LP, Wilding W et al. Factors affecting capture myopathy in white-tailed deer. *J Wildl Manage* 1996;60(2):373–380.
42. Windingstad RM, Hurley SS, Sileo L. Capture myopathy in a free-flying greater sandhill crane (*Grus canadensis tabida*) from Wisconsin. *J Wildl Dis* 1983;19(3):289–290.
43. Fowler ME. *Restraint and Handling of Wild and Domestic Animals.* Ames, Iowa: Iowa State University Press, 1995.
44. Rubec PJ, Cruz F, Pratt V et al. Cyanide-free net-caught fish for the marine aquarium trade. *Aquarium Sci Conserv* 2001;3:37–51.
45. Cato JC, Brown CL. *Marine Ornamental Species: Collection, Culture, and Conservation.* Ames, Iowa: Iowa State Press, 2003.

46. IUCN. *2008 IUCN Red List of Threatened Species*. Gland, Switzerland, and Cambridge, UK: IUCN—The World Conservation Union, Species Survival Commission (SSC), 2008.

47. Howell K. Mortality in Tanzania's bird trade. In: Leader-Williams N, Tibanyenda RK, eds. *The Live Bird Trade in Tanzania*. Gland, Switzerland: IUCN Species Survival Commission, 1996;63–66.

48. RSPCA. *Shell Shock: The Continuing Illegal Trade in Tortoises*. Horsham, UK: RSPCA, 2001;1–11.

49. IATA. *Live Animal Regulations 2008/2009*. Montreal, Canada: International Air Transport Association, 2008.

50. LASA. Guidance on the transport of laboratory animals: Report of the transport working group established by the laboratory animal science association (LASA). *Lab Anim* 2005;39:1–39.

51. Chomel BB, Belotto A, Meslin F-X. Wildlife, exotic pets, and emerging zoonoses. *Emerg Infect Dis* 2007;13(1):6–11.

52. Coblentz BE. Exotic organisms: A dilemma for conservation biology. *Conserv Biol* 1990;4(3):261–265.

53. Boyle DB. Disease and fertility control in wildlife and feral animal populations: Options for vaccine delivery using vectors. *Reprod Fertil Dev* 1994;6(3):393–400.

54. Martin RD. *Primate Origins and Evolution: A Phylogenetic Reconstruction*. London: Chapman and Hall, 1990;804, xiv.

55. Mayer J. The importance of understanding the natural history of novel species used in research. *Lab Anim* (NY) 2004;33(9):32–33.

56. Jones TA, Waitt CD, Dawkins MS. Water off a duck's back: Showers and troughs match ponds for improving duck welfare. *Appl Anim Behav Sci* 2009;116(1):52–57.

57. Gaskill BN, Rohr SA, Pajor EA et al. Some like it hot: Mouse temperature preferences in laboratory housing. *Appl Anim Behav Sci* 2009;116(2–4):279–285.

58. Garner JP. Perseveration and stereotypy: Systems-level insights from clinical psychology. In: Mason G, Rushen J, eds. *Stereotypic Animal Behaviour: Fundamentals and Applications to Welfare*. Wallingford, UK: CABI, 2006;121–152.

59. O'Regan HJ, Kitchener AC. The effects of captivity on the morphology of captive, domesticated and feral mammals. *Mamm Rev* 2005;35(3–4):215–230.

60. Nelson NJ, Thompson MB, Pledger S et al. Egg mass determines hatchling size, and incubation temperature influences post-hatching growth, of tuatara *Sphenodon punctatus*. *J Zool* 2004;263(01):77–87.

61. Schmidt-Nielsen K. *Animal Physiology: Adaptation and Environment*. 3rd ed. Cambridge: Cambridge University Press, 1983;619, xii.

62. Hernandez-Divers SJ. Clinical aspects of reptile behaviour. *Vet Clin North Am Exot Anim Pract* 2001;4(3):599–612.

63. Judah V, Nuttall K. *Exotic Animal Care and Management*. New York: Thomson Delmar Learning, 2008;268, xiii.

64. Wolfensohn SE, Honess PE. *Handbook of Primate Husbandry and Welfare*. Oxford, UK: Blackwell Publications, 2005.

65. Moe MA. *The Marine Aquarium Reference: Systems and Invertebrates*. Plantation, FL, USA: Green Turtle Publications, 1992;512.

66. Boness DJ. Water quality management in aquatic mammal exhibits. In: Kleiman DG, Allen ME, Thompson KV et al., eds. *Wild Mammals in Captivity: Principles and Techniques*. Chicago: University of Chicago Press, 1996:231–242.

67. Moe MA. *The Marine Aquarium Handbook: Beginner to Breeder*. 2nd ed. Plantation, FL, USA: Green Turtle Publications, 1992;320.

68. Clutton-Brock TH, Harvey PH. Species differences in feeding and ranging behaviour in primates. In: Clutton-Brock TH, ed. *Primate Ecology: Studies of Feeding and Ranging Behaviour in Lemurs, Monkeys and Apes*. London: Academic Press, 1977:557–579.

69. Gore MA. Effects of food distribution on foraging competition in rhesus monkeys, *Macaca mulatta*, and hamadryas baboons, *Papio hamadryas*. *Anim Behav* 1993;45(4):773–786.

70. Boccia ML, Hijazi AS. A foraging task reduces agonistic and stereotypic behaviours in pigtail macaque social groups. *Laboratory Primate Newsletter* 1998;37(3):1–5.

71. Chamove AS, Anderson JR, Morgan-Jones SC et al. Deep woodchip litter: Hygiene, feeding, and behavioural enhancement in eight primate species. *Int J Study Anim Probl* 1982;3:308–318.

72. Bloomsmith M, Laule G, Thurston R et al. Using training to modify chimpanzee aggression. In: *Proceedings, American Association of Zoological Parks and Aquariums Central Region Conference*. Dallas, USA. 1992.

73. Young RJ. Environmental enrichment for captive animals. In: Kirkwood J, Hubrecht R, Roberts E, eds. UFAW animal welfare series, ed. Oxford, UK: Blackwell Science Ltd, 2003;228, xii.

74. Mellen J, MacPhee MS. Philosophy of environmental enrichment: Past, present, and future. *Zoo Biol* 2001;20(3):211–226.

75. Kennedy BW, Compton S, Turner JG et al. Editorial: Can you hear me now? *J Am Assoc Lab Anim Sci* 2007;46(1):9.

76. Meredith A. Chipmunks. In: Meredith A, Redrobe S, eds. *BSAVA Manual of Exotic Pets*. Gloucester, UK: British Small Animal Veterinary Association, 2002.

77. Bearder SK. Lorises, bushbabies and tarsiers: Diverse societies in solitary foragers. In: Smuts B, Cheney D, Seyfarth R et al., eds. *Primate Societies*. Chicago, USA: University of Chicago Press, 1987.

78. Gregory N. Physiology and behaviour of animal suffering. In: Kirkwood J, Hubrecht R, Roberts E, eds. *UFAW Animal Welfare Series*. Oxford, UK: Blackwell Scientific Ltd, 2004;268, xii.

79. de Waal FBM, Aureli F, Judge PG. Coping with crowding. *Sci Am* 2000;282(5):76–81.

80. Bloomsmith MA, Else JG. Behavioral management of chimpanzees in biomedical research facilities: The state of the science. *ILAR J* 2005;46(2):192–201.

81. Swaisgood R, Shepherdson D. Environmental enrichment as a strategy for mitigating stereotypies in zoo animals: A literature review and meta-analysis. In: Mason G, Rushen J, eds. *Stereotypic Animal Behaviour: Fundamentals and Applications to Welfare*. Wallingford. UK: CABI, 2006:256–268.

82. Maki S, Alford PL, Bloomsmith MA et al. Food puzzle device stimulating termite fishing for captive chimpanzees (*Pan troglodytes*). *Am J Primatol* 1989;19(Suppl. 1):71–78.

83. McGrew WC, Brennan JA, Russell J. An artificial "gum-tree" for marmosets (*Callithrix j. Jacchus*). *Zoo Biol* 1986;5:45–50.

84. Maple TL, Perkins LA. Enclosure furnishings and structural environmental enrichment. In: Kleiman DG, Allen ME, Thompson KV et al., eds. *Wild Mammals in Captivity: Principles and Techniques*. Chicago: The University of Chicago Press, 1996;212–222.

85. Meredith A, Johnson-Delany C, eds. *BSAVA Manual of Exotic Pets*. 5th ed. Gloucester, UK: British Small Animal Veterinary Association, 2010:424.

86. Van de Harst JE, Spruijt BM. Tools to measure and improve animal welfare: Reward-related behaviour. *Anim Welf* 2007;16(S):67–73.

87. Honess P, Gimpel J, Wolfensohn S et al. Alopecia scoring: The quantitative assessment of hair loss in captive macaques. *Altern Lab Anim* 2005;33(3):193–206.

88. Shively CA, Friedman DP, Gage HD et al. Behavioral depression and positron emission tomography–determined serotonin 1a receptor binding potential in cynomolgus monkeys. *Arch Gen Psychiatry* 2006;63:396–403.

89. Soulsbury CD, Iossa G, Kennell S et al. The welfare and suitability of primates kept as pets. *J Appl Anim Welf Sci* 2009;12(1):1–20.

90. de Haro L, Pommier P. Envenomation: A real risk of keeping exotic house pets. *Vet Hum Toxicol* 2003;45(4):214–216.

91. Nyhus PJ, Tilson RL, Tomlinson JL. Dangerous animals in captivity: Ex situ tiger conflict and implications for private ownership of exotic animals. *Zoo Biol* 2003;22(6):573–586.

92. Alterman L. Toxins and toothcombs: Potential allospecific chemical defenses in *Nycticebus* and *Perodicticus*. In: Alterman L, Doyle GA, Izard MK, eds. *Creatures of the Dark: The Nocturnal Prosimians*. New York: Plenum Press, 1995:413–424.

Index